T0304754

PROCESS EVALUATION FOR PUBLIC HEALTH INTERVENTIONS AND RESEARCH

PROCESS EVALUATION FOR PUBLIC HEALTH INTERVENTIONS AND RESEARCH

Allan Steckler

Laura Linnan

Editors

Foreword by Barbara A. Israel

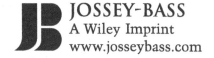

JOSSEY-BASS
A Wiley Imprint
www.josseybass.com

Published by Jossey-Bass
A Wiley Imprint
One Montgomery Street, San Francisco, CA 94104-4594   www.josseybass.com

Jossey-Bass books and products are available through most bookstores. To contact Jossey-Bass directly call
our Customer Care Department within the U.S. at 800-956-7739, outside the U.S. at 317-572-399386 or
fax 317-572-4002.

Jossey-Bass also publishes its books in a variety of electronic formats. Some content that appears in print
may not be available in electronic books.

Library of Congress Cataloging-in-Publication Data
Process evaluation for public health interventions and research / Allan
Steckler, Laura Linnan, editors ; foreword by Barbara Israel. — 1st ed.
     p.   ;   cm.
   Includes bibliographical references and index.
    ISBN 978-1-119-02248-0
    1. Public health—Research—Methodology.   2. Health
promotion—Evaluation.   3. Medicine, Preventive—Research—Methodology.
    [DNLM: 1. Health Services Research.   2. Process Assessment (Health
Care)   3. Public Health.   W. 84.3 P963   2002]   I. Steckler, Allan B.   II.
Linnan, Laura.

RA440.85 .P76   2002
362.1'07'2—dc21   2002012702

CONTENTS

Contents

FOREWORD

The need for systematic evaluations of public health interventions aimed at promoting health and preventing illness has been recognized for many years. Emphasis has been placed on conducting multiple types of evaluation, including outcome evaluation, which focuses on the results, health effects, or outcomes of an intervention, impact evaluation, which focuses on changes in targeted mediators or intermediate objectives considered essential to achieving the outcome, and process evaluation, which focuses on the extent to which the intervention was implemented with the content, accuracy, coverage, and quality that was planned. Although there has been growing emphasis on the combined use of these multiple types of evaluation within any given intervention, there remains in the literature a dearth of conceptual underpinnings and methodologies for conducting process evaluations.

Over the last several decades, there has also been increasing research evidence of the complex set of factors associated with health status—for example, individual behaviors, social, economic, cultural, ethnic, political, and physical environmental factors, and genetic and biologic characteristics, as well as the growing health disparities that exist between rich and poor and white and nonwhite populations. Accompanying these research findings, there have been increasing calls for more comprehensive approaches to public health interventions that address this complex set of determinants at multiple levels of practice—for example, the individual, family, organization, community, and policy levels. The implementation and evaluation of such comprehensive approaches has a number of challenges, and it is particularly important to gain a better understanding not only of the outcomes and effectiveness of the interventions involved but also of how and why they have had the effects that they have had. This increased understanding is best attained through conducting process evaluations.

This diverse set of determinants of health and comprehensive approaches to public health interventions necessitates the use of multiple conceptual and methodological approaches for carrying out process evaluations. There is no one set of process evaluation questions or evaluation methods that is going to be the most appropriate for all situations. However, the editors of this volume recommend following a *systematic* approach for developing a process evaluation effort that can be applied to most research and practice settings. Each process evaluation question must be selected because it is feasible and useful for addressing an important implementation issue. Each question suggests different methods—both quantitative and qualitative—that can be used to collect the information needed. In addition, the context, nature of the health problem, staffing, program participants, and many other factors need to be taken into account in designing and conducting a process evaluation.

Thus, process evaluation data provide information that is critical to helping intervention researchers and public health practitioners better understand how, why, and among which participants intervention aims have been achieved. Process evaluations can be conducted *formatively*—that is, either as part of the development of an intervention or to ensure that an intervention is implemented as intended, or they can be conducted *summatively*—that is, to examine the extent to which an intervention was implemented as it was intended. In the former instance, process evaluation data need to be collected on an ongoing basis and fed back regularly to the staff and participants involved in order to identify the strengths of the program and to determine the areas of the program that are not working well and therefore need to be improved. In this way, the program staff members can take advantage of opportunities to make changes in the intervention that will enhance program effectiveness. The results of process evaluations are also useful for dissemination of information that can be applied in replicating interventions that are deemed worthy. Here again, although outcome evaluations do provide information about whether intervention objectives have been met, they do not provide information on what produced the identified results—or lack of results. Therefore, process evaluations are most helpful when carried out in conjunction with impact and outcome evaluations.

Process evaluations need to be an ongoing and integral part of the evaluation of any public health intervention, whether it is conceived as intervention research or as public health practice. Funding sources need to recognize the benefits of process evaluations and should provide the resources necessary to conduct them.

Researchers and practitioners alike need the knowledge and skills necessary to conduct process, as well as impact and outcome, evaluations. This volume, *Process Evaluation for Public Health Interventions and Research*, provides a valuable resource both for those just beginning to learn about process evaluation and for those in the field who have been engaged in conducting process evaluations and want to enhance their expertise.

In this book, the editors provide a helpful history and review of the process evaluation literature, identifying what is known and where the gaps are in knowledge, theory, and practice. They discuss the key considerations that need to be addressed when conducting process evaluations—for example, the types of questions that need to be asked as well as the conceptual, methodological, and resource issues that need to be resolved.

Based on the firsthand experiences of the contributing authors, each of the chapters provides a wealth of knowledge on a specific case example of a process evaluation. These chapters are particularly useful in their diversity of settings (such as community, worksite, and school settings), levels (local, state, and national), participants (such as adolescents, adults, blue-collar or rural women, and elementary school-age children), health concerns (such as skin cancer prevention, injury prevention, prevention and cessation of drug and tobacco use, and the consumption of healthy foods), methods of data collection and analysis (quantitative and qualitative), and reporting mechanisms (such as presentations, published writings, and feedback documents). Each chapter has a section titled "Lessons Learned About Process Evaluation," which makes an important contribution to the process evaluation literature. The descriptions of the process evaluation cases involved, the inclusion of, for example, specific documentation forms, interview protocols, observation tools, tracking databases, and questionnaires, and the analysis of lessons learned all provide a much-needed addition to the process evaluation literature.

The editors and authors of this book have provided information and materials that are useful to researchers and practitioners alike who are engaged in conducting process evaluations. At a time when public health interventions are becoming more complex and comprehensive, with much still unknown about their implementation strategies and effectiveness, this volume serves to foster their value, offering multiple approaches to the conducting of process evaluations. The enhanced understanding gained through such evaluations will in turn serve to improve the quality and success of interventions aimed at promoting health, preventing disease, and reducing the health disparities that exist throughout the world.

September 2002   Barbara A. Israel
                                                                                           Ann Arbor, Michigan

Thanks to Stephen for bringing great joy to my life! *L.L.*

Thanks to Barbara, Tim, and Adam for putting up with me. *A.S.*

PREFACE

We have learned that solving social problems is difficult and exacting and calls for large resources of money, time, will, and ideas. Most social problems that this nation and other nations face are beyond the reach of easy solutions. No magic bullet is going to end crime, poverty, illness, or the degradation of the environment. People will continue to worry about education, violence, and community cohesiveness. Progress will be made in gradual stages, by incremental improvements, and it will take careful, systematic evaluation to identify which modes of intervention have better outcomes. With the information and insight that evaluation brings, organizations and societies will be better able to improve policy and programming for the well-being of all.
—CAROL H. WEISS (1998)

We take comfort and direction in reflecting on these wise words from a true leader in evaluation research. As coeditors of this book, we each have had the experience of collaborating on large, multisite, public health intervention trials. Specifically, each of us has had the good fortune to work on transdisciplinary teams that plan, implement, and analyze process evaluation efforts undertaken as part of these large multisite trials. As subcontractors, we have worked together to create process evaluation components for studies in which colleagues wanted to work with "outside" evaluators. In addition, we both teach about research and evaluation methods as well as advise public health graduate students in the School of Public Health at the University of North Carolina (UNC), Chapel Hill.

Why This Book Now?

Through these activities and through our collaboration with a number of excellent colleagues—both at UNC and nationally, we have been inspired to create a resource for those who might want to benefit from what we (and others) have learned about process evaluation over the years. The resource we have created is this book focused on process evaluation applied to public health interventions and research.

Over the past two decades, interest in evaluation applied to public health interventions (generally) and process evaluation (specifically) has grown. We trace the expanded interest in process evaluation in the first chapter of this book. We argue that an increase in the complexity of public health interventions has been a primary driver of an increased interest in process evaluation. Clearly, improvements in the knowledge and skills to do theory-driven intervention planning have led to the desire to evaluate more systematically why these intervention efforts are effective (or ineffective), for whom they are effective, and under what conditions they are effective. Process evaluation is integral to understanding why interventions achieve the results they do, and it also gives important insights into the quality and fidelity of the intervention effort.

However, despite the growth in published process evaluation literature in recent years, barriers to creating effective process evaluation efforts remain. For example, the political will to conduct a comprehensive process evaluation effort is often lacking. Specifically, funders (and some investigators) may be more interested in the outcomes of the work (for example, did the intervention achieve the desired effects?) than they are in how well the planned interventions were developed or implemented. Process evaluation may be an afterthought in a comprehensive evaluation effort. In some cases, process evaluation efforts are undertaken *after* data collection instruments have been created or, worse, after the intervention has been developed and implemented. A lack of commitment to doing process evaluation early in a project or study is a serious barrier to effective process evaluation.

Another important barrier to effective process evaluation is a lack of expertise in planning, developing, implementing, and assessing process evaluation efforts. Where do public health professionals and researchers learn how to do effective process evaluation? In our view, there is clearly a need for more comprehensive training in process evaluation methodology. We believe that when more individuals are adequately trained, they will not only serve an important role in public health intervention programs and research but will also become advocates for removing the barriers that exist.

A single book cannot hope to overcome all of these barriers, but it is not unrealistic to believe that the chapters included in this text will at least shed some light on a particularly important issue—process evaluation, which is needed if we are to advance our understanding of how and why public health interventions work effectively.

This book was also inspired by the fact that though a number of excellent resources are available that focus on both the planning and the evaluation of a wide range of health, education, and social programs, we were unable to identify a resource that addresses the issue of process evaluation specifically. We believe that as the complexity of our intervention efforts increases, planning for, implementing, and assessing process evaluation efforts are critical to moving the field forward. In other words, we agree with Weiss (1998) that progress will be made gradually, "and it will take careful, systematic evaluation to identify which modes of intervention have better outcomes." This book should help fill a gap in resources for those who are interested in looking specifically at the issue of process evaluation and the contribution it can make to progress in applied public health intervention research and practice.

Who Should Read This Book?

This book should appeal to several audiences. First, a primary intended audience for this book is students, especially those at the graduate level. We have had the experience of recruiting and orienting students to get involved in process evaluation efforts that we have under way for various intervention studies or other practice-based work. Most students have had a course in planning and evaluation, but we have yet to find a student who has had more than a lecture or two on process evaluation. Typically, students are asked to join the evaluation team and learn "on the job." We think this book will give students an additional, important resource to help guide their learning about process evaluation. It will give them a brief history of process evaluation and a review of the many purposes of process evaluation, and it will recommend an approach for designing an effective process evaluation effort. We believe that this book will facilitate the learning process and will serve as a useful reference for students who are invited to be involved in process evaluation efforts. To that end, faculty members who teach about evaluation (generally) or process evaluation (specifically), or who advise students who are involved in process evaluation efforts, are another important audience for this book.

We also believe that this book will prove useful to experienced researchers and practitioners who evaluate behavioral and social interventions in public health. For experienced researcher-practitioner-evaluators, we expect the contributed chapters to serve as practical guides for creating the next generation of process evaluation efforts. We have learned a great deal from the authors contributing to this book. They have generously shared their successes with process evaluation but have also shared key lessons learned from their experiences. We have found these insights to be extremely helpful. It is rare that we have the opportunity to learn from each other about what we should avoid (not just about the things that have worked). In each chapter, our contributing authors have laid out a series of practical, useful lessons that they have learned. Moreover, they have each shared key forms, sample reports, and other tools that both experienced and novice evaluators will find helpful. Rather than reinventing the forms and systems each time a new process evaluation effort is designed, readers should look carefully at the examples provided in this book. Each form will need to be modified to fit the context and audience of a new study, but the time and resources saved in starting with a proven tool can be impressive. We hope readers find these sample tools and forms useful and cost-effective.

There is another, perhaps less obvious, audience who might benefit from this book. We are referring to authors who write about applied research and evaluation methodology. For this group, we hope the book serves as a snapshot of the current state of the art of process evaluation that will be useful in the further development of this methodology. We see this book as extending the dialogue about process evaluation and we invite readers to share their questions, experiences, and opinions with us.

Why Did We Invite These Contributors?

Many colleagues have made generous, thoughtful contributions to this book, being willing to give detailed descriptions of their process evaluation efforts and to share their lessons learned about what has worked and about what has not worked very well in the planning and implementation of their process evaluation projects. We specifically invited these contributors for several reasons. First, we pursued process evaluation efforts that had variation in size, setting, and scope. In this book are chapters about process evaluation efforts that were staged at the local level, the state level, and the national level. This variation reflects the kind of process evaluation that typically occurs in the "real world" of program evaluation efforts. Although the approach to process evaluation is often the same at each of these levels, the resources available (people and money), as well as the complexity, may vary dramatically.

For this book, in addition to variation in the size of process evaluation efforts, we specifically looked for process evaluation efforts that vary in the scope of the work undertaken as part of the process evaluation. Thus, we pursued chapter contributions that feature variation in the types of questions being answered, in the methods being used (qualitative and quantitative), and in the analytic procedures being adopted. Some chapters focus on formative research efforts and some focus on summative research. We also pursued process evaluation "stories" that varied with regard to participants—focusing in turn on children, teens, adults, and health professionals. We also sought diversity in populations, to include minority, low-income, and rural populations. And we pursued variation in the type of setting. We have included three projects that took place in schools, two that were situated in worksites, and seven that were carried out in various other community settings, such as local cities, churches, and parks and recreation departments. The book is divided into four sections, according to the settings in which process evaluations took place. Because all evaluation is context-specific, variation in projects by setting seems essential. As readers appreciate the nuances of working in a particular setting, they will benefit from looking within each section to see how setting-specific projects overcame certain obstacles. Moreover, readers can look across settings in this book to see how a particular issue—such as data collection strategies or the encouragement of high response rates—was successfully handled in worksite settings and how this handling might also be applicable to a community or school setting. Wrestling with the intricacies of conducting process evaluations within and across settings has provided us with interesting insights, and we hope that this wisdom will benefit readers working across a variety of public health settings.

In selecting the authors contributing to this book, we chose researchers who were doing state-of-the-art work on process evaluation, had already published (or were close to publishing) the final results of their particular intervention study, were able to write clearly about their successes and difficulties in process evaluation efforts, and were generous about sharing specific tools and resources that they found particularly useful.

Chapter Features

There are thirteen chapters in this book, with an overview chapter and four sections that address community, worksite, school, and national or state process evaluation efforts. The introductory chapter, written by the coeditors, gives an overview and brief history of process evaluation linked to public health interventions. It attempts to clarify some common terms and offers a stepwise approach to designing a process evaluation effort. Each section of the book begins with a summary that clarifies the key highlights of the process evaluation efforts as reported in each chapter in that section. Each chapter provides background on the project or study, describes the intervention efforts, identifies the staff members involved in the process evaluation, and summarizes the strengths and limitations of the overall effort.

Another important feature of each of the chapters is the section entitled "Lessons Learned About Process Evaluation," in which the contributing authors detail what they believe are the most important lessons they have learned from their process evaluation efforts. And we invited authors to include as an appendix one to three process evaluation instruments that they used in their study, which most of them have done. It is our hope that readers will be able to use some of these instruments in their future process evaluation efforts.

Acknowledgments

We sincerely thank the contributing authors, whose work is represented here. The authors worked hard to represent their work in ways that are practical for the multiple audiences we are hoping to serve, and they have met rigorous deadlines without delay. Having worked on several books previously, we have been impressed with the quality and timeliness with which our contributing authors have produced these important chapters. Moreover, our contributing authors encouraged us and helped refine our ideas for the book, and a few provided support during the final editing process as well. Special thanks go to Deborah Helitzer and Erin Kobetz for providing excellent feedback on the first draft of the overview chapter, and we also thank Barbara Israel for writing a thoughtful Foreword for this book. For all of these wonderful contributions, we are very grateful.

We'd also like thank the Health Series team at Jossey-Bass for their encouragement and help throughout the process. Editor Andy Pasternack has been a delightful and positive supporter of our initial and evolving ideas for this book. And we'd like to acknowledge our colleagues—graduate students, administrative staff members, and faculty members—in the Department of Health Behavior and Health Education at UNC, Chapel Hill, who provided encouragement for undertaking this project and have created a collegial environment that abounds with ideas and opportunities.

In addition, Laura Linnan thanks colleagues who have helped shape her thinking about process evaluation efforts over the past twenty years: Glorian Sorensen, Mary Kay Hunt, Carol Weiss, Beti Thompson, Gwen Glaefke, Kate Lapane, Mary Lynne Hixson, David Abrams, Karen Emmons, Lois Biener, Sheila Jacobs, Suzanne Moriarty, Mike Guertin, and David Vampola. Allan thanks Ken

McLeroy, Bob Goodman, Michelle Kegler, Joel Gittelsohn, Deborah Helitzer, June Stevens, Deborah Rohm Young, and David Murray.

September 2002   Allan Steckler
Chapel Hill, North Carolina   Laura Linnan

Reference

Weiss, C. H. *Evaluation*. (2nd ed.) Englewood Cliffs, N.J.: Prentice-Hall, 1998, p. ix.

THE EDITORS

Allan Steckler is a professor of health behavior and health education in the School of Public Health at the University of North Carolina (UNC), Chapel Hill. He teaches qualitative evaluation methods, models of health education practice, organizational change, and diffusion of innovations to graduate students. For the past twenty years, Steckler has been involved in research and evaluation of school and community health promotion programs. He was coinvestigator for a federal rural health initiative-funded study to evaluate school and community medical self-care programs in Appalachian West Virginia, and he was principal investigator for a four-year project to evaluate drug and pregnancy prevention curricula in middle schools in North Carolina, funded by the Centers for Disease Control and Prevention and North Carolina's health department. He was also principal investigator for a five-year National Cancer Institute (NCI) funded project to study the process of disseminating smoking prevention curricula to middle schools. With his colleague Robert Goodman, he conducted an evaluation of the NCI's Data-Based Intervention Research program in state health departments. Recently, Steckler was involved in a National Heart, Lung, and Blood Institute (NHLBI) project that studied, through schools, obesity prevention among Native American youth. Currently, he is a coinvestigator for Trial of Activity for Adolescent Girls, an NHLBI-funded project to develop and test interventions for increasing physical activity among adolescent girls. In addition, Steckler is a coinvestigator for the Youth Empowerment Study, which is evaluating youth empowerment as an approach to reducing smoking among adolescents. He is also a coinvestigator for the Reconnecting Youth (RY, 2001–2006) study, a five-year National Institute on Drug Abuse-funded project designed to study methods of alcohol and drug prevention among high school students. Steckler is the codirector of TARGET, a reproductive health training program in association with the School of Public Health at Mahidol University in Bangkok, Thailand.

Laura Linnan is a certified health education specialist and assistant professor of health behavior and health education in the School of Public Health at UNC, Chapel Hill. She earned her doctorate from Harvard University's School of Public Health and served for six years as a research associate faculty member at Brown University in Providence, Rhode Island. Linnan has conducted applied worksite and community-based intervention research for more than thirteen years at Memorial Hospital of Rhode Island, working with the Pawtucket Heart Health Program in Pawtucket, Rhode Island, from 1988 to 1990 and with Miriam Hospital's Center For Behavioral and Preventive Medicine from 1990 to 1999. From 1989 to 1994, Linnan was project director/coinvestigator for the Brown Study Center of the Working Well Trial—the largest federally funded worksite-based intervention trial—and was co-principal investigator for Working Healthy Project 2, a five-year, NCI-funded follow-up study. As part of the Working Well Trial, Linnan was an active member of the Working Well Process Evaluation Working Group, which developed the tracking system that has been the basis of process evaluation systems adapted for use in several subsequent worksite and community-based trials. Prior to her research career, she planned, delivered, and evaluated health promotion programs in both private and public settings—at Metropolitan Life Insurance Company, at the NCI's Office of Cancer Communications, at the Massachusetts Department of Public Health, and at Michigan's Macomb County Health Department.

THE CONTRIBUTORS

Robert C. Addy is a data manager at the Center for Health Promotion and Prevention Research in the School of Public Health at the University of Texas (UT) Health Science Center in Houston.

Alice Ammerman is an associate professor in the Department of Nutrition in both the School of Public Health and the School of Medicine at the University of North Carolina (UNC), Chapel Hill.

Tom Baranowski is a professor of pediatrics in the Department of Pediatrics at the Baylor College of Medicine in Houston and is leader of the behavioral nutrition group at the U.S. Department of Agriculture-funded Children's Nutrition Research Center.

Karen Basen-Engquist is an associate professor in the Department of Behavioral Science at UT's M. D. Anderson Cancer Center in Houston.

Salli Benedict is assistant director for community development, implementation, and dissemination at the Center for Health Promotion and Disease Prevention at UNC, Chapel Hill.

Therese M. Blaine serves as a project director in the Division of Epidemiology at the University of Minnesota (UM), Minneapolis.

Marci Kramish Campbell is an associate professor in the Department of Nutrition in the School of Public Health at UNC, Chapel Hill, and is also program leader for cancer prevention and control at UNC's Lineberger Cancer Center.

Karin K. Coyle is director of research at ETR (Education, Training and Research) Associates in Santa Cruz, California.

Carolyn E. Crump is a research assistant professor in the Department of Health Behavior and Health Education in the School of Public Health at UNC, Chapel Hill.

Katherine Lyon Daniel is an epidemiologist and behavioral scientist who leads the Prevention and Health Communication Team of the National Center on Birth Defects and Developmental Disabilities at the Centers for Disease Control and Prevention (CDC).

Marsha Davis is an associate clinical professor in the Department of Human and Organizational Development at Vanderbilt University in Nashville.

Carl de Moor is an assistant professor in the behavioral science department and the biostatistics department of UT's M. D. Anderson Cancer Center in Houston.

Becky Ethlebah was the Apache field site coordinator for Johns Hopkins University's School of Public Health. She continues to collaborate with Johns Hopkins faculty members on American Indian-related health research.

David C. Fenn was the process evaluation field site coordinator at the Native American Research Center of the School of Medicine at the University of New Mexico (UNM) during the Pathways project.

Jean Forster is a professor in the School of Public Health at UM and is program director of prevention and policy studies at the University Cancer Center.

Allan Geller is a research associate professor in the Department of Dermatology at Boston University's School of Medicine.

Joel Gittelsohn is an associate professor in the Department of International Health at Johns Hopkins University.

Karen Glanz is professor and director of the Social and Behavioral Sciences Program at the Cancer Research Center of Hawaii at the University of Hawaii in Honolulu.

D. Knight Guire served as Statewide Endowment Process Evaluation System (STEPES) coordinator in the Division of Epidemiology at UM, Minneapolis, for one year. She is currently completing a Psy.D. degree program in clinical psychology.

Deborah L. Helitzer is a research associate professor of program evaluation and is director of the Office of Evaluation in the Department of Family and Community Medicine in the School of Medicine at UNM.

Marilyn Hughes is a faculty member working as research project director in the Department of Foods and Nutrition in the College of Foods and Consumer Sciences at the University of Georgia, Athens.

May Rose L. Isnec is a project manager in the Social and Behavioral Sciences Program at the University of Hawaii's Cancer Research Center of Hawaii.

Michelle C. Kegler is an assistant professor in the Department of Behavioral Sciences and Health Education in the Rollins School of Public Health at Emory University in Atlanta.

Erin N. Kobetz is a doctoral student in the Department of Health Behavior and Health Education in the School of Public Health at UNC, Chapel Hill.

Robert J. Letourneau is a social research associate at UNC's Injury Prevention Research Center in Chapel Hill.

Christine M. Markham is a senior research associate at the Center for Health Promotion and Prevention Research in the School of Public Health at UT's Health Science Center in Houston.

Catherine Jane Martin is a clinical psychologist in private practice in Tucson, Arizona.

Rebecca M. Mullis is professor and chair in the Department of Foods and Nutrition at the University of Georgia, where she teaches nutrition intervention.

Guy S. Parcel is the John P. McGovern Professor of Health Promotion at UT's Health Science Center in Houston, where he teaches behavioral sciences.

Marla Nahmabin Pardilla is a member of the national Native American Women's Cancer Control and Research Initiative, a program funded by the National Cancer Institute.

Christine E. Prue is a health communication training and research specialist with the CDC.

Sharon Rodine directs the HEART of OKC (Health, Empowered and Responsible Teens of OKC), a project coordinated by the Oklahoma Institute for Child Advocacy.

Mary Smyth is a licensed Minnesota educator and former teacher and is a public health specialist in the Division of Epidemiology of UM's School of Public Health in Minneapolis.

Kathy J. Spangler is the national programs director at the National Recreation and Park Association.

Dawn D. Stewart is a senior biostatistician at the Biostatistics Collaborative Coordinating Center, School of Public Health, UNC, Chapel Hill.

Elaine J. Stone was the senior National Heart, Lung, and Blood Institute (NHLBI) staff person assigned to the Pathways project. She was also the NHLBI staff person primarily responsible for the well-known and well-regarded Child and Adolescent Trial for Cardiovascular Health (CATCH) study.

Irene Tessaro is an assistant professor in the Department of Community Medicine at West Virginia University, where she teaches qualitative research methods and intervention design.

Beti Thompson is a member of the Fred Hutchinson Cancer Research Center and is a professor of health services in the School of Public Health and Community Medicine at the University of Washington.

Michele Volansky is a research associate at Westat in Rockville, Maryland.

Maihan B. Vu is a doctoral candidate in the Department of Health Behavior and Health Education in the School of Public Health at UNC, Chapel Hill.

Carla L. Warneke is a statistical analyst in the Department of Behavioral Science at UT's M. D. Anderson Cancer Center in Houston.

Vicki Harris Wyatt is an assistant professor of research in the Department of Health Promotions at the University of Oklahoma Health Sciences Center.

Soo-Jin Yoon is a program evaluator and a research scientist at the Health Sciences Center at UNM.

PROCESS EVALUATION FOR PUBLIC HEALTH INTERVENTIONS AND RESEARCH

CHAPTER ONE

Process Evaluation for Public Health Interventions and Research

An Overview

Laura Linnan and Allan Steckler

Improving and sustaining successful public health interventions relies increasingly on the ability to identify the key components of an intervention that are effective, to identify for whom the intervention is effective, and to identify under what conditions the intervention is effective. The published literature includes a plethora of reports about interventions that have successful outcomes. A limited number of studies, however, disentangle the factors that ensure successful outcomes, characterize the failure to achieve success, or attempt to document the steps involved in achieving successful implementation of an intervention. To truly advance science and our understanding of applied interventions, we must learn a great deal more about public health intervention successes and failures. Process evaluation efforts can assist in making these discoveries.

In the last decade, the literature on process evaluation related to public health interventions has grown considerably. In the late 1990s and in early 2000, there has been an explosion in the number of published studies that include extensive process evaluation components. There are several plausible explanations for this noticeable increase in the use of process evaluation. Social and behavioral interventions have become increasingly complex, making it important for researchers to know the extent to which all intervention components are actually implemented. This complexity stems from the fact that projects are often implemented at multiple locations, so that process evaluation becomes essential for ensuring that planned interventions are carried out equally at all sites. Complexity also results when interventions are implemented at multiple levels and with multiple audiences. Many contemporary studies use ecological approaches that intervene among individual, dyadic, group, organization, community, and population levels (McLeroy, Bibeau, Steckler, and Glanz, 1988). Accounting for the extent to which the intervention occurs at each level of influence (and among different subgroups) becomes increasingly complicated. As we attempt to eliminate inequalities in income and education level, we can, with thoughtful process evaluation efforts, obtain important clues about the influence of interventions among selected subgroups.

Another plausible explanation for why process evaluation efforts have proliferated is that we are looking for ways to explain why certain results were achieved. Specifically, when interventions lead to significant outcomes, it is important to understand which components of the intervention contributed to the success. Similarly, when large sums of taxpayer money are allocated to conduct multilevel community trials and the primary outcomes are insignificant (or the magnitude of the effect is small), there is an increased demand among researchers, funders, and members of the general public to understand why these interventions did not produce their intended effect (Fisher, 1995; Susser, 1995). Thus, process evaluation can help explain positive, modest, and insignificant results.

Process evaluation also provides important links to understanding and improving theory-informed interventions. Because more programs are developing theory-informed interventions, there is a greater need to understand which theoretical constructs make a difference (Glanz, Lewis, and Rimer, 1997). Process evaluation efforts can provide a link between theoretical constructs thought to be essential for intervention success and the final study outcomes. Understanding the mechanisms for how and why these constructs produce successful change (or fail to produce change) is key to refining theory and improving intervention effectiveness. Understanding under what conditions certain mediators are more (or less) influential in the achievement of certain study outcomes will inform the next and future generations of theory-informed interventions (Baranowski, Anderson, and Carmack, 1998; Baranowski and others, 1997).

Process evaluation efforts also help us understand the relationships among selected intervention or program components. In a comprehensive multimethod intervention, one might offer group classes, self-help programs, individual counseling sessions, and print materials. Process evaluation can help disentangle the effects of each method singly, and it can clarify the possible interactions that can occur to produce a synergistic effect. Few studies have attempted to reach into the "black box" of intervention effectiveness to explore which program components have been more or less effective, yet doing so is a powerful option within a comprehensive process evaluation effort (Harachi and others, 1999).

Assessing the quality and accuracy of the intervention delivered to program participants can also be achieved with process evaluation, which is another reason why these studies have proliferated. Increasingly, funders and program participants at all levels want assurances that the intervention being delivered is of a high quality and is highly accurate. In addition, attention to the cost-effectiveness of interventions is an increasingly important component of intervention planning and evaluation. Process evaluation efforts can assist with each of these requirements.

Finally, we contend that another reason for the rise in the use of process evaluation is the increasing recognition of the value of qualitative research methods (National Institutes of Health, 2001). Process evaluation frequently uses both quantitative and qualitative methods. Qualitative methods such as field site visits, structured observations of interventions, and open-ended interviews are often employed in conducting process evaluations. As the value attached to qualitative methods has increased, opportunities for publishing these findings and learning from their results have increased as well. Integrating different methods—such as qualitative and quantitative methods—yields rich detail about study outcomes that neither method could achieve alone (Tashakkori and Teddlie, 1998; Steckler and others, 1992).

Taken together, the recent increase in published literature on process evaluation results reflects the complexity of public health interventions today, and it reflects the many ways in which thoughtful, comprehensive process evaluation efforts can shed light on questions that will inform improvements in theory, intervention design, and methods in the future.

The remainder of this chapter presents a brief overview of the history of process evaluation as it relates to public health. After identifying current gaps in knowledge and clarifying barriers to effective process evaluation, the chapter presents definitions of key process evaluation terms and describes an approach that program planners, researchers, and evaluators may find helpful when planning and conducting process evaluation efforts.

Brief History and Review

Process evaluation is not a new concept. As early as during the 1960s, an explanation of process evaluation appeared in a widely used textbook on program evaluation (Suchman, 1967), although Suchman does not label it "process evaluation" per se. Suchman writes:

> In the course of evaluating the success or failure of a program, a great deal can be learned about how and why a program works or does not work. Strictly speaking, this analysis of the process whereby a program produces the results it

does is not an inherent part of evaluative research. An evaluation study may limit its data collection and analysis simply to determining whether or not a program is successful. . . . However, an analysis of process can have both administrative and scientific significance, particularly where the evaluation indicates that a program is not working as expected. Locating the cause of the failure may result in modifying the program so that it will work, instead of its being discarded as a complete failure [p. 66].

This early definition of process evaluation includes the basic framework that is still used today; however, as is discussed later in this chapter, the definitions of the components of process evaluation have been further developed and refined.

Few references to process evaluation were made in the literature during the 1970s. In evaluation research, the 1970s were devoted to the issues of improving evaluation designs and measuring program effects. For instance, Struening and Guttentag's *Handbook of Evaluation Research* (1975) does not contain any reference to process evaluation (see also Glass, 1976; Guttentag and Saar, 1977; Green, 1977).

In their influential book, Green, Kreuter, Deeds, and Partridge (1980) define process evaluation in a somewhat unusual way: "In a process evaluation, the object of interest is professional practice, and the standard of acceptability is appropriate practice. Quality is monitored by various means, including audit, peer review, accreditation, certification, and government or administrative surveillance of contracts and grants" (p. 134).

The emphasis on professional practice as the focus of process evaluation as suggested by Green, Kreuter, Deeds, and Partridge (1980) faded as attention returned to the idea of assessment of program implementation. By the mid-1980s, the definition of process evaluation had expanded. Windsor, Baranowski, Clark, and Cutter (1984) explain the purpose of process evaluation in the following way:

Process produces documentation on what is going on in a program and confirms the existence and availability of physical and structural elements of the program. It is part of a formative evaluation and assesses whether specific elements such as facilities, staff, space, or services are being provided or being established according to the given program plan. . . . Process evaluation involves documentation and description of specific program activities—how much of what, for whom, when, and by whom. It includes monitoring the frequency of participation by the target population and is used to confirm the frequency and extent of implementation of selected programs or program elements. Process evaluation derives evidence from staff, consumers, or outside evaluators on the quality of the implementation plan and on the appropriateness of content, methods, materials, media, and instruments [p. 3].

McGraw and others (1989) write that "'process' or 'implementation' evaluation is not a new concept. . . . Yet in the broad field of social experimentation, it is only recently—since the late 1970s, that this aspect of program evaluation is accorded more formal recognition" (p. 460). This historical assessment appears to be accurate. Starting in the mid- to late 1980s, we can see the beginnings of contemporary process evaluation theory and methods and their application to applied public health interventions.

One of the key publications in the mid-1980s that laid the groundwork for modern process evaluation was an article titled "Avoiding Type III Errors in Health Education Program Evaluations: A Case Study" (Basch and others, 1985). Researchers are familiar with a Type I error (for example, rejecting a "true" null hypothesis) or a Type II error (for example, failing to reject a "false" null hypothesis), but a Type III error ensues from "evaluating a program that has not been adequately implemented" (p. 316). Although the idea of the Type III error was not new in 1985 (Dobson and Cook, 1980; Rezmovic, 1982), our research suggests that this was the first time this idea appeared in the public health literature. The article argues that measuring program implementation is critical to avoiding a Type III error and thus drawing incorrect conclusions about the effectiveness of a given intervention. That is, in addition to answering the evaluation question Did the program work? evaluators must first answer the question Was the program actually carried out as planned?—and if it was not carried out as planned, they must answer the question How did the program vary from the original plan?

The community-based cardiovascular disease prevention (CVD) demonstration studies funded by the National Heart, Lung, and Blood Institute (NHLBI) in the early 1980s through the next decade represented an important step forward in planning, implementing, and evaluating community-based public health interventions. Investigators from the Stanford Five-City Program, the Pawtucket Heart Health Program, and the Minnesota Heart Health Program had the foresight to get together periodically and look for ways to collaborate on the development of research questions, data collection, interventions, and program evaluation. The program evaluation units in each of the studies were independent (Pirie and others, 1994), but as studies evolved, investigators began to realize the importance of developing a consistent approach to assessing the *dose* of intervention delivered by the program staff in each of the communities. As a result, the three demonstration studies combined key components of their process tracking systems so that they could compare the extent of their activities by targeted risk factors (smoking, nutrition, physical activity, blood pressure, and blood cholesterol levels) over time. It was a big effort to join components of the three tracking systems that were already in the field, but the benefits of this effort were significant. The intervention staff of each project obtained feedback on whether they were meeting expectations for program delivery. Corrective feedback was possible, based on the results.

In addition, these studies were among the first intervention studies to conceptualize and measure the importance of the dose received by program participants. Previously, program evaluators were content to measure the extent to which the intervention was delivered as planned. However, investigators were aware that many interventions were delivered that participants never received. For example, programs were scheduled and offered, but no one attended them. It was important to recognize that if programs were not received, important corrective action needed to be taken to improve the intervention or marketing of these programs. Moreover, when interpreting results, one must take into account the fact that participants may not have received what was delivered. As a result, the CVD demonstration studies advanced the field by collecting data from community members (through surveys) to assess participation in recently sponsored programs and exposure to various media messages. Pirie and others (1994) have published a detailed descriptive paper on program evaluation strategies of the demonstration studies which underscores the numerous contributions made by these investigators to conceptual thinking and the operationalization of key program evaluation components. The individual projects also published numerous papers that offer great insights about developing and implementing process evaluation efforts that will benefit process evaluators today. Of the many articles published, we recommend the one by Finnegan, Murray, Kurth, and McCarthy (1989), which describes the tracking of program implementation for the Minnesota Heart Health Program, the one by McGraw and others (1989), which describes the process evaluation system of the Pawtucket Heart Health Program, and the one by Flora and others (1993), which describes the community education monitoring system of the combined demonstration studies.

Because these demonstration projects were the largest federally funded trials, many beginning investigators received their training in public health interventions and evaluations by getting involved with these projects. By the early 1990s, investigators who had worked on these studies were now publishing papers on components of the process evaluation data and were conducting community-based studies of their own. A number of investigators from the CVD demonstration studies were collaborators on the next large, federally funded multi-institute trial. Corbett, Thompson, White, and Taylor (1991) describe the process evaluation used in the National Cancer Institute (NCI)-funded Community Intervention Trial for Smoking Cessation (COMMIT) (1988–1991). For this large community-based intervention study, they applied what they learned from the limitations of the CVD demonstration study tracking system and state in their 1991 article that process evaluation addresses what the intervention program consists of, how activities serve short-term objectives, how activities are carried out, and what other factors contribute to outcomes. It may entail "implementation evaluation," "quality control," "quality assurance review," "program utility assessment," "process analysis," and other assessments. Process evaluation can have a "formative" role during the development and unfolding of a program as well as a "summative" function. Quantitative process objectives along a timeline are often employed to facilitate evaluation of program delivery. Process evaluation may be designed to provide information to feed back suggestions to program designers, for mid-course corrections. For some researchers, process evaluation may also refer to qualitative assessment of the dynamics of program operation. Ultimately, what is needed is to know what specific results were and how they came about [p. 293].

The early 1990s represented an important period of growth in the number and complexity of community- and school-based intervention studies. At approximately the same time as the COMMIT study, the NCI funded the national Working Well Trial (1989–1994)—the largest federally funded worksite-based intervention trial (Abrams and others, 1994; Heimendinger and others, 1995; Sorensen and others, 1996) (see Chapter Six for a description of the process evaluation efforts of Working Well)—and an NHLBI-funded school-based study titled CATCH (Child and Adolescent Trial for Cardiovascular Health) (1986–1994) was conducted. The study design had been published earlier (Stone, McGraw, Osganian, and Elder, 1994), but the main process evaluation results were published in 1997 (Perry and others, 1997). The CATCH intervention had been implemented in fifty-six schools in four states. The process evaluation had four main objectives: (1) *participation*—Did teachers, food service personnel, and PE specialists attend the training sessions? (2) *dose*—Were prescribed components of the CATCH program implemented? (3) *fidelity*—Were the prescribed intervention components implemented according to protocol? and (4) *compatibility*—Did the CATCH programs fit the context of the schools as well as the needs, expectations, and values of the staff members and teachers? Because of its extensive process evaluation, the CATCH study made important contributions to the development of process evaluation theory and methods (Perry and others, 1997). McGraw and others (1994) describe the overall model for the CATCH process evaluation, which includes the measurement of student characteristics, intervention activities, student outcomes, the exogenous and competing effects, and school characteristics/outcomes. In addition, the interventions were based on principles of organizational change and social cognitive theory. The CATCH process evaluation data were used to describe program implementation, quality control and monitoring, and program effects. The CATCH process evaluation data were also used to assess the environmental context in which the interventions took place (Elder and others, 1994).

By 2000, the design and implementation of process evaluation efforts became quite complex, reflecting, in part, the complexity of the interventions they sought to monitor (Bartholomew, Parcel, Kok, and Gottlieb, 2001). Important conceptual work on process evaluation has been the hallmark of recent published reports on process evaluation. Perhaps the most thorough explanation of the components of process evaluation is offered by Baranowski and Stables (2000), who list eleven components of process evaluation:

1. *Recruitment*—attracting agencies, implementers, or potential participants for corresponding parts of the program
2. *Maintenance*—keeping participants involved in the programmatic and data collection
3. *Context*—aspects of the environment of an intervention
4. *Resources*—the materials or characteristics of agencies, implementers, or participants necessary to attain project goals
5. *Implementation*—the extent to which the program is implemented as designed
6. *Reach*—the extent to which the program contacts or is received by the targeted group
7. *Barriers*—problems encountered in reaching participants
8. *Exposure*—the extent to which participants view or read the materials that reach them
9. *Initial use*—the extent to which a participant conducts activities specified in the materials
10. *Continued use*—the extent to which a participant continues to do any of the activities
11. *Contamination*—the extent to which participants receive interventions from outside the program and the extent to which the control group receives the treatment

This list provides a useful beginning framework for organizing conceptual thinking about process evaluation and for developing consistent definitions to be used in the measurement of key process evaluation components.

Gaps in Current Knowledge

A number of gaps in current knowledge about process evaluation must be addressed if the field is to move forward. We review a number of these gaps, particularly focusing on (1) the lack of clear, consistent definitions for key process evaluation components and (2) the lack of a systematic process for planning and developing a process evaluation effort.

A selected review of recent process evaluations revealed an impressive array of process measures. For example, process evaluation efforts have measured the fidelity of the intervention implementation (that is, the quality of the program implementation), its reach, the time spent on program activities, the use of intervention materials, the level of participation, the dose delivered, the external factors, the program's penetration, its quality measures—such as the accuracy of the information and services provided, its impact, the relationships among program components, the training results, and the costs. At this point, there appears to be considerable overlap in how key terms like fidelity, dose, exposure, and reach are defined. Because of the diversity of process evaluation measures, methods used to collect the data, and ways of reporting results, it is difficult to compare findings across studies, and all but the most experienced evaluators may be overwhelmed by it. Creating clear, consistent definitions of existing process evaluation outcome measures would fill an existing gap in knowledge about process evaluation.

The lack of a systematic approach to guiding process evaluation efforts causes another serious gap in current knowledge about process evaluation. Most published literature describes the process evaluation for a single project or research effort. Few resources that take a systematic approach to designing a process evaluation effort are available in the current literature. Without guides for the planning and development of a process evaluation effort, project staff members are often left to reinvent an approach as well as the forms and systems needed to carry out the evaluation effort. Thus, a gap in current knowledge about process evaluation results from the lack of a stepwise approach to creating and implementing a process evaluation effort.

Independent of the approach used are key components that evaluators must consider when planning and carrying out a comprehensive process evaluation effort. First, the role of theory is unclear in many of the most recent process evaluation efforts (Weiss, 1998). When theory guides intervention development, process evaluation efforts that measure the implementation of each intervention component will also be theory-linked. If evaluators fail to specify the underlying theory upon which interventions are developed, they will miss the opportunity to advance our understanding of likely mechanisms of change and how theory—and interventions—can be improved to reflect that new understanding.

Second, in view of the resource intensity of comprehensive process evaluation efforts, researchers should attempt to strike a practical balance between the data that is clearly needed and the data that is merely "nice to have." A "less is more" approach to data collection may be preferable to collecting all possible data. The burden on the project staff (for collecting and managing the data) and on participants (for providing data) can often be a big barrier to collecting all the required data and for maintaining the quality of the collected data. Embedded in the larger stepwise approach to process evaluation must be a process for prioritizing the research questions that are addressed, thus giving priority to the type and amount of data collected and the methods used to collect data.

Process evaluation typically yields a wealth of information—particularly because a wide range of methods are used to collect data. Typical quantitative data collection methods include surveys, reports, checklists, attendance logs, self-administered forms, project archives, and community profiles. Qualitative data collection methods include observations, structured interviews, focus groups, and content analysis of audiotapes and videotapes. These lists are by no means exhaustive, but very little is known about which methods are more (or less) appropriate in certain situations. For example, when is it best to use qualitative versus quantitative methods? Which methods are more successfully used in middle schools than in elementary schools? Which methods are quite appropriate in faith-based settings but are not appropriate in worksites? Although using a mixture of the qualitative and quantitative methods brings the strengths of both approaches to an evaluation effort, limited resources often require deciding which method is the most cost-effective for answering a particular question. Little information is presently available to guide the decision-making process.

Wide variation in analytic strategies for presenting process evaluation results exists, yet it is fair to say that most process evaluation analyses employ descriptive statistics. As powerful analytic strategies for assessing study outcomes are developed, it is desirable to employ these same techniques, when appropriate, to the process evaluation data. For instance, McGraw and others (1994) and Baranowski, Anderson, and Carmack (1998) clarify the role and benefits of mediator analyses by using process evaluation data. Process evaluation is often focused on the mechanisms of change, and because new analytic strategies are being developed on a regular basis to deal with these mediator questions, evaluators are encouraged to explore the full range of analytic strategies available to answer prioritized questions.

Finally, related to a lack of guidance about how to plan, develop, and implement process evaluation efforts is the fact that there are few training opportunities available for students or professionals who want this expertise. In typical public health training programs, one course on program planning and evaluation may be required. With the many essential topics that must be covered in that type of course, process evaluation may be covered in one or two lectures. Even with advanced training, unless a student works on a project or study in which a process evaluation effort is being designed, there are simply few opportunities to learn about how to build effective process evaluation efforts. On many projects, an outside consultant may be hired to assist with the process evaluation effort. Yet when time and resources are spent getting the evaluator "up to speed" on a particular set of intervention goals, less time and money are available to focus on the process evaluation effort itself. In general, most public health professionals would benefit from additional training on program evaluation—including process evaluation— to build a larger pool of professional resources with expertise in this area.

Advancing Future Public Health–Linked Process Evaluation Efforts

Like Patton's utilization-focused evaluation (1997), process evaluation will be most effective when it takes into account the needs, wants, and concerns of the potential users of the system. Key stakeholders in designing an effective process evaluation effort include all the project staff members who deliver services or handle data, project managers and investigators who have been involved in designing an intervention or project evaluation effort, and participants who may be asked to collect data and review reports. We view the development process as highly iterative—trying out various techniques, revising them, and reaching consensus on key forms and tools to be used to collect the data, the questions to be answered with these process evaluation data, and reports generated to inform stakeholders about progress and problems. In addition to using a collaborative process, including extensive pretesting, reaching consensus on a set of terms that can be universally recognized and applied to process evaluation efforts is desirable.

Defining the Components of Process Evaluation

As shown in Table 1.1, *context* refers to the larger physical, social, and political environment that either directly or indirectly affects an intervention program. Since process evaluation is concerned with answering how and why an intervention was successful or not, an understanding of the context is often necessary. To assess the context, process evaluators determine which environmental factors might influence program implementation and then determine how the appropriate data might be collected. For instance, in a program designed to increase physical activity among young people, access to recreational facilities would be an important contextual factor to take into account. Even if the intervention to increase physical activity was not successful overall, perhaps certain subgroups of young people—for example, those with greater access to recreational facilities—were more likely to experience increases in physical activity, whereas young people with little access to such facilities might be less likely to experience such positive outcomes. Brainstorming a list of potentially important contextual factors prior to

TABLE 1.1.   KEY PROCESS EVALUATION COMPONENTS.

Component	Definition
Context	Aspects of the larger social, political, and economic environment that may influence intervention implementation.
Reach	The proportion of intended target audience that participates in an intervention. If there are multiple interventions, then it is the proportion that participates in each intervention or component. It is often measured by attendance. Reach is a characteristic of the target audience.
Dose delivered	The number or amount of intended units of each intervention or each component delivered or provided. Dose delivered is a function of efforts of the intervention providers.
Dose received	The extent to which participants actively engage with, interact with, are receptive to, and/or use materials or recommended resources. Dose received is a characteristic of the target audience and it assesses the extent of engagement of participants with the intervention.
Fidelity	The extent to which the intervention was delivered as planned. It represents the quality and integrity of the intervention as conceived by the developers. Fidelity is a function of the intervention providers.
Implementation	A composite score that indicates the extent to which the intervention has been implemented and received by the intended audience.
Recruitment	Procedures used to approach and attract participants. Recruitment often occurs at the individual and organizational/community levels.

intervention delivery is the ideal situation. Sometimes, existing archival data can be used retrospectively to understand contextual influences.

Reach concerns the degree to which the intended audience participates in an intervention (Glasgow, Vogt, and Boles, 1999; Glasgow, McCaul, and Fisher, 1993). Reach is often measured as the percentage or proportion of the target audience that attends a given intervention or part of an intervention. Effective intervention programs aim to reach as many participants as possible; therefore, measurement of reach is critical for estimating total program implementation.

Knowing which subgroups of the intended target population actually participate is also critically important. For example, if overall reach is moderately high but only the healthiest subgroup of individuals participates, evaluators would be interested in taking corrective action to extend the reach among the entire population. At a minimum, evaluators typically assess certain characteristics of the population, such as health status or health risk level, age, race/ethnicity, gender,

and income and education level. In calculating the reach, it is sometimes difficult to know precisely what the correct denominator is for determining the percentage of a target audience that has participated. For example, in faith-based
settings, the church membership may change on a weekly basis. How one deter-
mines the actual membership may be determined by averaging attendance over
an eight-week period or through some other reasonable estimating procedure. Or
if the goal of a program is to reach senior citizens in a community, census data
from government agencies may be available to estimate how many community
members fifty-five years of age and older reside in a given community.

  Dose delivered is a term that is commonly used in the process evaluation literature and it refers to the amount or proportion of the intended intervention that is
actually delivered to program participants. Dose delivered is directly related to
program implementation. By this we mean that dose is usually determined by the
actions or behaviors of those who deliver the intervention. The process evaluation question that dose delivered answers is, What proportion of the intended
intervention was actually delivered to the intended audience? For instance, how
many lessons from the curriculum were actually delivered by the trained teachers
to the fifth-grade students? Related to dose delivered is the concept of *dose received*.
Baranowski and Stables (2000) term dose received as "exposure," or a measure of
the extent to which participants receive and use educational materials or other
recommended resources. Like Pirie and others (1994), we prefer to think about
dose delivered and dose received as two important, conceptually similar, yet different process evaluation components. To measure dose received, evaluators would
ask the question What proportion of the educational materials did participants
actually receive? and What proportion was read, viewed, or otherwise used by participants? Pirie and others (1994) suggest that surveys of participant program
awareness, message awareness, or other surveillance/monitoring strategies are
common methods for ascertaining dose received.

  Of the process evaluation components shown in Table 1.1, perhaps the most
difficult to measure is fidelity. *Fidelity* refers to the quality of the implementation
of an intervention. Although it appears fairly straightforward, devising appropriate measures is often difficult because quality may appear to be a subjective
notion (Dusenbury, Brannigan, Falco, and Hansen, 2001). Measures of fidelity
include addressing whether the intervention is carried out according to a prespecified plan and whether it is carried out in both the manner and the spirit in
which it was intended. It is the manner and the spirit that often prove difficult to
assess. Some projects develop checklists of core intervention components or minimum requirements that an intervention must include in order to receive a high
fidelity rating (Baranowski and Stables, 2000). Fidelity may be assessed by observations of intervention implementation by a trained observer using a structured

observation guide (Resnicow and others, 1998). A less expensive method is to have program implementation staff members fill out some type of survey or questionnaire to assess how an intervention was implemented. For example, they indicate whether all the components of the intervention were carried out and rate how well they were carried out. Of course, the problem with this approach is the possibility of biased response or recall. Identifying multiple indicators of fidelity may strengthen convictions about results. Balancing cost considerations with creative thinking about efficient, unobtrusive ways to collect data on fidelity is an area of ongoing research.

Program *implementation* includes a combination of reach (who participated), dose (what the program delivered), dose received (what participants received), and fidelity (the quality of the intervention delivered). Whereas fidelity is often a difficult process evaluation component to measure, program implementation is difficult to operationalize (or calculate). Program implementation relies on accurate measurement of the four components and must then add a weighting factor to determine the final implementation score. Some authors have recommended that implementation be the result of the product of reach, dose, and fidelity (Baranowski and Stables, 2000; Glasgow, Vogt, and Boles, 1999). An alternative approach would be to average the four to assess implementation. Using the multiplicative approach, if 75 percent of the audience is reached, with 75 percent dose delivered, 75 percent dose received, and 75 percent fidelity, then a program implementation "score" would be 0.32 (for example, $0.75 \times 0.75 \times 0.75 \times 0.75$). Using the averaging approach, such as $0.75 + 0.75 + 0.75 + 0.75/4$, the program implementation score would be 0.75—for example, the average of the four process measures. Program evaluators should decide a priori what method of calculating implementation will be used in a given project and what the acceptable levels of implementation will be. For instance, is an implementation rate of 75 percent desirable? If not, then what is the acceptable rate? If intervention staff members have a realistic implementation score to aim for, they are in a much better position to achieve the objectives. In establishing realistic implementation score objectives, researchers should take into account evidence on participation rates linked to certain intervention dose levels available in the literature, or they should talk with colleagues who are attempting similar interventions.

Baranowski and Stables (2000) argue that *recruitment* is a key process evaluation component. Recruitment refers to the procedures used to approach and attract prospective program participants. Examining the resources that were employed and the reasons for nonparticipation among individuals and/or organizations that were approached can be used as measures of recruitment effectiveness. Typical process evaluation questions related to recruitment include: Which subgroups of individuals or organizations were more (or less) likely to be successfully recruited? Why were certain groups of individuals or organizations more (or less) likely to be recruited? Was the recruitment process consistently applied across all individuals or organizations? If recruitment efforts yield a biased sample, it is important to understand the implications of the bias on the final outcomes. With appropriate process-related recruitment results, evaluators/ investigators will avoid overgeneralizing findings to all subgroups or attributing widespread success to a project that was not truly tested in all populations.

Thus, we contend that at the very least, process evaluators should collect data to determine the context (including documentation of recruitment efforts), the reach, the dose (delivered and received), and the fidelity of the intervention. In addition, accurate information should be gathered to describe the context in which the intervention occurred, decisions should be made early in the study about how to determine an implementation score for the intervention, and recruitment procedures should be documented.

In addition to these minimum requirements, a host of additional process evaluation variables may be collected, including changes in intermediate outcomes that lead to hypothesized changes in final outcomes, training results, program-specific results (embedded within the larger study outcomes), formative/pretesting procedures, and various quality assurance measures. Because there are often limits in terms of resources, time, and personnel to collect these data, difficult decisions must be made about which process evaluation data are to be collected and analyzed. The remainder of this chapter focuses on a stepwise approach that evaluators may use to plan for, prioritize, and implement a successful process evaluation effort.

Designing and Implementing Process Evaluation Efforts

A clear definition of terms, a collaborative process that includes the evaluator and all key stakeholders, assurance that pretesting will occur, and an effort to use the following systematic approach will assist program evaluators in designing and implementing effective process evaluation efforts.

Clarify theory. Figure 1.1 represents a recommended process for designing and implementing process evaluation efforts. Building on the guidance of Weiss (1998), McGraw and others (1989), and Helitzer and Yoon (Chapter Four), we begin with theory. Specifically, evaluators are asked to specify the theory that underlies the intervention being delivered. Often, it is useful to draw a conceptual model of the intervention (Earp and Ennett, 1991), or logic model, clarifying the specific theoretical constructs of interest, those expected to change, and possible mediators of the change process. From those conceptual plans, *interventions that influence specified theoretical constructs of interest can be developed* and pretested with

FIGURE 1.1. A PROCESS FOR DESIGNING AND IMPLEMENTING EFFECTIVE PROCESS EVALUATION EFFORTS.

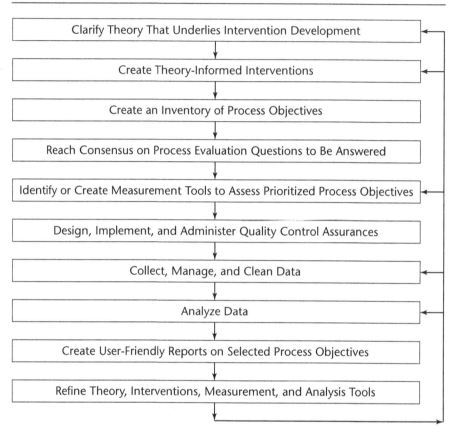

Note: It is recommended that key stakeholders be involved in all aspects of this process.

intended audiences. The role of theory does not end at this first step. Process evaluation results can be used to test theory (or parts of theory) as well as to create new theory. This process encourages the use of theory to guide the planning and implementation of a process evaluation effort.

Create an inventory of process objectives. For any public health intervention, there are likely to be several important intervention components. For example, in a comprehensive tobacco control worksite-based intervention, one might offer smoking cessation classes, self-help quitting programs, print materials with information about the dangers associated with environmental tobacco smoke, and a twenty-four-hour quit challenge. The program developers are in the best position to write realistic, measurable process objectives for each intervention component. Using theory and evidence from previous (and similar) interventions, program developers have the required expertise to know what to expect from an intervention of a certain intensity, frequency, and duration.

Following the flow diagram (Figure 1.1), the program developers would write one or more process objectives for each key intervention component. Like all objectives, these should be measurable and time-sensitive, and they should include information about what will specifically be delivered, who will receive the intervention, by when will they receive it, and what method will be used. If the first three steps of the process are followed, the process objectives will provide a measurable and theoretical link to the intervention. The process objectives will also help guide the evaluation effort.

Reach consensus on process evaluation questions to be answered. Once an inventory of process objectives is compiled, the team has provided a great deal of clarity about the intervention plan and its theoretical and conceptual links. Next, the team should reach consensus on the process evaluation questions to be addressed. As mentioned previously, the tendency will be to try to answer all possible questions, but this is not recommended in most cases.

Instead, consider brainstorming a list of possible process evaluation questions. To create the list of possible questions, start with the key components of a process evaluation that are defined in this chapter. For example, at a minimum, the team should consider placing a priority on getting answers to questions about reach, dose, and fidelity. In addition, if possible, get answers to questions about the context in which the intervention is taking place, as well as some information about the recruitment process.

As the team reviews the full inventory of process objectives, they might be tempted to create questions that address all of them. However, prioritizing the questions and performing a good measure of a few process objectives is likely to yield far more meaningful results than trying to measure all possible objectives. The burden on staff members and participants to collect and manage enormous amounts of data can become prohibitive. Thus, evaluators should prioritize by establishing criteria (a priori) for selecting which questions will yield the most valuable information for a particular study. The priority list of evaluation questions to be answered should be determined by using a consensus-building process with the project team. For example, if the intervention project is focused on a required training, there may be less focus on recruitment and much more focus on the costs and quality of the training approach. Here, the project team will make decisions based on consideration of the intervention, organizational demands or barriers, funding agency requirements, research study aims, available resources, and potential burden to the participants or study staff. In other words, decisions about what evaluation questions should be prioritized represent an effort to match the art and the politics with the science of developing effective process evaluation efforts. A collaborative process using a team approach to prioritize all possible questions will help focus the process evaluation effort. Moreover, this process will help ensure that all team members have the same expectations about what the process evaluation effort will achieve.

Creating a number of decision rules—or criteria for selecting priority questions up front—may make the process easier for all concerned. For example, theory may be a guide for prioritizing among particular questions. Alternatively, if the evaluation budget is very tight, the team may agree to assess the cost of answering each question as part of the decision rules for prioritizing evaluation questions. Another method for prioritizing among all possible research questions could follow the approach offered by Green and Kreuter (1999) in the third phase of the PRECEDE planning process. They inventory all possible behavioral and environmental determinants influencing a specific public health problem and then prioritize both within and between those categories of determinants. Applying that notion to the evaluation effort, a grid could be used to rate each question by the changeability and importance of the question to the overall process evaluation effort. Thus, the project staff would consider all possible process evaluation questions and would follow a systematic approach for prioritizing the questions to be answered. The bottom line is that the team decides on the decision rules up front and has all the stakeholders who are involved in the process prioritize the key questions.

Identify measurement tools. All process objectives should be measurable so that well-written objectives will indicate how the objective is to be measured. Once process evaluation questions are prioritized, the evaluator reviews the process objectives that line up with a particular research question and either *identifies* or *creates* measurement tools to assess them. It is possible that no appropriate tools are available—or easily constructed. In this case, that particular evaluation question may be reprioritized and another from the inventory may be moved forward. Clarifying the ways in which the data will be collected to assess a particular process objective must take into account (1) the type of data collection required (paper and pencil forms, electronic forms, or some other technology), (2) the frequency of data collection, (3) who is responsible for data collection, (4) the reliability and validity of the data collection measures, (5) the cost, and (6) the potential burden to participants and staff members. These are not simple issues. The evaluator is encouraged to review sample forms (like those found in this book) to reduce development time. It is a good idea to talk with other process evaluators about potential problems encountered with a particular data collection method, as well as talk with potential end users for the measurement tool—and get their input early in the process. When the measurement tools for each process objective are identified, it is imperative to pretest the use of these tools under "real-world" conditions. An iterative process of testing, revising, retesting, and improving these forms is ideal. Allowing enough time to accomplish a thorough pretest of the data collection tools cannot be stressed enough. The time taken up front should be viewed as an investment that will reap great returns when it comes time to analyze and make sense of the data.

Quality assurance. Quality assurances about the data collection, coding, and management steps should be built into the process evaluation effort early and should be monitored throughout the study implementation period. In the Working Well Trial (see Chapter Six), several quality assurance steps were instituted by the data coordinating center at the Fred Hutchinson Cancer Research Center. First, field staff at all four study centers were required to complete a standardized training and certification program for using the study-wide process tracking system before they engaged in data collection. If staff members did not "pass" the certification test, they were asked to repeat the test until they met proficiency requirements. Second, process tracking coordinators at each study center reviewed the printed data collection forms and screened them for missing information and potential coding errors before the data were entered into the database locally. A majority of errors were identified through this local checking process. Third, the local database was then uploaded to the data coordinating center and the staff there did a second quality assurance check to identify missing data, potential coding errors, or any other systematic errors that might occur. Fourth, a monthly conference call between the data coordinating center staff and the local process tracking coordinator identified problems, provided updates on new coding information, and offered ongoing training and collaboration on the use of the tracking system. Fifth, reports were generated on a regular basis for the process tracking coordinator and the project directors/principal investigators at each study center to keep them apprised of the status of the process evaluation effort. These reports also served as a quality assurance check when problems were identified and solved.

It may not be realistic to assume that in all projects it will be possible to establish the extensive quality assurance steps undertaken in a large national trial like Working Well, but a series of quality assurances must be in place to ensure that the process data collected is meeting established quality standards and that project staff members are aware of and committed to the quality assurance process. Having a project staff person dedicated to the data management task is an ideal situation. This individual is responsible for troubleshooting problems, upholding quality standards, and monitoring/reporting on the status of the process evaluation effort over time. Technology has advanced at a fast pace, and the tools available to manage large datasets typically found in a process evaluation effort are becoming more readily available.

Although cost and complexity are always important considerations, using a relational database that allows evaluators to link different sources of data by unique identifiers is recommended. Flexibility is also essential when selecting either the technology to collect the data or the software packages to manage the data. Often, a process evaluation effort will be modified over the course of a project or study. If the system one is using to manage the data is inflexible, or if the software is so rigid that modifications are not possible (without great expense to the project), then data management efforts can become difficult. Evaluators are encouraged to talk with colleagues who have managed process evaluation data on similar projects to get an idea of what has worked well—or not so well. Blaine, Guire, and Forster (Chapter Eleven) review the steps required to develop and revise a statewide data management tool for tracking local smoking control efforts in Minnesota. This chapter offers useful insights and practical tips about how to create these systems and what to avoid in the process.

Data analysis and reporting. The analysis and reporting of process evaluation data does not typically receive much attention in the published literature. A few important points are worth consideration as evaluators face these steps in a process evaluation effort. First, evaluators should consider moving beyond descriptive statistics when analyzing process evaluation data. In some cases, this will be impossible—or unnecessary, but in the cases where sample size allows for multivariate statistics, it is critical to apply the most powerful analytic strategies available when reporting results. Moreover, to fully understand the mediating mechanisms of change, structural equation modeling techniques might prove particularly useful. Most evaluators are beginning to recognize the importance of using mixed methods and mixed analytic strategies for making sense of available process evaluation data.

Report generation is an essential component of a comprehensive process evaluation effort. If key stakeholders are involved in prioritizing the process evaluation questions to be addressed, it makes sense to discuss what type of reports they would like to see generated at that same point in the process. Getting end users involved in the process of creating practical reports will increase buy-in for all aspects of the data collection process. Evaluators typically have flexibility in the format and "look" of the report. End users can help clarify the best ways to create practical, easy-to-use reports.

Reports can be generated to assist with project management tasks, to motivate the staff to collect and enter data on a timely basis, and to identify possible problems in collecting or coding data. In addition, reports may be shared with study participants to help them stay involved in the study or to meet data collection timelines. Moreover, timely feedback on participation, or the extent to which the intervention has been delivered as planned, can generate great enthusiasm for the project among participants and other key stakeholders. Corrective feedback when problems are identified is also possible when reports are generated on a timely basis. Reports are also great tools for sharing success stories; everyone involved will benefit if reports are used to share good news, progress, or special achievements that would have gone unrecognized otherwise.

Summary

Process evaluation is a growing and important component of a comprehensive evaluation effort. This overview has briefly reviewed the history of process evaluation as it has been applied to public health interventions, has identified gaps in knowledge concerning process evaluation, has recommended definitions and the consistent use of key process evaluation components, and has presented a strategy for designing and implementing effective process evaluation efforts. Improvements in the conceptual thinking about process evaluation will drive changes in the design, measurement, data collection, analysis, and timely reporting of the process evaluation data. Process evaluation data can be used to answer important questions that advance understanding of how and why public health interventions work, which has positive implications for both research and practice.

References

Abrams, D. B., and others. "Cancer Control in the Workplace: The Working Well Trial." *Preventive Medicine*, 1994, *23*, 15–27.

Baranowski, T., and Stables, G. "Process Evaluation of the 5-a-Day Projects." *Health Education and Behavior*, 2000, *27*(2), 157–166.

Baranowski, T., Anderson, C., and Carmack, C. "Mediating Variable Framework in Physical Activity Interventions: How Are We Doing? How Might We Do Better?" *American Journal of Preventive Medicine*, 1998, *15*(4), 266–297.

Baranowski, T., and others. "Theory as Mediating Variables: Why Aren't Community Interventions Working as Desired?" *Annals of Epidemiology*, 1997, *7*(S7), S89–S95.

Bartholomew, L. K., Parcel, G. S., Kok, G., and Gottlieb, N. H. *Intervention Mapping: Designing Theory and Evidence-Based Health Promotion Programs*. Mountain View, Calif.: Mayfield, 2001.

Basch, C. E., and others. "Avoiding Type III Errors in Health Education Program Evaluations: A Case Study." *Health Education Quarterly*, 1985, *12*(4), 315–331.

Corbett, K., Thompson, B., White, N., and Taylor, R. "Process Evaluation in Community Intervention Trial for Smoking Cessation (COMMIT)." *International Quarterly of Community Health Education*, 1991, *11*(3), 291–309.

Dobson, D., and Cook, T. J. "Avoiding Type III Errors in Program Evaluation: Results from a Field Experiment." *Evaluation and Program Planning*, 1980, *3*, 269–276.

Dusenbury, L., Brannigan, R., Falco, M., and Hansen, W. B. Unpublished manuscript. Tanglewood Research, Greensboro, N. C., November 2001.

Earp, J. A., and Ennett, S. T. "Conceptual Models for Health Education Research and Practice." *Health Education Research*, 1991, *6*(2), 163–171.

Elder, J. P., and others. "Process Evaluation of Environmental Factors and Programs." *Health Education Quarterly*, 1994 (supp. 2), S107–S128.

Finnegan, J. R., Murray, D. M., Kurth, C., and McCarthy, P. "Measuring and Tracking Education Program Implementation: The Minnesota Heart Health Program Experience." *Health Education Quarterly*, 1989, *16*, 77–90.

Fisher, E. B. "The Results of the COMMIT Trial." *American Journal of Public Health*, 1995, *85*, 159–161.

Flora, J. A., and others. "A Community Education Monitoring System: Methods from the Stanford Five-City Project, the Minnesota Heart Health Program, and the Pawtucket Heart Health Program." *Health Education Research*, 1993, *8*, 81–95.

Glanz, K., Lewis, F. M., and Rimer, B. K. "Linking Theory, Research, and Practice." In K. Glanz, F. M. Lewis, and B. K. Rimer (eds.), *Health Behavior and Health Education: Theory, Research, and Practice*. San Francisco: Jossey-Bass, 1997.

Glasgow, R. E., McCaul, K., and Fisher, K. J. "Participation in Worksite Health Promotion: A Critique of the Literature and Recommendations for Future Practice." *Health Education Quarterly*, 1993, *20*(3), 391–408.

Glasgow, R. E., Vogt, T. M., and Boles, S. M. "Evaluating the Public Health Impact of Health Promotion Interventions: The RE-AIM Framework." *American Journal of Public Health*, 1999, *89*(9), 1322–1327.

Glass, G. V. (ed.). *Evaluation Studies Review Annual*. Vol. 1. Thousand Oaks, Calif.: Sage, 1976.

Green, L. W. "Evaluation and Measurement: Some Dilemmas for Health Education." *American Journal of Public Health*, 1977, *67*, 151–156.

Green, L. W., and Kreuter, M. W. *Health Promotion Planning: An Ecological Approach*. Mountain View, Calif.: Mayfield, 1999.

Green, L. W., Kreuter, M. W., Deeds, S. G., and Partridge, K. B. *Health Education Planning: A Diagnostic Approach*. Mountain View, Calif.: Mayfield, 1980.

Guttentag, M., and Saar, S. (eds.). *Evaluation Studies Review Annual*. Vol. 2. Thousand Oaks, Calif.: Sage, 1977.

Harachi, T. W., and others. "Opening the Back Box: Using Process Evaluation Measures to Assess Implementation and Theory Building." *American Journal of Community Psychology*, 1999, *27*, 715–735.

Heimendinger, J., and others. "The Working Well Trial: Baseline Dietary and Smoking Behaviors of Employees and Related Worksite Characteristics." *Preventive Medicine*, 1995, *24*, 180–193.

McGraw, S. A., and others. "Methods in Program Evaluation: The Process Evaluation System of the Pawtucket Heart Health Program." *Evaluation Review*, 1989, *13*, 459–483.

McGraw, S. A., and others. "Design of Process Evaluation Within the Child and Adolescent Trial for Cardiovascular Health (CATCH)." *Health Education Quarterly*, 1994, *2* (supp.), S5–S26.

McLeroy, K. R., Bibeau, D., Steckler, A., and Glanz, K. "An Ecological Perspective on Health Promotion Programs." *Health Education Quarterly*, 1988, *15*, 351–377.

National Institutes of Health. *Qualitative Methods in Health Research: Opportunities and Considerations in Application and Review.* Washington, D.C.: National Institutes of Health. Office of Behavioral and Social Sciences Research, 2001.

Patton, M. Q. *Utilization-Focused Evaluation.* (3rd ed.) Thousand Oaks, Calif.: Sage, 1997.

Perry, C. L., and others. "The Child and Adolescent Trial for Cardiovascular Health (CATCH): Intervention, Implementation, and Feasibility for Elementary Schools in the United States." *Health Education and Behavior,* 1997, *24*(6), 716–735.

Pirie, P. L., and others. "Program Evaluation Strategies for Community-Based Health Promotion Programs: Perspectives from the Cardiovascular Disease Community Research and Demonstration Studies." *Health Education Research,* 1994, *9*(1), 23–36.

Resnicow, K., and others. "How Best to Measure Implementation of Health Curricula: A Comparison of Three Measures." *Health Education Research,* 1998, *13,* 239–250.

Rezmovic, E. L. "Program Implementation and Evaluation Results: A Reexamination of Type III Error in a Field Experiment." *Evaluation and Program Planning,* 1982, *5,* 111–118.

Sorensen, G., and others. "Worksite-Based Cancer Prevention: Primary Results from the Working Well Trial." *American Journal of Public Health,* 1996, *86,* 939–947.

Steckler, A., and others. "Toward Integrating Qualitative and Quantitative Methods: An Introduction." *Health Education Quarterly,* 1992, *19*(1), 1–8.

Stone, E. J., McGraw, S. A., Osganian, S. K., and Elder, J. P. "Process Evaluation in the Multicenter Child and Adolescent Trial for Cardiovascular Health (CATCH)." *Health Education Quarterly,* 1994 (supp. 2), 1–148.

Struening, E. I., and Guttentag, M. (eds.). *Handbook of Evaluation Research.* Thousand Oaks, Calif.: Sage, 1975.

Suchman, E. A. *Evaluative Research: Principles and Practice in Public Service and Social Action Programs.* New York: Russell Sage Foundation, 1967.

Susser, M. "Editorial: The Tribulations of Trials—Interventions in Communities." *American Journal of Public Health,* 1995, *85,* 156–158.

Tashakkori, A., and Teddlie, C. *Mixed Methodology: Combining Qualitative and Quantitative Approaches.* Thousand Oaks, Calif.: Sage, 1998.

Weiss, C. *Evaluation.* (2nd ed.) Englewood Cliffs, N.J.: Prentice Hall, 1998.

Windsor, R. A., Baranowski, T., Clark, N., and Cutter, G. *Evaluation of Health Promotion and Education Programs.* Mountain View, Calif.: Mayfield, 1984.

PART ONE

Community-Related Process Evaluation Efforts

The four chapters included in this section illustrate the great diversity of public health interventions conducted in community settings. One characteristic that all of the chapters have in common is that the intervention was carried out at multiple sites. In Chapter Two, Kegler, Wyatt, and Rodine chronicle the involvement of a number of neighborhoods in a teen pregnancy prevention program. In the skin cancer prevention program described by Glanz, Isnec, Geller, and Spangler in Chapter Three, the education program was conducted at a number of public swimming pools. In Chapter Four, Helitzer and Yoon describe an intervention to prevent alcohol and other drug use by adolescents, which was conducted in numerous sites in Albuquerque, New Mexico. In Chapter Five, Ammerman presents a nutrition education program designed to prevent certain cancers, which was conducted in sixty African American churches in rural North Carolina.

Such diversity in the health problems addressed, the target audiences, and the settings places unique demands on those involved in designing process evaluation efforts for community-based programs. For instance, in the project Kegler, Wyatt, and Rodine describe in Chapter Two, the process evaluation was part of a larger evaluation of the HEART of OKC project. The purpose of the Heart of OKC was to reduce teen pregnancies by developing and implementing neighborhood and community action plans through a collaborative process that involved piloting promising interventions and embedding the interventions in a lead agency or organization for long-term sustainability. The process evaluation was designed to answer two major evaluation questions: (1) What are the factors that facilitate or inhibit neighborhood mobilization around a positive youth development approach to teen pregnancy prevention? and (2) Are neighborhood and community-level action plans implemented as intended? The first evaluation question, which concerns the factors that facilitate or inhibit neighborhood mobilization around a positive youth development approach to teen pregnancy prevention, was answered using a multiple case study design with cross-case comparisons. Three methods of data collection were used: (1) semistructured personal interviews with key informants, (2) observation of task force meetings, and (3) review of existing documents.

In Chapter Three, Glanz, Isnec, Geller, and Spangler report on the methods and findings of process evaluation across two distinct phases of the Pool Cool program, a sun safety program implemented by project and local staff members at swimming pools. The first phase (the main trial phase) involved developing and testing the efficacy of the Pool Cool program in a randomized trial at twenty-eight swimming pools in two geographic locations. The second phase was a pilot study of nationwide dissemination of the Pool Cool program (the pilot dissemination phase) in 186 pools in the United States and Canada. During the main trial phase, the process evaluation was designed to help determine the extent of program implementation, the amount of time spent on the program, whether environmental changes were implemented, whether children and the lifeguards were exposed to the program components, and how they rated program components. It also identified unanticipated circumstances that helped explain program implementation or outcomes as well as ascertaining whether the experimental (sun protection) and the control (injury prevention) pool sites had equal levels of program implementation. The process evaluation for the main trial assessed the *reach* of the Pool Cool intervention (that is, how many people received how much of the intervention) and the satisfaction of persons exposed to it.

Process evaluation data sources in Pool Cool included monitoring forms completed by lifeguards and aquatics instructors (Chapter Three, Appendix A), project staff logs of what occurred in their contacts and visits with participating pools, observations, and selected items on the postprogram surveys. These data sources were intended to allow triangulation of the data and to pick up a range of intended and unintended occurrences and situations. The quantitative instruments—monitoring forms, observation records, and posttest surveys—had all been pretested and refined during the pilot study. Among the notable process evaluation findings was that statistical analysis revealed a *dose-response* relationship with recommended sun protection behaviors; in other words, those who received more of the program had better sun protection practices. These data indicate that the sun protection program was successfully implemented and well received in swimming pools, as was the parallel control program, injury prevention. During the dissemination phase of the Pool Cool study, a number of process measures were used to determine the extent to which swimming pools had actually implemented the intervention program. These process evaluation methods may be of interest to those who are trying to assess program dissemination, adoption, and implementation.

In Chapter Four, Helitzer and Yoon describe the Adolescent Social Action Program (ASAP), which had two primary long-term goals. The first was to prevent risky behaviors from resulting in morbidity and mortality—specifically such behaviors as tobacco and alcohol abuse among low-income minority youth in high-risk communities. The second was to empower the young people to become leaders who were capable of promoting changes in their communities' behaviors, social values, and environmental policies and norms. The theoretical foundation of the program was based on protection motivation theory and Freire's empowerment dialogue method.

ASAP operated in over thirty multiethnic (predominantly Hispanic and Native American) communities in New Mexico, served nearly sixteen hundred middle- and high school students, and trained over four hundred adult facilitators. The program was eventually expanded to serve twenty-seven hundred elementary school children through the program's peer education activities with younger students. An important part of the ASAP program was the group of adult facilitators who worked with the young people during the six-week hospital and detention-center sessions. Most of the facilitators were recruited through university classes and received university credit for their involvement. The ASAP program is an example of an intervention that serves as a bridge between school and community settings. We decided to include this chapter with the other community-based programs primarily because the program itself was conducted outside of schools by trained facilitators who were not school personnel. Also, one of the key purposes of ASAP was to have students return to their communities to act as initiators of community change.

The purpose of the ASAP process evaluation was to document fidelity to the program (tracking students and documenting participation, attendance, and exposure), thereby enhancing the interpretation of the program's results. This check for fidelity (to determine whether the program was implemented as intended) was designed not only for the summative purpose of determining if Type III error had occurred but also for the formative purpose of reducing the possibility of such error occurring, through the program's constant monitoring of its implementation and by its conducting appropriate activities to correct insufficient implementation.

In Chapter Five, the final chapter in the community section, Ammerman describes the design, implementation, and findings from the process evaluation of a five-year faith-based intervention that was designed to reduce cancer risk through dietary change: Partnership to Reach African Americans to Increase Smart Eating (PRAISE!). In this study, sixty churches were randomized to receive either the nutrition intervention immediately (Group I) or a delayed intervention (Group II), which received an interim nonnutrition intervention. Follow-up outcome data were collected after twelve months, and then Group II received the delayed intervention.

Project outcomes were measured at the individual level and included a baseline psychosocial, health, and demographic questionnaire administered by trained telephone interviewers. Dietary intake was also assessed by telephone interviews, using a food frequency instrument modified to reflect the Southern diet. All of these measures were repeated at the twelve-month follow-up.

Researchers attempted to design an intervention that was culturally sensitive and sustainable within the study churches and that could be disseminated to other churches. In addition, PRAISE! developers wanted to test this intervention within a true research partnership between the university and faith-based communities. The PRAISE! process evaluation was designed to address three areas: (1) *intervention implementation*—the fidelity of the intervention, the perceived "fit" in the church, and organizational/leadership factors that facilitated or inhibited implementation, (2) the *research partnership*—the degree to which church members and leaders were comfortable with the research process and felt that they were research partners rather than "research subjects," and, (3) the *potential for sustainability and diffusion*—the degree to which intervention implementers at the church level perceived the intervention as sustainable at each church and whether they thought it could be shared with other churches. Process measures included participant tracking, event surveys, county coordinator checklists, pastor surveys, and Health Action Team leader surveys, which were collected both during and following the intervention (Chapter Five, Figure 5.1).

With regard to variation in implementation of the program among churches, Ammerman, in Chapter Five, writes, "Although we feel that this is a strong approach to community-based interventions, it raises specific challenges regarding the use of process measures to determine the fidelity of the intervention. It may be more appropriate to describe it as the spirit and intent of the intervention." Ammerman is suggesting that fidelity should be assessed not by whether implementers rigorously followed prespecified content and methods but rather whether the resulting intervention met the "spirit and intent" of the intervention as planned. This approach to implementation fidelity is somewhat different from what is usually described in the literature.

As these chapters illustrate, of all the settings in which behavioral interventions are conducted, those in community settings are perhaps the most varied in terms of study design and intervention methods. As a result, process evaluation in community settings is likely to be highly variable in terms of the specific process evaluation measures used. A consistent planning approach that allows for the prioritizing of process evaluation questions is critical under conditions in which wide variation is likely.

CHAPTER TWO

Process Evaluation of an Asset-Based Teen Pregnancy Prevention Project

Healthy, Empowered, and Responsible Teens of Oklahoma City

Michelle C. Kegler, Vicki Harris Wyatt, and Sharon Rodine

The teen birth rate declined dramatically in the United States during the 1990s, due to a combination of decreased sexual activity among adolescents and their increased use of contraceptives—particularly condoms—at first intercourse (Flanigan, 2001; Hogan, Sun, and Cornwell, 2000; Ventura, Curtin, and Mathews, 1998). Experts are still debating what motivated these changes. Possible explanations include more cautious attitudes about sex, improved contraceptives, economic prosperity, and welfare reform (Flanigan, 2001). Despite this significant progress, over eight hundred thousand adolescents become pregnant each year in the United States.

Adolescent pregnancy and childbearing are associated with adverse health and social consequences for teen mothers and their children (Hogan, Sun, and Cornwell, 2000; Hatcher and others, 1994; Hoffman, 1998). Negative health consequences include increased risk of low birth weight, sudden infant death syndrome, and infant mortality (Annie E. Casey Foundation, 1998; Babsin and Clark, 1983; MacDorman and Atkinson, 1998). In addition, children born to adolescent mothers are more likely to live in poverty, have difficulties in school, and suffer from abuse and neglect (Annie E. Casey Foundation, 1998; Hardy, Welcher, and Standly, 1987; Connelly and Strauss, 1992). Teen pregnancy also significantly decreases a young woman's chances of finishing high school, thereby contributing to ongoing economic challenges (Hechtman, 1989; Annie E. Casey Foundation, 1998). For these reasons, adolescent sexual behavior—specifically adolescent childbearing—continues to be an important concern for public health (Centers for Disease Control and Prevention, 2001).

In 1995, the Centers for Disease Control and Prevention (CDC) funded thirteen communities in a new initiative to demonstrate that community partners could mobilize and organize community resources to prevent teen pregnancy (Centers for Disease Control and Prevention, 2001). Community eligibility criteria included a population base of two hundred thousand and a teen birth rate at least 50 percent higher than the national average, which was 56.8 per thousand women aged fifteen to nineteen in 1995 (Ventura, Mathews, and Curtin, 1999). Oklahoma City successfully competed to become one of the demonstration project sites. For the targeted central Oklahoma City intervention area, the birth rate for women aged fifteen to nineteen was 145.1 per thousand in 1995.

The Oklahoma City initiative—Healthy, Empowered, and Responsible Teens of Oklahoma City, called HEART of OKC—selected an asset-based approach to youth development as its overarching prevention strategy, with the goal of reducing teen births by increasing the asset base in families, neighborhoods, schools, and the central city as a whole (Rodine, 1998; Kegler, Rodine, McLeroy, and Oman, 1998). During the needs assessment phase, nine key assets were identified by young people and adults in the project area as being critical to prevention: (1) aspirations for the future, (2) constructive use of time, (3) respect for culture, (4) skills for meaningful employment, (5) decision-making skills to promote good health, (6) healthy family communication, (7) positive peer role model, (8) positive relationships with nonparent adults, and (9) service to others.

There is growing interest in a positive youth development approach to preventing teen pregnancy; however, the theoretical underpinnings to this approach are still formative (Philliber and Namerow, 1995; Pittman and Irby, 1999; Bogenschneider, 1996; Benson, 1997). Recent empirical work examining the relationship of assets to adolescent risk behavior lends support to this approach. For example, the constructive use of time—which is the case when, according to HEART of OKC, a teen participates in out-of-school and in-school programs and activities—helps prevent adolescent engagement in risky behavior, encourages the development of positive attributes, and assists young people in developing positive skills (Scales and Leffert, 1999). Studies show that teen participation in out-of-school and in-school programs, including sports for girls, helps to lower risk-taking behavior and pregnancy (Scales and Leffert, 1999; Sabo and others, 1999). Similarly, almost all of the HEART of OKC assets have at least limited empirical support linking them to decreased risk behavior, including sexual behavior (Scales and Leffert, 1999; Pick and Palos, 1995; Letson, Hammerton, Miller, and Lembitz, 2000; Liebowitz, Castellano, and Cuellar, 1999; Scales and Gibbons, 1996).

Larger Evaluation of the HEART of OKC Program

The process evaluation reported here was part of a larger evaluation of the HEART of OKC, which began in 1995 with funding through 2002. The members of the process evaluation team varied over time but generally consisted of a full-time doctoral-level evaluator, an evaluation consultant, and a .5 FTE research assistant, all originally affiliated with the Department of Health Promotion Sciences in the College of Public Health at the University of Oklahoma (UO) Health Sciences Center. The evaluation team was funded through a subcontract with the Oklahoma Institute for Child Advocacy, the lead or hub agency for the Oklahoma City-based, CDC-funded demonstration project.

The purpose of the demonstration project was to reduce teen pregnancies by developing and implementing neighborhood and community action plans through a collaborative process involving young people and adults, the piloting of promising interventions, and the embedding of the interventions in a lead agency or organization for long-term sustainability (Centers for Disease Control and Prevention, 2001). Funds could be used for needs and asset assessments, for the building of partnerships across community sectors, for training, for the field-testing of promising interventions, and for evaluation, but not for direct service delivery. Thus, the focus was largely on collaboration and the coordination of existing community resources to address teen pregnancy. During the implementation phase, HEART of OKC focused on four inner-city zip code areas where the teen birth rates were the highest and racial and ethnic diversity was the greatest.

By design, the project was both neighborhood-based and population-based. In the proposal development stage, state health department staff members, in collaboration with the Oklahoma Institute for Child Advocacy (OICA) and UO's College of Public Health, contacted community-based organizations (CBOs) that served the needs of diverse racial and ethnic groups in central Oklahoma City—primarily Native American, Hispanic, African American, and Asian (primarily Vietnamese). Once funded, the OICA, the hub agency, subcontracted with these community-based organizations to select priority inner-city neighborhoods and recruit neighborhood residents and organizational representatives to outline plans to address teen pregnancy by using a youth development approach. Both young people and adults were involved in the information-gathering and planning activities.

The first two years of the effort were spent selecting the priority neighborhoods, forming adult and youth task forces, conducting neighborhood and population-based needs and assets assessments, identifying a core set of assets on which to focus the interventions, and developing neighborhood and community action plans. The remaining five years were spent implementing the action plans, with specific interventions being reviewed and revised annually as new opportunities emerged, existing interventions expanded, and the initial pilot activity was completed.

The process evaluation reported here complements the outcome evaluation designed to examine the relationships between the nine key assets identified in the planning phase and several risk behaviors—including sexual activity—among young people in the targeted neighborhoods (Oman and others, 2002; Atkins and others, 2002; Oman and others, 2001). In-depth data were collected from over thirteen hundred parent-teen dyads randomly selected from households in the priority neighborhoods of Oklahoma City and a comparison community. Additional outcome evaluation activities include organizational network interviews conducted with youth-serving organizations in the intervention and comparison communities before and after intervention. And information from the organizational network interviews was used to assess changes in the level and type of collaboration around youth development.

The process evaluation was designed to answer two major evaluation questions: (1) What are the factors that facilitate or inhibit neighborhood mobilization around a positive youth development approach to teen pregnancy prevention? and (2) Are neighborhood- and community-level action plans implemented as planned? The rest of this chapter describes evaluation efforts to answer these two questions.

Neighborhood Mobilization

Methods

The first evaluation question, which focuses on the factors that facilitate or inhibit neighborhood mobilization around a positive youth development approach to teen pregnancy prevention, was answered by using a multiple case study design with cross-case comparisons (Yin, 1993). Three methods of data collection were used: (1) semistructured personal interviews with key informants, (2) observation of task force meetings, and (3) review of existing documents. The research design and data collection instruments were reviewed and approved by UO's Health Sciences Center Institutional Review Board.

During the planning phase, five neighborhoods participated in the project. Each of these neighborhoods was selected, in part, because of a priority racial/ethnic population. These included neighborhood A (Vietnamese), neighborhood B (white), neighborhood C (Hispanic), neighborhood D (African American), and neighborhood/community E (Native American). All of these were neighborhood-based except for the Native American initiative, which covered the central city area.

The case studies described the mobilization process in the neighborhoods for the planning phase (years one and two) and the first part of the intervention phase (years three and four). In most of the neighborhoods, HEART of OKC, under the auspices of the OICA, contracted with community-based organizations with ties to particular populations or geographic areas to recruit residents to engage in planning activities focused on positive youth development and teen pregnancy prevention.

Interviews. Twenty-one semistructured interviews were conducted with key informants during the planning and intervention phases of the project. During the planning phase, interviews were conducted with two lead agency staff members, one evaluator, one state health department staff member, and five neighborhood coordinators. Early in the intervention phase, interviews were conducted with two lead agency staff members, four neighborhood coordinators, and an adult and youth task force participant from each active neighborhood (three youth and three adult volunteer interviews). Interview guides containing open-ended questions were developed for each major category of key informant. All interviews were tape-recorded and transcribed. Planning phase interview guides covered respondent background, community/needs assessment, selection of neighborhoods, staffing and leadership, and general satisfaction and dissatisfaction with the project to-date. Implementation phase interview guides covered staffing, organizational structure, leadership, membership and recruitment, decision making, communication, tension (conflict), participation, capacity building, and general satisfaction and dissatisfaction with the project to-date.

Observation. Four of the neighborhood task forces were observed by evaluation staff members during the planning phase and three were observed again during the implementation phase. In two communities, there were no active task forces at the time of the observation. An observation guide was used for both rounds of observations, based on instruments used in previous research (Kegler, Steckler, Malek, and McLeroy, 1998; Goodman and Wandersman, 1994). The major sections of the guide covered room arrangement, attendance, agenda, organizational climate, meeting organization, leadership style, staff's role, decision-making process, community action plan awareness, group input into the planning process, group cohesiveness, tension/conflict, interaction between staff members and chairs of the task force, time spent working versus listening to presentations, general participation level, balance of task to process activities, meeting productivity, mechanism to involve task force members, and overall meeting effectiveness. In addition, the coordinators were asked several open-ended questions to solicit their views on the effectiveness of the meeting.

Documents. The documents collected for each case included needs and assets assessment reports, meeting minutes and agendas, action plans, and progress logs (implementation phase only). These documents were helpful in developing meeting chronologies and in writing case descriptions for each neighborhood.

Mobilization Measure

The main outcome of interest was the extent to which a neighborhood was mobilized to address positive youth development and teen pregnancy prevention. The primary measure was whether an adult or youth task force was formed and, if formed, whether it remained active into the second intervention year. Secondary measures of mobilization included the number of meetings held during the planning phase and average attendance at the meetings. Based on these measures, the neighborhoods were classified into high, medium, and low levels of mobilization.

Case Study Analysis

Content analysis was performed on all case study materials (Patton, 1990). A codebook was developed to aid in the content analysis of the interview transcripts and observation notes. For the first round of interviews and observations, two evaluators coded the data independently. The two sets of codes were then compared and discrepancies were resolved through discussion. For the second round of data collection, two evaluators coded three of the transcripts to develop a common understanding of the coding scheme. Following this, one evaluator coded the remaining transcripts and the second evaluator reviewed the codes.

All transcripts and field notes were entered into NUD*IST, a qualitative data analysis software package. Codes were entered into NUD*IST and then reports were generated for each of the factors covered in the case study questions. These reports contained all comments related to a particular code. Matrices were then created to assess the related text from each category of respondent (Miles and Huberman, 1994). These matrices were used to prepare the case descriptions, which were reviewed by the neighborhood coordinators and lead agency staff members for accuracy. A series of site-ordered matrices were then prepared to aid in the identification of patterns across cases, and neighborhoods were ordered by level of mobilization.

Findings Related to Neighborhood Mobilization

The cross-site analysis was based largely on site-ordered matrices using mobilization as the primary concept of interest (Table 2.1). Neighborhood A, which focused on the Vietnamese community, evidenced the highest degree of mobilization. Youth and adult task forces were formed early in the project and were still active

TABLE 2.1. SITE-ORDERED MATRIX ON NEIGHBORHOOD MOBILIZATION BY CHARACTERISTICS OF THE COMMUNITY-BASED ORGANIZATION (CBO), COORDINATION, AND LEADERSHIP.

Rank Based on Level of Mobilization (1 = highest)	Neighborhood	CBO Had Prior Ties to Neighborhood	Coordinator(s) from Neighborhood	Coordinator Experience in Community Organizing	Staff Time Devoted to Project*	Leadership Positions	Leadership in Running Meetings
1	A	Yes	Yes	High	Full-time	No formal positions; rotated by activity	Coordinator Community Leader
2	C	Yes	No	Low	Full-time	Formal positions	Coordinator
3	E	No	No	Low	Part-time	None	Coordinator
4	B	No	Yes	Low	Part-time	None	Coordinator
5	D	Yes	No	High	Part-time	None	Coordinator

*All coordinators were part-time initially; some shifted to full-time later in the planning phase.

in the third year of intervention. Average attendance was higher than for the other neighborhoods and more meetings were held. Member input into the action plans was significant, and implementation of the action plans was high in intervention years one and two. Neighborhood C (Hispanic focus) had the next-highest degree of mobilization, although mainly with young people rather than with adults. The coordinator developed the action plan with little input from the task force, but young people were very involved in implementing activities and helped plan a variety of specific activities. The youth task force was still active in the third year of intervention.

Neighborhood B, a predominantly white area of the city, was not able to sustain over time its resident involvement in a youth development planning project. Because no CBO was present in the neighborhood and devoted to addressing youth-related issues in this part of the city, the HEART of OKC hub agency provided the organizational base for this initiative. Although interest among residents appeared high initially, it diminished over time. No action plan was developed, and HEART of OKC did not keep this area as a high-priority neighborhood in the intervention phase of the seven-year project.

Similarly, Neighborhood D, a heavily African American community, was not successfully mobilized around teen pregnancy prevention from a positive youth development perspective. The neighborhood association that was approached to form the core of a planning group was primarily interested in safety and crime prevention activities, especially in relation to gangs. Moreover, the coordinator did not feel that an extensive planning process was necessary. She had worked in the neighborhood for several years, had strong ties to the neighborhood youth, and felt that she knew their needs. Near the end of the planning phase, however, she experienced several major life changes and left the project. As there was no agency physically located in the neighborhood, there seemed little on which to anchor the project. Unfortunately, there was not enough left in place, such as a task force, committed residents, or needs assessment findings, and there were too few indications of readiness to justify continued efforts to address teen pregnancy as a neighborhood concern.

The effort in neighborhood/community E, which focused on Native American youth, was not able to find a geographic area with a large enough concentration of Native American residents to justify a neighborhood-based effort. Native American tribal governments are located in other areas of the state rather than in central Oklahoma City. Therefore, this effort evolved to focus on Native Americans living within the central city area (and not in one particular neighborhood). This initiative had a modest level of community mobilization, which was not sustained into the third year of intervention. Thus, the order of neighborhood mobilization from highest to lowest was Neighborhood A, C, E, B, and D.

Across these five neighborhoods, three of the dimensions that emerged as critical to mobilization were staffing, leadership, and recruitment. Table 2.1 presents a site-ordered matrix listing several characteristics of the staff and the CBOs managing the neighborhood mobilization efforts. Neighborhood A was the only project whose coordinator was from the community and whose organizing CBO, like the coordinator, had strong ties to the community. This coordinator also put in the greatest number of hours and had extensive community organizing experience. None of these factors by themselves, however, appeared sufficiently strong to guarantee successful mobilization. For example, Neighborhood B had coordinators from the general neighborhood but still had a low level of mobilization. Neighborhood D had a coordinator with significant community organizing experience and similarly did not mobilize around positive youth development. It appears that strong connections to the neighborhood and its residents, in combination with a significant commitment of time and relevant experience, were essential to successful neighborhood mobilization. Moreover, the coordinators in the most successful neighborhood efforts had credibility in the community, an aptitude for community development, and the ability to articulate a vision and purpose for the project that was consistent with the needs and aspirations of neighborhood residents. They also exhibited skills in fostering relationships with key people and organizations, building ownership in the project, and balancing planning activities with tangible, concrete progress.

It was also beneficial to anchor the mobilization activities with CBOs that had an established presence in the neighborhoods and that viewed positive youth development as compatible with their mission. The mobilization also appeared more successful when the leadership, both of the task forces and of the CBOs, believed in the value of planning and did not feel that they already knew the needs of the young people in their neighborhoods and could therefore eliminate many of the planning phase activities.

In all of the neighborhood task forces formed through the HEART of OKC, the coordinators were the primary leaders (see Table 2.1). The coordinators led the task force meetings across all the neighborhoods. However, in the two neighborhoods with the greatest mobilization—neighborhoods A and B, there were opportunities for leaders to emerge. Leadership responsibility rotated among the members for various activities in neighborhood A, and in neighborhood B, the youth task force had formal leadership positions.

Across neighborhoods, there were several recurring themes related to recruitment. One was the difficulty of rallying people around teen pregnancy prevention. In some communities, it was difficult because of the sensitivity of the topic or because it touched on religious and moral issues associated with premarital sex and contraception. In other communities, it was seen as a problem for "other" groups, not for the young people in their neighborhood or community. In certain racial/ethnic groups, teen pregnancy was not necessarily seen as a "problem." In other neighborhoods, it was not a top priority in terms of needs. HEART of OKC was careful to define itself as a positive youth development initiative, in part, to provide a way to reengage adults with young people and help adults understand that everyone has a role to play in helping young people navigate through adolescence in a safe and healthy way. The goal was to place the issue of teen pregnancy within the context of the whole person and not just within one risk behavior. Early in the project, however, some of the coordinators explained the project as being solely about teen pregnancy prevention, and this may have affected community willingness to become involved—especially if there were other issues that were seen as having a higher priority for time and resources (as in neighborhoods C and E).

Another finding across neighborhoods was that it was easiest to recruit people and organizations with whom the coordinators already had positive relationships. A corollary to this is that the coordinators who lived in the general areas and were already well connected were better able to engage people in the process (see Table 2.1). It was also easier to recruit professionals and people already involved in adolescent health and development. In almost all of the projects, there was difficulty in engaging parents and residents in the planning process, and several project participants mentioned having particular difficulty in involving men. Again, this is not unusual in high-need, high-poverty neighborhoods with mobile populations and a great array of challenges in daily life.

Finally, mobilization around prevention through positive youth development appeared to have the greatest success in the central city areas of Oklahoma City, where the neighborhood (or ethnic community) itself had an established sense of identity, some degree of existing cohesion and connection, a shared vision, and a history of working together. When artificial boundaries were used, or when there was not some form of visible community identity with a particular neighborhood or area (as with the Native Americans living in Oklahoma City or the multiple neighborhoods in the area designated as neighborhood B), mobilization proved very difficult.

Reporting and Using the Findings

The findings from the case studies were shared through a formal case study evaluation report (Kegler and Wyatt, 2000). This report on neighborhood mobilization included five- to fifteen-page descriptions of each of the five HEART of OKC neighborhood initiatives. For each neighborhood, the description included the following sections: (1) neighborhood mobilization, (2) task force maintenance and support, (3) participant views of the planning phase, (4) action plan description and implementation, and (5) summary. These descriptions were followed by a discussion of findings based on a cross-site analysis. The report was shared with each of the twelve other CDC-funded projects and with the CDC. Its primary purpose was to document what happened in each of the neighborhood-based efforts and to identify keys to success as well as challenges to help other communities go through a similar process more smoothly. Since dissemination of the report itself was limited to those involved with the CDC initiative, the evaluators are also planning to disseminate the findings through other channels (Kegler and Wyatt, 2001).

These case studies were used primarily for program accountability purposes, in part, because they were produced well into the intervention phase. HEART of OKC had advocated a neighborhood-based—as opposed to citywide—approach, and it was useful for the funder and for those involved in similar community projects to understand the feasibility of mobilizing inner-city neighborhoods around positive youth development as a prevention strategy as well as the factors that both facilitate and inhibit such efforts.

Action Plan Implementation

Methods

The second major evaluation question asked whether neighborhood and community-level action plans were implemented as planned. One of the deliverables required by the CDC was a community action plan; however, because these projects were to be largely community-driven, the CDC did not specify a format for these plans. In Oklahoma City, project staff members had varied backgrounds and most were not familiar with writing measurable objectives that tied logically to a goal, with detailed tasks, time lines, and responsible parties specified. Without this—or some form of written plan, it would have been very difficult to document the progress made by the project. Therefore, one of the first evaluation tasks was to provide a format and technical assistance on how to write an action plan.

Evaluation staff members developed action plan worksheets that included the intervention name, the related HEART of OKC goal, relationships to program model and targeted assets, the rationale underlying the intervention, intervention-specific objective(s), the organizations to involve, the number of young people to reach, and a detailed listing of tasks, deadlines, and responsible parties (see Figure 2.1 for a sample action plan worksheet from the Teen Outreach Program [TOP]) (Kirby, 2001). The evaluation staff then held a series of meetings with

FIGURE 2.1. SAMPLE ACTION PLAN WORKSHEET HEART OF OKC INTERVENTION AREA: CENTRAL CITY OKC.

Intervention: Teen Outreach Program (TOP)

Related HEART of OKC Goal

[Goal 1] Decrease teen pregnancies and related risk behaviors to enable central OKC youth to increase their chances for good health, school completion, and economic self-sufficiency as adults.

[Goal 2] Increase the proportion of youth in central OKC who report having assets that are related to the avoidance of teen pregnancy.

Program Model Strategy and Associated Assets

Prime pregnancy prevention	Decision making related to good health
Health promotion	Positive peer role models
Positive peer influences	Service to others
Community involvement	

Rationale

In terms of teen pregnancy prevention programs, the Teen Outreach Program (TOP) is one of the most evaluated programs in the country. TOP has a twelve-year evaluation record that shows significant outcomes in terms of fewer school course failures, suspensions, dropouts, and teen pregnancies. The best results are shown at the high school grade levels. It can be used in school or community settings and offers an interactive format for youth at varying academic and developmental levels. The St. Louis Junior League developed the original program. The OKC Junior League is an active community partner with the HEART of OKC project and will be implementing this program at two inner-city high schools. The volunteer service component is a match with the school district's plan to include service-learning experiences as part of the regular curriculum.

Intervention/Activity Specific Objective

To integrate the Teen Outreach Program (TOP) at High School 1 (HS1) and High School 2 (HS2) during the 2000–2001 school year, under the program coordination and sponsorship of the OKC Junior League. The initial program will be designed to involve at least 100 male and female students. The curriculum will be integrated into the life skills classes at both schools.

Organizations To Involve

HEART of OKC (OICA)

OKC Public Schools (High School 1 and High School 2)

Junior League of OKC

Other community partners

Number of Youth to Reach

Participants: 100 male and female students (50 per school) with a comparison group of 100 male and female students

Planning Adults: 12 adults

Tasks	Timeline	Responsible Party
• TOP classroom and community service components implemented at High Schools 1 and 2	10/00–09/01	Names deleted
• Junior League planning meetings re: community service, guest speaker scheduling, classroom parties, end-of-the-year banquet, etc.	10/00–09/01	
• Classroom Parties	11 & 12/00; 2 & 4/01	
• Planning for the End of the Year Banquet	11/00–04/01	
• End of the Year Banquet	04/01	
• Planning for 2001–2002 TOP Implementation	05/01–08/01	
• New TOP class begins	08/01	
• TOP classroom and community service components implemented at High Schools 1 and 2	08/01–09/01	

neighborhood coordinators, both in groups and individually, to complete the work-sheets. This process was repeated annually and provided the basic framework for assessing program implementation.

Documentation of program implementation was recorded by the program staff in intervention-specific monthly progress logs. These logs have three major sections (see Figure 2.2 for a sample progress log from TOP). The first section focuses on planning activities and solicits descriptions of the planning activity (for example, meeting, phone call, key event), organizations and individuals involved as planners and/or participants, and the number of adults, young people, and organizations involved in planning or as participants. The second section focuses on resources—including a general description—and the type of resource (money, free/reduced price service, equipment, space, food, adult volunteer time, youth volunteer time, and other). The third section focuses on contextual factors, and in it coordinators had enough space to describe the contextual factors that facilitated or impeded achievement of the desired community change. They were encour-aged to document events—such as another organization obtaining a grant, staff turnover in a key position, change in neighborhood leadership, a critical issue or event that emerged in the neighborhood, positive (or negative) press coverage, or anything else that was believed to have an impact on their ability to move an intervention forward.

These logs were collected monthly and then were used by evaluation staff members to prepare semiannual summary reports and resource summary logs that were submitted to the CDC as part of the progress reports. In preparing these summary reports, evaluation staff members met individually with the project staff people responsible for the implementation of specific interventions, reviewed the documentation submitted, and gave feedback on progress toward achieving objectives. When necessary, changes were made to accurately document the events and activities that occurred during the particular reporting period when the logs were incomplete.

Findings Related to Implementation

Table 2.2 shows findings related to implementation for the first several years of the intervention phase. Interventions were developed in response to the needs that emerged during the two-year needs and assets assessment phase. They addressed one or more of the "9 Key Assets" that were identified by young people and adults in the central city neighborhoods as protective factors important to positive youth development and teen pregnancy prevention. The interventions were designed to test promising prevention messages and program models. Each included a lead agency or organization that might provide long-term leadership and support for

FIGURE 2.2. SAMPLE PROGRESS FROM HEART OF OKC PROJECT.

Progress Logs

HEART of OKC Process Evaluation

Year 6: October 2000–September 2001

Descriptive Title of Program/Intervention: Teen Outreach Program (TOP)

Neighborhood/Community: Central City

Month: October   Year: 2000

SECTION I - Planning Activities. Use this space to describe actions and planning activities that are related to the design and implementation of the intervention. Include key meetings, telephone conversations, and other activities and events that you believe will (or did) contribute to the intervention.

Date	Brief Description	1. List the **Organizations (O)** involved.
		
		2. If youth and/or adults were involved in planning the activities, indicate by writing **YI** for *youth involved* or **AI** for *adults involved.*
		
		3. If youth and/or adults were participants in the activities, indicate by writing in **YP** for *youth participants* or **AP** for *adult participants.*
			Number Involved
			1. **O** =
			
			2. **YI** =
			   AI =
			
			3. **YP** =
			   AP =

Oct	TOP Junior League Planning Meeting at OICA.	Community Coordinator, 8 Junior League Volunteers, 2 TOP classroom teachers	O = 4
Oct	Coordinated with Junior League volunteers to recruit and schedule local professional speakers and community service placements for the school year.	Community Coordinator and 8 Junior League Volunteers	O = 2
Oct	Worked with High School Teacher 1 and Junior League Volunteer to coordinate plans for High School 1. TOP students to participate in Junior League video to be taped November 1, 2000.	Community Coordinator	O = 3
Oct	Junior League Volunteer forwarded names of members from the Junior		

(Continued)

FIGURE 2.2. SAMPLE PROGRESS FROM HEART OF OKC PROJECT. (CONTINUED)

League Community Advisory Board interested in participating in the TOP project. The community coordinator will contact.	Community Coordinator	
Oct	Continued working with High School teachers 1 and 2 to outline plans for TOP for the school year.	O = 4

SECTION II—Resources. Use this space to describe resources mobilized for the intervention. Be sure to include the acquisition of funding through grants, donations, gifts in-kind, etc. Resources can include volunteer time, material goods, and reduced prices in services, space, and money.

Date	Brief Description	Types of Resources *(Please list resources for all that apply.)*
Oct	Continued financial commitment from the Junior League for TOP—They allocated almost $11,000.00 for the year. TOP speakers who are not charging.	Money: *$11,000* Free/Reduced Price Services: *free speakers* Equipment: Space: Food: Adult Volunteer Time: Youth Volunteer Time: Other (describe):

SECTION III—Contextual Factors: Use this space to describe contextual factors that facilitated or impeded achieving the desired community change. This can include things like another organization getting a grant, staff turnover, negative press coverage, etc. These factors can be removed from HEART of OKC activities but must be thought to have an influence on the community change.

Date	Brief Description
Oct	The administration for the High Schools 1 and 2 are pleased to have the TOP program implemented at their high schools.

the expansion and replication of the intervention. The CDC initiative provided no funding for direct services, so any direct service funding needed for each intervention had to be secured from another source.

During the first three years of the implementation phase, twenty interventions were initiated by HEART of OKC or its community partners (see Table 2.2). Ten were still being implemented in year four of the five-year intervention phase and two were completed without transfer to a partner organization. Five interventions were successfully institutionalized by a partner organization, with reduced support from HEART of OKC. Two were still in a pilot phase and one was more of a needs assessment activity.

The major intervention strategies fall into six general categories: (1) sexuality education, (2) academic success and development, (3) employment skills, (4) service programs, (5) parent-child communication, and (6) community awareness. The largest number of interventions falls under the sexuality education category, and these interventions tend to take place in the schools and reach the largest number of young people. HEART of OKC and its community partners also implemented many programs in the intervention categories focusing on academic success and service programs. These tended to be the types of interventions that best engaged community partners, such as the local universities and churches. In examining the current status of the programs, it appears that programs focusing on academic success were most easily institutionalized by partner organizations. Analyses of the various assets addressed by these interventions show that positive peer role models and relationships with nonparent adults are receiving significant programmatic effort. Fewer interventions target cultural respect, parent-child communication, and employment skills, although at least four interventions address each of these assets.

Using the Evaluation Findings on Implementation

The evaluation staff prepared summary reports every six months to illustrate the progress made toward completion of identified action plan interventions, and these reports serve as the primary measure of implementation. The resource summary logs were also created from the progress logs to document the organizations involved, the young people and adults involved in the planning of the activities, and the young people and adults actually participating in the intervention activities. Both were used primarily for accountability purposes and were included in progress reports to the CDC. These progress reports serve as a major data source for the cross-site evaluation currently under way by the CDC and several contractors.

TABLE 2.2. SUMMARY OF COMMUNITY PARTNER INTERVENTIONS, HEART OF OKC PROJECT, OKLAHOMA INSTITUTE FOR CHILD ADVOCACY.

Interventions by Program Type	Major Assets Addressed[1]									Current Status[2] as of 6/01
	Aspir	Time	Culture	Employ	Dec-mkg	Fam	Peers	Adults	Service	
Sexuality Education										
Are We Almost There?— middle school sexuality education prior to PSI					X		X			O
Postponing Sexual Involvement (PSI) for Young Teens—middle school abstinence promotion program					X		X			O
Wise Guys—male involvement program					X		X			O
Teen Outreach Program (TOP) - high school prevention program					X		X		X	P/O—a 3-year pilot
Health-to-Work—Health education and prevention for recipients of TANF (Temporary Assistance to Needy Families)	X				X	X				P/O—refining pilots & replicating
Older Adolescent Initiative (18–19 yr.-olds)—focus groups; designing pilot intervention	X				X		X	X		Pre-P
Academic Success and Development										
Youth Leadership and Personal Enhancement—educational enrichment program		X			X		X	X	X	O
Supporting Kids in Independent Living (SKIL)	X	X		X	X		X	X		I
21st-Century Learning Centers—academic/prevention programs during nonschool hours	X	X	X	X	X	X	X	X	X	I

Program	Aspir	Time	Culture	Employ	Dec-mkg	Fam	Peer	Adults	Service	Current Status
Emerson Partners—Academic support/mentoring for pregnant & parenting students at alternative school provided by St. Luke's United Methodist Church								X		I
Employment Skills										
Health Careers—partnered with Health Sciences Center	X			X	X			X	X	C
Employment Training—partnership with Home Depot	X			X	X			X	X	C
Service Programs										
UCO Community Partners—partnership with University of Central Oklahoma	X							X		I
Community/Neighborhood Service Activities		X					X	X	X	O
Intergenerational Service Learning/Health Education			X			X		X	X	O
Uniting Congregations for Youth Development—expanding youth programs	X					X		X	X	O
Parent-Child Communication										
Plain Talk for Parents—parent education						X	X	X		O
Parent-Teen Communication Workshops					X	X		X	X	O
Youth Forum (media/regular newspaper feature re: youth)			X		X	X		X	X	O
Community Awareness										
Child Watch Tours			X					X	X	I

[1]*Codes for Assets:* Aspir = Aspirations for the future, Time = Constructive use of time, Culture = Respect for culture, Employ = Skills for meaningful employment, Dec-mkg = Decision-making skills to promote good health, Fam = Healthy family communication, Peer = Positive peer role model, Adults = Positive relationships with nonparent adults, Service = Service to others

[2]*Codes for Current Status:* P = Still in pilot status, C = Completed, O = Ongoing, I = Institutionalized or transitioned to partner organization

In addition, the evaluation staff developed flowcharts from the monthly progress logs to provide a visual summary of the various activities implemented (see Figure 2.3 for a six-month flowchart for TOP). The original intent of the flowcharts was to provide feedback to the coordinators on their level of effort in implementing particular interventions and their progress toward meeting objectives. A second purpose was to share the steps taken, or give "how to" information, across neighborhoods. As the project shifted to more of a central city focus (rather than being neighborhood task force-based), there was less need for sharing information across neighborhoods, and so the utility of the flowcharts decreased, although they are still included in reports to the CDC.

Though the goals, objectives, target audiences, activities, time lines, community partners, and program settings varied from intervention to intervention, the process evaluation format provided a common structure and frame of reference for the design and tracking of the interventions and the analysis of their effectiveness. According to the project staff, evaluation findings related to planning and implementation were useful in several ways. First, the various components of the process evaluation—such as action plans, progress logs, and flowcharts—enabled the staff to reflect on the major factors affecting movement toward meeting objectives, thereby aiding in identifying adjustments that needed to be made in future program design and implementation. The project staff and community partners expanded their knowledge regarding the relationship of a quality planning process, to the ultimate success of an intervention. The evaluation also provided a workable and common framework for ongoing intervention design, implementation, analysis, program refinement, and evaluation. In addition, the evaluation provided deeper understanding of the factors, opportunities, or challenges that influenced the planning and implementation of the interventions.

Another major way the evaluation aided the project was in providing a foundation and rationale for decisions regarding changes in the intervention design and implementation. The evaluation information helped the staff determine whether the intervention needed an additional pilot in the same format, needed to be refined before testing an additional pilot, was ready to be expanded in its current form, or could be brought to closure as a pilot intervention and transitioned to a community partner for ongoing support. Finally, the evaluation enabled the staff to track critical events or issues that may be important to consider when determining strategies for the successful replication of the intervention design and implementation process. To summarize themes and lessons learned in a user-friendly manner that had a tangible, practical application to the intervention was also viewed as beneficial by the project staff.

FIGURE 2.3. SAMPLE FLOWCHART, HEART OF OKC.

Central City Community—Teen Outreach Program (TOP)

Objective: To integrate TOP at High School 1 & High School 2 during 2000–2001 school year, sponsored by Junior League; involving 100 male/female students in Life Skills classes.

Year 6: October 2000–September 2001

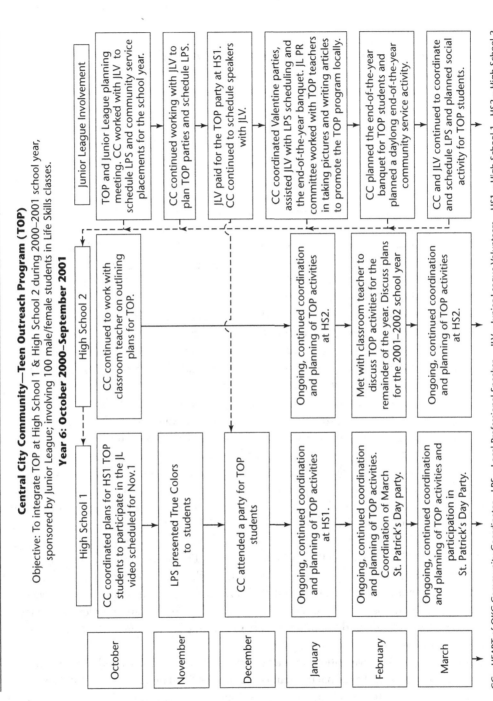

CC = HEART of OKC Community Coordinator   LPS = Local Professional Speaker   JLV = Junior League Volunteers   HS1 = High School 1   HS2 = High School 2

Lessons Learned About Process Evaluation

LESSON 1. *A close working relationship between evaluators and stakeholders is important.*

One of the most important lessons learned from this process evaluation was the value of a close working relationship between the evaluators and the primary stakeholders—in this case the hub staff and the major community partners. This evaluation underscores the need for evaluators and practitioners to spend time together. A common language needs to be developed as well as a shared understanding of the purpose of the evaluation. By having a close working relationship, the evaluators were able to provide some structure to the interventions so that progress toward their implementation could be tracked. Without a good relationship, this may have been perceived as threatening. It also helped to have the hub agency serve as an intermediary between the evaluation team and the coordinators responsible for the interventions. When the evaluators used language others could not understand, the hub agency staff members were able to step in and help bridge any misunderstanding. Clear expectations, trust, and open communication were essential to the positive working relationship developed between the evaluation team and the program staff. This strong working relationship provided stability to the project and was critical to the professionalism and productivity of the evaluation and the program team throughout the project.

Patton's utilization-focused approach to evaluation (1997) emphasizes the critical role of stakeholders through the entire evaluation process. He defines this approach as "evaluation done for and with specific, intended primary users for specific, intended primary uses" (p. 23). Throughout the entire evaluation process, including initial conceptualization of the project, the program staff and the evaluation team had frequent and ongoing dialogues on the general programmatic approach, specific intervention activities, and the evaluation process. All instruments were developed with the assistance of the project staff members, who carefully reviewed all the evaluation reports. The project was neither program-driven nor evaluation-driven but was a truly collaborative effort between the evaluation team and the primary stakeholders, focused on finding practical, user-friendly methods for linking science with practice at the community level. The faculty in academia and the practitioners in community settings worked as partners, with conversations occurring regularly.

The evaluation literature discusses the advantages and disadvantages of internal and external evaluators (Patton, 1997). The HEART of OKC process evaluation technically used external evaluators, characterized as having no long-term position within the organization or program being evaluated. The primary benefit of an outside evaluator is the ability to be objective and independent, thereby providing credibility to the evaluation. In this demonstration project, the CDC strongly encouraged an outside independent evaluator. Because of the collaborative nature of the evaluator-stakeholder relationship, typical advantages of an inside evaluator were also realized, the most notable being knowledge of the nuances of the local situation.

LESSON 2. *Process evaluations need to be flexible to adapt to program changes.*

A second lesson learned was that process evaluations need to be flexible enough to adapt to a program's evolutionary changes. The HEART of OKC project was more fluid than many public health initiatives, adopting what the project director labeled a "network of opportunities" approach. This approach enabled the project staff to support community organizations whose agendas evolved to include positive youth development and to respond to other local initiatives. However, with this approach the evaluation staff encountered many challenges, such as having to determine which major interventions should be tracked in any given program year. By developing the action plan worksheets and encouraging staff members to identify priority interventions to be piloted, the evaluators were able to set some basic parameters for the process evaluation. A related strength of this process evaluation, as identified by the project staff, was the ability to plan, implement, and analyze intervention action plans annually (short-term) yet track them over a multiyear period (long-term). In this community, few community partners and program providers working with young people—whether in schools, congregations, or youth-serving agencies—have a history of working together on collaborative interventions that are monitored and evaluated over time.

LESSON 3. *Qualitative methods, including case studies, can make valuable contributions to process evaluation.*

A third lesson learned was the value of qualitative methods for understanding how programs are implemented in various contexts. The case study methodology allowed the evaluators to document neighborhood-based project activities and systematically identify common themes across projects in very different environments and with very different populations (Yin, 1993; Patton, 1990). A case study approach also allowed the evaluators to describe community context and how that related to progress. Similarly, the largely qualitative progress logs worked across varying types of interventions implemented in a wide variety of settings with diverse partners. The logs accommodated varying levels of effort and allowed the staff to describe facilitating and inhibiting factors. In addition, progress, accomplishments, and barriers were documented in a nonthreatening way. The progress logs allowed the project staff to "capture their successes," however they defined them, and they also helped keep the staff focused on their priority interventions in environments where they could easily be pulled in numerous directions. This ultimately aided the project in being accountable to the funding agency—the CDC.

LESSON 4. *Some process evaluation methods can be very labor-intensive.*

The fourth lesson learned was that certain process evaluation techniques are very labor-intensive. Transcribing and coding interview transcripts is time-intensive but only the first step in qualitative analysis. Because of the large amount of data analysis and writing involved in preparing the case study report described here, the report was produced well after the planning and mobilization phase of the project. As a result of this delay, the main purpose of the document was to share what happened with the other funded communities. Had the report been produced in a more timely manner or in phases, it may have had more relevance for the coordinators working in each of the neighborhoods. The most likely benefit for the HEART of OKC staff was the opportunity to step back and critically reflect on the process they had gone through during the actual interviews.

The progress logs were also extremely labor-intensive—and more from the project staff perspective. Although the evaluators eventually received logs from all staff members, some were completed retrospectively and probably suffered from recall bias. Other biases likely resulted from the collection of logs from only one staff person, as opposed to documenting progress from the perspective of partner organization staff members, task force members, and, when appropriate, program participants. The reports produced from the logs evolved over time, because it was initially difficult to determine the best way to synthesize the data from the logs. Again, the evaluation staff primarily used the logs to complete reports to the CDC, and the project staff perceived them as having little day-to-day use.

LESSON 5. *Process evaluations that disentangle the "black box" of large community interventions are needed.*

The HEART of OKC implemented or supported twenty interventions in the four years of the implementation phase. Conducting tailored process (and short-term outcome) evaluations for each of these interventions was beyond the scope of the current evaluation, although this was done for several of the more innovative or promising interventions—typically those using a pre- or posttest design. In theory, an outcome evaluation would assess the cumulative impact of all of these interventions implemented simultaneously. It would be beneficial to sort out which specific programs or program components contributed to any observed change in youth assets or risk behaviors resulting from HEART of OKC. A very common follow-up question to the exclamation It worked! is *What* worked? Although the process evaluation documented most of the activity associated with HEART of OKC interventions, it will be hard to answer the What worked? and Why? questions in any meaningful or succinct way. This may be the focus of future evaluation efforts as the interventions are embedded within community partner agencies and organizations for long-term sustainability.

Contribution

The HEART of OKC process evaluation contributes to both practice and evaluation methods. HEART of OKC is one of the first community efforts to address teen pregnancy by using a positive youth development approach. Careful documentation of the successes and barriers associated with organizing inner-city, high-poverty neighborhoods to better support young people through multiple case study methods will aid in successful replication elsewhere. Although findings from this evaluation should not be generalized to all neighborhoods, those interested in starting a similar effort should consider working with "real" communities (as opposed to neighborhoods delineated by census or zip code boundaries) and should tap into existing networks such as this demonstration project was able to do with the Vietnamese community. Hiring staff members who have ties to particular communities and who possess the right qualities—such as being an effective communicator, being trustworthy, having the ability to facilitate the work of others, and being generous enough to share credit with others—for community organizing work is also essential. In addition, documentation of the steps taken to implement each major intervention will also aid in replicating and disseminating this innovative model for preventing teen pregnancy. Sharing progress logs and flowcharts with others doing similar work will broaden the understanding of how to implement these interventions as well as provide insight into the resources and level of effort required.

Community-wide prevention initiatives with multiple and simultaneous interventions are notoriously difficult to evaluate (Mittelmark, 1999). Secular trends (as in the case of teen pregnancy), unit of analysis issues, synergistic effects of multiple interventions, and dispersion of program participants all contribute to these challenges. Although the HEART of OKC process evaluation does not overcome these challenges, it does address some of these challenges and illustrates alternative methodologies that may be better suited to community-driven prevention initiatives.

References

Annie E. Casey Foundation. *When Teens Have Sex: Issues and Trends: KIDS COUNT Special Report.* Baltimore, Md.: Annie E. Casey Foundation, 1998.

Atkins, L. A., and others. "Adolescent Tobacco Use: The Protective Effects of Developmental Assets." *American Journal of Health Promotion,* 2002, *16*(4), 198–205.

Babsin, C., and Clark, M. "Relationships Between Infant Death and Maternal Age." *Journal of Pediatrics,* 1983, *103,* 391–393.

Benson, P. *All Kids Are Our Kids.* San Francisco: Jossey-Bass, 1997.

Bogenschneider, K. "An Ecological Risk/Protective Theory for Building Prevention Programs, Policies and Community Capacity to Support Youth." *Family Relations,* 1996, *45,* 127–138.

Centers for Disease Control and Prevention. *Interim Progress Report: The CDC Community Coalition Partnership Demonstration Programs for the Prevention of Teen Pregnancy.* Atlanta, Ga.: Centers for Disease Control and Prevention, 2001.

Connelly, C., and Strauss, M. "Mothers' Age and Risk for Physical Abuse." *Child Abuse and Neglect,* 1992, *16,* 709–718.

Flanigan, C. *What's Behind the Good News: The Decline in Teen Pregnancy Rates During the 1990s.* Washington, D.C.: The National Campaign to Prevent Teen Pregnancy, 2001.

Goodman, R., and Wandersman, A. "FORECAST: A Formative Approach to Evaluating Community Coalitions and Community-Based Initiatives." *Journal of Community Psychology,* CSAP Special Issue, 1994, pp. 6–25.

Hardy J., Welcher, D., and Standly, J. "Long-Range Outcome of Adolescent Pregnancy." *Clinical Obstetrics and Gynecology,* 1987, *21,* 1215–1232.

Hatcher, R., and others. *Contraceptive Technology.* New York: Irvington, 1994.

Hechtman, L. "Teenage Mothers and Their Children: Risks and Problems: A Review." *Canadian Journal of Psychiatry,* 1989, *34,* 569–575.

Hoffman S. "Teenage Childbearing Is Not So Bad After All . . . or Is It? A Review of the New Literature." *Family Planning Perspective,* 1998, *30,* 236–239.

Hogan, D., Sun, R., and Cornwell, G. "Sexual and Fertility Behaviors of American Females Aged Fifteen to Nineteen Years: 1985, 1990, and 1995." *American Journal of Public Health,* 2000, *90*(9), 1421–1425.

Kegler, M., and Wyatt, V. *A Multiple Case Study of Neighborhood Mobilization Around Positive Youth Development and Teen Pregnancy Prevention in Oklahoma City.* HEART of OKC Evaluation Report, Oklahoma City, 2000.

Kegler, M., and Wyatt, V. "Factors Associated with Successful Neighborhood-Based Partnerships to Prevent Teen Pregnancy Through Positive Youth Development." Unpublished manuscript, 2001.

Kegler, M., Rodine, S., McLeroy, K., and Oman, R. "Combining Quantitative and Qualitative Techniques in Planning and Evaluating a Community-Wide Project to Prevent Adolescent Pregnancy." *International Electronic Journal of Health Education,* 1998, *1*(1), 39–48.

Kegler, M., Steckler, A., Malek, S., and McLeroy, K. "A Multiple Case Study of Implementation in Ten Local Project ASSIST Coalitions in North Carolina." *Health Education Research, Theory, and Practice,* 1998, *13*(2), 225–238.

Kirby, D. *Emerging Answers: Research Findings on Programs to Reduce Teen Pregnancy* (Summary). Washington, D.C.: National Campaign to Prevent Teen Pregnancy, 2001.

Letson, G., Hammerton, S., Miller, D., and Lembitz, D. "Teen Pregnancy Reduction in Program with Peer Staff." *Journal of Adolescent Health*, 2000, *26*(4), 240–241.

Liebowitz, S., Castellano, D., and Cuellar, I. "Factors That Predict Sexual Behaviors Among Young Mexican American Adolescents: An Exploratory Study." *Hispanic Journal of Behavioral Sciences*, 1999, *21*(4), 470–479.

MacDorman, M., and Atkinson, J. "Infant Mortality Statistics from the 1996 Period-Linked Birth/Infant Death Data Set." *Monthly Vital Statistics Report*, 1998, *46*(12, supp.).

Miles, M., and Huberman, A. *An Expanded Sourcebook: Qualitative Data Analysis.* Thousand Oaks, Calif.: Sage, 1994.

Mittelmark, M. "Health Promotion at the Community-Wide Level: Lessons from Diverse Perspectives." In N. Bracht N. (ed.), *Health Promotion at the Community Level.* Thousand Oaks, Calif.: Sage, 1999.

Oman R., and others. "Reliability and Validity of the Youth Asset Survey (YAS)." Unpublished manuscript, 2001.

Oman, R. F., and others. "An Adolescent Age Group Approach to Examining Youth Risk Behaviors." *American Journal of Health Promotion*, 2002, *16*(3), 167–176.

Patton, M. *Qualitative Evaluation and Research.* Thousand Oaks, Calif.: Sage, 1990.

Patton, M. Q. *Utilization-Focused Evaluation: The New Century Text.* (3rd ed.) Thousand Oaks, Calif.: Sage, 1997.

Philliber, S., and Namerow, P. *Trying to Maximize the Odds: Using What We Know to Prevent Teen Pregnancy.* New York: Philliber Research Associates, 1995.

Pick, S., and Palos, P. "Impact of the Family on the Sex Lives of Adolescents." *Adolescence*, 1995, *30*(119), 667–675.

Pittman, K., and Irby, M. "Beyond Prevention: Linking Teenage Pregnancy Prevention to Youth Development." Paper presented to the Centers for Disease Control and Prevention 5th annual Technical Assistance Workshop: "Building with Communities Toward a New Millennium," Feb. 1999.

QSR NUD*IST, Version 4, Qualitative Solutions and Research, Pty., Ltd., 1997. Software.

Rodine, S. "Teen Pregnancy Prevention: A New Approach." *Pregnancy Prevention for Youth: An Interdisciplinary Newsletter*, 1998, *1*(2), 4–5.

Sabo, D., and others. "High School Athletic Participation, Sexual Behavior and Adolescent Pregnancy: A Regional Study." *Journal of Adolescent Health*, 1999, *25*(3), 207–216.

Scales, C., and Leffert, N. *Developmental Assets: A Synthesis of the Scientific Research on Adolescent Development.* Search Institute, 1999.

Scales, P., and Gibbons, J. "Extended Family Members and Unrelated Adults in the Lives of Young Adolescents: A Research Agenda." *Journal of Early Adolescence*, 1996, *16*, 365–389.

Ventura, S., Curtin, S., and Mathews, T. *Teenage Births in the United States: National and State Trends, 1990–1996.* Hyattsville, Md.: National Center for Health Statistics, Centers for Disease Control, 1998.

Ventura, S., Mathews, T., and Curtin, S. "Declines in Teenage Birth Rates, 1991–1998: Update of National and State Trends." *National Vital Statistics Reports*, 1999, *47*(26), 1–12.

Yin, R. *Applications of Case Study Research.* Thousand Oaks, Calif.: Sage, 1993.

CHAPTER THREE

Process Evaluation of Implementation and Dissemination of a Sun Safety Program at Swimming Pools

Karen Glanz, May Rose L. Isnec, Allan Geller, and Kathy J. Spangler

Skin cancer is the most common form of cancer in the United States, and it accounts for an estimated 1.3 million new cases of cancer each year (American Cancer Society, 2000). The incidence rate of melanoma, the most deadly form of skin cancer, has more than doubled since the early 1970s (National Cancer Institute, 1999; American Cancer Society, 2000) and continues to rise (Jemal, Devesa, Fears, and Hartge, 2000). Mortality from melanoma has increased by 30 percent over the past two decades (Howe and others, 2001).

Exposure to ultraviolet radiation from the sun is the most important known cause of skin cancer. Lifelong protection from the sun's rays can prevent most skin cancers (Gilchrest, Eller, Geller, and Yaar, 1999). Because sun exposure during childhood accounts for an estimated 80 percent of the total lifetime exposure (Preston and Stern, 1992) and children in elementary school receive more solar exposure than secondary school students do (Diffey, Gibson, Haylock, and McKinlay, 1996), young children can benefit substantially from preventive actions.

Skin cancer is the most common cancer, but it is also one of the most preventable. For primary prevention of skin cancer, one should limit time spent in

The work reported here was funded by the Centers for Disease Control and Prevention, grant U56-CCU 914658.

the sun, avoid the sun during peak hours (10 a.m. to 4 p.m.), use sunscreen with a sun protection factor (SPF) of 15 or higher when outside, wear protective cloth-ing (hats, shirts, and pants) and sunglasses, seek shade when outdoors, and avoid sunburn (American Cancer Society, 2000; Hill and Ferrini, 1998). Skin cancer is most common in fair-skinned individuals, and persons who lived in tropical, sunny climates when they were young are also at increased risk (Gilchrest and others, 1999; Department of Health and Human Services, 1996).

Although awareness about skin cancer is growing, the practice of preventive behaviors remains low in the United States (Robinson, Rigel, and Amonette, 1998). Preventive interventions have demonstrated modest success, with the majority of programs being delivered in school settings (Buller and Borland, 1999). Another, especially promising, setting for skin cancer prevention activities is outdoor recre-ation settings (Rosenberg, Mayer, and Eckhardt, 1997; Glanz and others, 1998; Glanz, Lew, Song, and Murakami-Akatsuka, 2000).

In particular, aquatics settings—such as swimming pools—are uniquely suited to sun safety programs, for several reasons: swimming lessons offer a structure for teaching sun safety skills, children and adults are minimally clothed, which in-creases the relevance of protective practices, families and communities often gather at swimming pools in the summer, lifeguards and aquatics instructors can serve as role models, and environmental changes and supportive policies can promote solar protection for pool users. The fact that most pool managers are willing to adopt skin cancer prevention curricula (Rosenberg, Mayer, and Eckhardt, 1997) suggests that such efforts can succeed. Up to now, only two studies of aquatics-based skin cancer prevention programs have been published (Mayer and others, 1997; Lombard, Neubauer, Canfield, and Winett, 1991). Both studies were novel and showed some positive effects, but they were constrained to small samples, in lim-ited geographic areas, and they emphasized either educational efforts (Mayer and others, 1997) *or* environmental-behavioral efforts (Lombard and others, 1991).

This chapter reports on the methods and findings of process evaluation across two distinct phases of the Pool Cool program, a sun safety program at swimming pools. The first phase (the main trial phase) involved developing and testing the efficacy of the Pool Cool program in a randomized trial at twenty-eight swimming pools in two geographic locations. The second phase was a pilot study of nationwide dissemination of the Pool Cool program (the pilot dissemination phase).

Evaluation of the combined main trial and pilot dissemination phases is based on the Reach, Efficacy, Adoption, Implementation, and Maintenance (RE-AIM) framework for evaluation (Glasgow, Vogt, and Boles, 1999; Glasgow, 2002). Process evaluation data also helped us interpret results of the efficacy trial. The main trial included a process evaluation addressing *reach* and an impact evaluation to assess *efficacy*. Reach is concerned with how many people received how much of the intervention. Efficacy is concerned with how much change occurred as a result of the intervention. For the pilot dissemination phase, process evaluation focused on *adoption* and *implementation*. Future work is planned to continue the sun safety program and evaluate *maintenance* as well as reevaluate the reach and efficacy of Pool Cool, comparing two different strategies to encourage its diffusion. We also used diffusion theory (Rogers, 1995) to help analyze and interpret the process evaluation findings from the pilot dissemination phase.

The project team responsible for process evaluation during each of the two phases of the program was closely integrated with the research, development, and core program implementation team. For the main trial phase, a total of twenty-two investigators and staff members were involved, including two behavioral scientists, four health educators, thirteen field research assistants, and three data management staff members. The pilot dissemination phase had a process evaluation team of ten, consisting of two behavioral scientists, four health educators, two data managers/statisticians, and two staff members from the National Recreation and Parks Association.

Context of the Larger Pool Cool Project

The skin cancer prevention program for aquatic settings was first systematically developed using formative evaluation methods and was then evaluated in a randomized controlled trial of its efficacy. After the efficacy of Pool Cool was demonstrated, we conducted a pilot study of dissemination at 186 pools across the United States and in Canada.

Program Development and Efficacy Trial: Intervention and Evaluation Methods

The aims of Pool Cool, a multicomponent skin cancer prevention program, were to improve sun protection (SP) behaviors and reduce sunburns among children who take swimming lessons and to provide sun safety environments and policies at swimming pools that would accept an SP program. Initial formative research was conducted in 1997, and it built on our previous formative research in outdoor recreation settings (Glanz, Carbone, and Song, 1999). We made site visits to swimming pools and conducted focus groups with pool managers, aquatics instructors, and lifeguards. The information collected during this period helped the project team understand both the opportunities and the practical challenges of implementing a skin cancer prevention program at swimming pools. According to focus group participants, the key considerations were easy implementation and the need to weatherproof any materials and environmental supports. Informants confirmed our expectation that a sun safety program was consistent with their organization's primary mission of promoting healthy, safe outdoor recreation and skill development.

The Pool Cool SP intervention was pilot tested at six pools (three in Hawaii and three in Massachusetts) during the summer of 1998. Results of the pilot testing showed high acceptance of the program by the site staff, including the willingness to attend orientation sessions and lead SP education during swim lessons. The program strategies were refined based on feedback from aquatics staff members.

During the pilot year, we also explored study design options for the main trial. We found that pools were increasingly providing on-site sunscreen, so it would not be possible to test the separate effects of environmental and educational strategies as we had done in a previous study (Glanz, Lew, Song, and Murakami-Akatsuka, 2000). The pilot test also revealed the importance of providing a program for *control sites,* as pool managers and community advisers felt that participation would be limited if people at the control group sites were asked to collect data but did not receive a program benefit. This was the basis for offering an injury prevention (IP) program at pools randomized to the control arm.

Pool Cool was evaluated in a randomized, controlled trial at a total of twenty-eight swimming pools in Hawaii and Massachusetts during the summer of 1999. The program was for children five to ten years of age (primarily those taking swimming lessons), their parents, and lifeguards and aquatics instructors. Participating pools included public municipal and suburban pools, YMCAs, and pools on military bases. The swimming pool site was the unit of randomization and intervention. Randomization was done separately in Hawaii and Massachusetts, using a blocking procedure to balance pool size and geographic location within regions.

Sites in the SP arm (n = 15 pools) received the Pool Cool SP intervention, which included a one-hour staff orientation/training by the study staff, as well as both educational and environmental components for the children, the parents, and the pool environment. The *educational* components included a series of eight sun safety lessons to be taught at the start of each swimming lesson (provided on waterproof laminated sheets), a *big book* to make lessons more interactive, on-site interactive activities, and incentives to reinforce the sun safety messages. The *environmental* components included providing sunscreen, shade, and signage, as well as promoting sun-safe environments. Research project staff members visited each pool about twice a week. Table 3.1 provides more detail about the intervention strategies used in the main trial phase.

TABLE 3.1.   POOL COOL SUN PROTECTION PROGRAM INTERVENTION COMPONENTS.

Lifeguard/Aquatic Instructor Training

Leader's Guide
- ➢ Skin cancer and sun safety basics
- ➢ How to include Pool Cool into swim lessons
- ➢ Other Pool Cool activities and incentives
- ➢ Evaluation Activities: Monitoring Forms and Surveys

Educational Components

Sun Safety Lessons
(1) Introducing Pool Cool: Rules for Sun Safety
(2) Water, Water Everywhere
(3) The Ins and Outs of Sunscreen, Part 1
(4) The Ins and Outs of Sunscreen, Part 2
(5) Covering Up with Protective Clothing
(6) Hats and Sunglasses
(7) Shady Deals
(8) Pool Cool Review

Big Book: Pool Cool Rules for Sun Safety (to use with lessons)

Activities
(1) The UV Index—Weather Watch
(2) Sun Jeopardy Game
(3) UV Light Machine (Dermascan)
(4) Colored Sunscreen Demonstration
(5) Sun Protective Clothing
(6) UV Solar Exposure Cards
(7) Skin Examination
(8) Pool Cool Review

Incentives

Sun-Safe Message Pens
Pool Cool Lanyards
Sunscreen Samples
T-Shirts
Hats
Pool Cool Refrigerator Magnets

Photosensitive Water Bottles
Glitter Sunscreen
Lip Balm
Pool Cool Insulated Lunch Sacks/
Can Holders

Environmental Components

Sunscreen—Pump Bottles
Shade Structure (tent, canvas/tarp cover, umbrella for lifeguard stands)
Sunscreen Tips Poster for Swimming Pools
Sun Signs—Official-Looking Metal Traffic Signs Adapted for Sun-Safe Messages (for fences)
Informal **Consultations** on Environmental and Policy Changes

Sites in the IP arm (n = 13 pools) received a parallel IP program, including lessons and activities on bicycling safety, rollerblading safety, fire safety, traffic and walking safety, playground safety, and poisoning and choking prevention.

The main evaluation was based on self-administered surveys completed at the beginning of the summer and approximately eight weeks later—by parents (for themselves and their children) and by lifeguards/aquatics instructors. Response samples were two independent cross-sections of parents accompanying or picking up their children at the pools. Measures for questionnaire items were selected or adapted from previous surveys on this topic that have been published in the literature (Newman, Agro, Woodruff, and Mayer, 1996; Weinstock, 1992; Arthey and Clarke, 1995) or have been used in earlier studies conducted by the project team (Koh, Bak, and Geller, 1997; Glanz and others, 1998). The main behavior outcomes—measures of SP behaviors—were assessed on a four-point ordinal scale ranging from 1 ("rarely or never") to 4 ("always"). The behaviors that were measured included using sunscreen, wearing a hat, wearing a shirt, seeking shade, and wearing sunglasses, and a composite sun protection habits index was made. Each survey took about ten minutes to complete.

Main Trial Results

The analyses of the efficacy trial used completed surveys from 1,010 parents at baseline and 842 parents at follow-up, as well as 220 aquatics staff members at baseline and 194 aquatics staff members at follow-up. Results showed significant positive changes—with children's increased use of sunscreen and shade, an overall improvement in their SP habits, and fewer sunburns among them, as well as improvements in parents' SP habits and reported pool SP policies. In the SP group, there was a reported 23 percent reduction in children's sunburns from the number that occurred in the preceding summer, with only a 1 percent reduction in sunburns from the previous summer in the IP group (p = 0.04). Effect sizes were small for child behavior changes and for sunburns (d = .17–.23) (Cohen, 1988). At follow-up, the SP group parents reported a 55.1 percent higher level of SP policies at their pools, compared with the IP group, on a scale of 0 to 4 (p < 0.001), for a medium effect size (d = .54). A *dose response* (as amount of intervention increases so does behavioral change) trend was found for exposure to Pool Cool lessons and activities. Observational indicators showed favorable changes in the availability of sunscreen, sun safety signage, and the use of shirts by lifeguards (Glanz and others, forthcoming). When the child and parent effect models were rerun using the random effects models to account for within-pool clustering, they remained virtually unchanged.

The Pool Cool SP program significantly increased children's sunscreen use, shade seeking, and total SP habits, compared with the effect of a control program, and it reduced sunburns in fair-skinned children. There was a clear dose response effect; that is, people who received more program components were more likely to be affected. This suggests that the magnitude of observed program effects is a conservative analysis of impact. Parents' sunscreen use, hat wearing, and total SP habits were also improved. And lifeguards' sunburns were reduced, though no improvements in lifeguards' behaviors were found (Geller and others, 2001). This may have happened because lifeguards were more rigorous about taking precautions during peak hours of sunshine and on the sunniest days, even though they were not consistent about improving their sun safety habits.

Of particular importance is the fact that reported pool SP policies increased substantially in the SP arm of the trial. These reports were corroborated by independent observations that showed significant improvements in sunscreen availability, sun safety signage, and lifeguards' wearing of hats. The effects were seen in two disparate ethnic and climactic locations.

From Main Trial to Pool Cool Dissemination Pilot Study

The effect sizes were modest, but this is to be expected with a relatively low-intensity public health approach to prevention. When multiplied across a large population, the impact on morbidity, and even mortality, can be substantial. We concluded that if the Pool Cool program could be widely disseminated, successfully implemented, and maintained over time, it could make an important contribution to preventing skin cancer. This was the basis for the pilot study of the nationwide dissemination of the Pool Cool program.

A key requirement for program dissemination was a partnership with an appropriate linkage agent with national ties to aquatics and recreation programs. Therefore, we approached the National Recreation and Park Association (NRPA), which is the professional organization for the recreation industry. The NRPA supports over five thousand parks and recreation departments nationwide, and these departments manage over sixty-five thousand public swimming pools. The NRPA has excellent communication/promotion channels, including monthly membership magazines, program catalogues, and a dynamic Web site. In addition, the NRPA has a history of collaborating with health promotion programs that have a natural place in recreation and leisure services, including a youth activity promotion program and a physical fitness program for older adults. Because the NRPA is responsible for training and professional certification in specialized skill areas, it is well positioned to collaborate on both the pilot dissemination and longer-term diffusion of the Pool Cool sun safety program.

After developing a memorandum of agreement that specified the respective roles and commitments of the NRPA and the Pool Cool program centers, the Pool Cool team worked with the NRPA to develop promotional efforts. The pilot dissemination was announced in a brochure and in "advertorials" in the NRPA program guide and magazine during Winter/Spring 2000. These materials invited interested pool managers to complete a mailed or Web-based application form to become *pilot sites* (basic) or *highlight sites* (enhanced). With modest publicity, the response was enthusiastic, and managers of 186 pools across the United States and in Canada participated in the year 2000 dissemination.

Program materials were adapted for dissemination as *tool kits* in either corrugated logo boxes or customized coolers on wheels and included leaders' guides, sun safety lessons, *mini-big books,* a decision maker's guide, a resource guide, sun safety signs and posters, and a Pool Cool zip disk for reproducing additional materials. And the project team provided support by telephone, e-mail, and fax. We conducted site visits and telephone interviews and analyzed various sources of process evaluation data at the end of the summer.

Main Trial Phase Goals and Methods

During the main trial phase, the process evaluation was designed to help determine the extent of program implementation, the amount of time spent on the program, whether environmental changes were implemented, whether children and the lifeguards were exposed to the program components, and how they rated the program components. The process evaluation was also intended to identify unanticipated circumstances that might explain program implementation or outcomes and to ascertain whether both experimental (SP) and control (IP) pool sites were equivalent in levels of program implementation. The process evaluation for the main trial assessed the *reach* (that is, the percent of intended audience who participated in Pool Cool) of the Pool Cool intervention and the satisfaction of persons exposed to it (Glasgow, Vogt, and Boles, 1999; Glasgow, forthcoming).

Data sources included *monitoring forms,* completed by lifeguards and aquatics instructors (see the example in Appendix A), *project staff logs* of what occurred in their contacts and visits with participating pools, *observations,* and *selected items on the postprogram surveys.* These data sources were intended to allow triangulation of the data and to pick up a range of intended and unintended occurrences and situations. The quantitative instruments—monitoring forms, observation records, and posttest surveys—had all been pretested and refined during the pilot study of the preceding summer.

Monitoring and staff logs were completed throughout the intervention period. The monitoring forms were designed to ascertain implementation of each of the eight sun safety (or IP) lessons, including the time spent on the lessons, components of the lessons taught, whether parents were present, and how each lesson was received. Survey items on the posttest surveys asked parents about their own or their child's participation, the incentives they received, and their reactions. At posttest, the survey asked aquatics staff members about the frequency with which they taught SP or IP lessons, the various teaching methods they used, and the incentives they received.

Data were collected at both the SP and the IP pools. All pools were included, and all lifeguards were asked to complete monitoring forms.

Results

We analyzed monitoring form data to ascertain the delivery of both the SP and the IP interventions at participating pools. Seventy-six percent of the aquatics instructors reported teaching the lessons, and 61.9 percent said that they taught the majority of the lessons (five or more). Monitoring forms (n = 615 forms) indicated that between 88 and 100 percent of aquatics instructors taught each lesson, that the average length of time per SP or IP lesson was five to six minutes, that about 40 percent of the children were "interested" or "very interested," and that more parents were present at the IP lessons than at the SP lessons (48 percent versus 10 percent). About two-thirds of the parents reported receiving SP or IP information and 57 percent said that their pool taught these health topics in swimming lessons, although activity participation was reported to be at a fairly low level. This finding led us to create a combined dose variable reflecting receipt of the SP intervention (in the experimental group only). Statistical analysis revealed a dose-response relationship with recommended SP behaviors. In other words, those who received more of the program had better SP practices. These data indicate that the SP program was successfully implemented and well received at swimming pools, as was the parallel IP program.

Staff posttest surveys showed that 87 percent of SP staff taught SP in swim lessons, nearly 66 percent used the Pool Cool leader's guide, and 60 percent used sunscreen provided in a dispenser. At IP pools, 83 percent of the staff reported that they taught child IP lessons, and 70 percent said that they used the Pool Cool leader's guide. Finally, because the response samples were not a cohort, we examined the association between the frequency of teaching Pool Cool lessons and the posttest SP habits. There was a trend toward higher SP habits scores with more frequent teaching of lessons and activities. This trend was not statistically significant, however.

Staff logs served dual roles—as ongoing quality assurance tools and to provide a check on any unanticipated results from the monitoring forms and surveys. They were used to help solve problems throughout the summer and revealed variable levels of distribution of incentives and aquatics staff participation. This finding was partly related to the size of the pool sites and their swimming lesson programs and was partly reflective of pool manager and staff enthusiasm for implementing the Pool Cool SP and IP programs. Another theme that emerged was related to the differential participation and implementation during rainy, cool, or cloudy weather, and this was seen more in Boston than in the Hawaii pool sites.

In summary, key findings in the main trial process evaluation were used to support and help interpret the efficacy findings. They showed a high level of implementation and satisfaction across both the SP and the IP arms, and they indicated that the program did not require a lot of time from the pool staff (lifeguards and managers). This information also provided a basis for publicizing the dissemination phase.

Pilot Dissemination Phase Goals and Methods

The aims of the Pool Cool dissemination pilot study were to (1) develop a program package, or tool kit, from the intervention evaluated in the efficacy trial, (2) assess the interest in, and acceptability of, Pool Cool being adopted in various locations without on-site project staff members, (3) assess the rate of decisions to adopt Pool Cool, and (4) determine rates of implementation and satisfaction with two versions of the adapted Pool Cool program package. The second, third, and fourth of these aims constitute the aims of the process evaluation during the pilot dissemination phase.

The research design included preimplementation data, data collected during the program period, and interviews and surveys conducted at the end of the summer. Data sources for the process evaluation included application forms (Web-based/paper forms), site visits, telephone interviews, evaluation forms, and checklists. Each instrument was intended to capture information about a different stage of dissemination, and each was designed to be relatively unobtrusive and low in respondent burden. We purposively sampled from a variety of locations and types of pools for the site visits and observations. For other methods, we sought to obtain data from as many pools as possible.

Two options were offered for the pilot dissemination phase: pools could either be a *highlight site* or a *pilot site*. The highlight sites would receive a more comprehensive tool kit, or package of materials, which included a big book and extra supplies and incentives, packed in a durable plastic cooler on wheels (a Pool Cool cooler). These sites also had to agree to a site visit by the project team. The pilot sites received a smaller tool kit with samples of supplies and incentives and with ordering forms for extra items (to be purchased at the pool's expense), packed in a rectangular corrugated logo box with a handle. Both highlight site pools and pilot site pools were expected to participate in evaluation forms completion and telephone interviews.

Pools that applied to be part of the Pool Cool dissemination pilot were asked to confirm their decision to adopt the program by signing a pool reply form. Application form data provided background information. Other instruments and methods used to determine rates of implementation and satisfaction were site visits, evaluation forms and checklists, telephone interviews, and surveys. Samples of selected forms are shown in Appendix B.

Results

Here we summarize findings for each aim, based on data received by September 2000.

Interest and Background Information

Application forms were completed either on written forms or on the Web. From twenty-one U.S. states and Ontario, Canada, 110 forms were received, representing 176 pools. The number per state ranged from one to twenty-three, with the most (twenty-three) from Ohio, nineteen from California, and thirteen from Illinois. On most of the application forms, respondents indicated that they would like to be either a highlight site (80.9 percent) or a pilot site (19.1 percent), and many respondents checked both options. Over 90 percent indicated that their pools were located in urban or suburban areas. Respondents were parks and recreation staff members (45.9 percent), aquatics coordinators (37.6 percent), or pool managers or directors (16.5 percent). About three-quarters were responsible for two or more pools, and most (57.3 percent) said that they made decisions about new programs themselves, whereas others (24.7 percent) indicated that they made these decisions with others. The most common pool sizes were twenty-five meters (67.3 percent), with 16 percent reporting fifty-meter lengths. New multisection pool sizes accounted for the remainder. Eighty percent of the pools had at least ten summer aquatics instructors, most of whom also worked as lifeguards. In addition, 80 percent of the pools expected at least a hundred five- to ten-year-old children in swimming lessons that summer, with the median number of children being 350 and the number of children ranging from forty to fifteen hundred. The most common schedule of swimming lessons (at 64.4 percent of pools) was two weeks, four to five times per week. Seventy-eight percent of pools were open only during the summer season.

The majority of pools reported providing sun safety advice (89.1 percent), sunscreen (74.5 percent), umbrellas (74.5 percent), and shirts and/or hats (87.3 percent) for their lifeguards and aquatics instructors. They also reported including SP information in in-service trainings (86.4 percent) and staff manuals (77.3 percent). More than 80 percent recommended that staff members use sunscreen and wear sunglasses and protective clothing. However, few pools reported providing sunscreen (25.5 percent), sun safety advice (29.1 percent), or sun safety signs (6.4 percent) for swimmers. It was more common for them to provide shade areas (69.1 percent) and to schedule swimming lessons to avoid peak sun hours (50.9 percent). Respondents at 71.8 percent of the pools recommended to pool users that they wear sunscreen, and respondents at 42.7 percent of the pools told pool users to seek shade, but only 20 percent recommended wearing a hat, only 14.5 percent recommended avoiding peak sun, and only 12.7 percent recommended wearing protective clothing.

Decision to Adopt

The project team originally planned to offer the dissemination pilot to a total of one hundred pilot sites and fifteen highlight sites. However, we decided instead to provide program materials and support to all pools that subsequently confirmed their decision to adopt the program. To formalize the decision to adopt the Pool Cool program, swimming pool managers who were interested in participating were asked to sign and return a pool reply form to confirm their continued interest and make a commitment to complete evaluation forms and/or allow a site visit by Pool Cool and/or the NRPA. The response exceeded 100 percent (106 percent), as some late requests arrived after the deadline for application forms. A total of 186 pools returned reply forms, including seventeen for highlight sites and 169 for pilot sites. As a result, this large number of pilot and highlight sites led to a delay in producing and shipping program materials (because of a limited staff to meet the demand). Materials were shipped in late June and early July.

Implementation and Satisfaction

We conducted site visits at eight highlight sites and five pilot sites in Hawaii, California, Colorado, Ohio, Massachusetts, Maryland, and Ontario. A site visit protocol included interview questions and forms. Pool Cool was being implemented at all but one of the sites visited, and at that pool, the local high school used the facility for swimming lessons and the aquatics coordinator had not reassigned the Pool Cool tool kit to another pool. Some tool kits shipped to Ontario were delayed in Canadian Customs. Interviews indicated that every pool that implemented the program was using the leader's guide (two-thirds had made additional copies), teaching the Pool Cool lessons, using the mini-big book, and displaying the sun safety signs. All pools had also used the pump bottle of sunscreen, and all but one site had conducted a training session for their swim instructors and looked at or used the decision maker's guide, the resource guide, and brochures. More than half of the sites had conducted the poolside activities. Only two pools had used the Pool Cool disk to produce additional materials. The majority of the sites were observed using Pool Cool materials such as signs, sunscreen, and incentives. All lifeguards were wearing protective clothing (mainly shirts), though few were observed using sunscreen. Reactions to the materials were very favorable; pool managers and swim instructors indicated that the materials were easy to use, attractive, and well received. Several pool managers were disappointed that the materials had arrived after the summer season had begun. They requested more materials and incentives, asked that the sun safety signs be made larger, and said that they shared the materials with other pools in their district. Several felt that the decision maker's guide would be useful for planning for the next year's swim season.

Evaluation forms, checklists, and telephone interviews were used to assess implementation, satisfaction, and environmental and organizational policies for SP at the end of the pilot dissemination phase. Telephone interviews were conducted during the first week of September to obtain information from pools that had not yet returned written forms. Some informants who were county/municipal liaisons responded for multiple pools in their districts. As a result, we were able to obtain information from a total of 144 out of the 186 swimming pools, or 77.4 percent. Ninety percent of the pool managers said that they taught the Pool Cool lessons, with a median of eight aquatics instructors teaching them at each pool. Ninety-seven percent gave lessons to children aged five to ten years, but about half of them gave lessons to children younger than five and older than ten. Seventy percent said that the kids liked the lessons moderately or a lot, and 96.8 percent said that they would either definitely (71 percent) or possibly (25.8 percent) teach the lessons the following summer. Two-thirds to three-quarters of the pools completed the poolside activities and most said the staff members and children liked them moderately or a lot. About half of the pools said that they made copies of the lessons, activities, leader's guides, and big book, and about one-third made extra copies of signs from the zip disk. Several pools adapted the activities using their own creative ideas, including making Pool Cool sun safety banners, creating a "Pool Cool wall," and publicizing the program through the local media. Some pools used the program activities for rainy-day alternative activities. The most frequent complaint from pool managers was that the materials arrived too late, and they said that they would have liked more items for the children and lifeguards. Some were concerned about "adding one more thing" to cover in swimming lessons and felt that environmental and policy changes would take more than one summer season to accomplish. We received letters with compliments and feedback from many pools.

We used checklist data to examine the internal consistency of measures of implementation and pool sun safety policies. Because of the small number of highlight sites, the preliminary implementation measure was limited to two items (teach lessons and display information), with a Cronbach alpha of 0.84. The pool sun safety policies measure used four items on policies directed toward swimmers (encourage shade, remind about sunscreen, remind parents to send sunscreen, provide sunscreen), and each was measured on a three-point scale. The resulting composite index has a Cronbach alpha of 0.88. A similar parent-reported policy measure yielded an alpha of 0.80, the same as in the efficacy trial.

Criterion validity indicates how well a new measure obtains the same result as that found from another available, highly credible measure or standard (Nunnally and Bernstein, 1994). To assess the criterion validity of the implementation measure, we examined narrative and quantitative site visit data in comparison with pool reports on checklists, evaluation forms, and telephone interviews. This was done by two or three independent raters for each of ten highlight pools and two pilot pools where site visits had been conducted. Raters were blinded to the database contents and had not been on any site visits. Raters gave each pool a score between one (lowest) and five (exemplary). Ratings were highly reliable, with only one pool receiving a rating discrepant by more than one point difference. Eighty-three percent of ratings were consistent with conclusions based on the quantitative data. We concluded that the implementation measure has high criterion validity.

We received seventy-one lifeguard surveys from nine pools. Eighty percent of the lifeguard respondents were white, with an average age of twenty-one years, and most (60.6 percent) reported having a sunburn the preceding summer. Among SP behaviors, they were most likely to report wearing sunglasses and sunscreen, followed by staying under an umbrella or wearing a shirt, and they were least likely to report wearing a hat. Most lifeguards reported taking part in Pool Cool activities and receiving at least one Pool Cool incentive item.

Lessons Learned About Process Evaluation

LESSON 1. *Process evaluation can serve different purposes in different phases of a study.*

During each of the two phases of the Pool Cool skin cancer prevention program, process evaluation was integral to the implementation and assessment of the intervention, but it played different roles in each of the two phases. During the efficacy trial, it mainly addressed reach, satisfaction, and level of implementation. During the pilot dissemination phase, process evaluation focused on the adoption and implementation of components of the program during the pilot dissemination phase. In each phase, the results of the process evaluation provided important information for understanding the program and interpreting the findings. Although some of the information obtained in the process evaluation might have emerged through ad hoc experiences of the staff working on Pool Cool, the use of systematic tools and strategies for data collection provided much richer and more dependable sources of information.

LESSON 2. *Site visits and structured observations are useful process evaluation tools.*

Site visits are very feasible and even welcomed by pool managers. Observations were useful both in the main trial phase and in the pilot dissemination phase. They corroborated information from interviews, checklists, and monitoring forms, which revealed individual approaches at the various swimming pools.

LESSON 3. *Process evaluation can help interpret the results of a randomized trial.*

During the efficacy trial phase, monitoring forms and staff surveys revealed a high level of implementation of both the SP and IP versions of Pool Cool by the aquatics staff. There were few major differences: the length of the lessons was similar, as was the perceived interest level of the children. The approximately equal levels of implementation allowed us to interpret group differences in key outcomes as being due to the different programs rather than the differential uptake of the program.

LESSON 4. *Process evaluation data can be used to examine a dose-response relationship.*

Although the staff surveys and monitoring forms showed consistent and fairly high implementation levels, and the log forms showed that all incentives were distributed, the parents' responses to postprogram surveys suggested that many of them and their children were not fully exposed to the intervention. This appeared to be most likely due to the repeated cross-sectional design, which meant that some children came to swimming lessons after some of the lessons or activities were carried out. Because of this, we created a dose measure based on the number of lessons and activities that the SP group children received. The finding of a clear dose response effect on SP habits for children receiving two or more lessons or activities, compared with those whose parents reported that they received zero or one, suggested a steady increment in SP habits scores between the least involved and the most involved respondents (Glanz and others, forthcoming). Similarly, the aquatics instructors' results showed a trend toward higher SP habits scores associated with teaching more lessons and activities (Geller and others, 2001). In this case, the process evaluation served two functions: (1) it helped interpret the study findings and supported the main effects and (2) it clearly revealed important limitations of the repeated cross-sectional study design.

LESSON 5. *Process evaluation can be used to identify intervention problems.*

One of the first key conclusions we made was that "there is nothing like a site visit." The study team learned more from being on-site, and in some cases attempting to find the program sites, than could ever have been learned from phone calls and self-administered forms and surveys. In a word, we learned what could go wrong and how easily things could slip through the cracks when dissemination is conducted over a wide geographic area. Also, we overreached during the pilot dissemination phase by agreeing to send materials to almost twice as many pools as we had originally anticipated. We were unable to match the pools' enthusiasm with a larger project staff and hence delivered materials much later than desirable to many of the pools. From this lesson, we learned how important it is to ship materials on time, and we completed materials shipping for nearly three hundred pools in the following year.

LESSON 6. *Process evaluation results can identify problems with data collection and possible solutions.*

With respect to data collection methods, we learned that efforts to collect surveys need to begin earlier, be more systematic, and include visible incentives. Without these efforts, response rates were too low for the data to be informative. Data collection can be most successful if aligned with seasonal events such as registration for swimming lessons.

LESSON 7. *Process evaluation results can be used to help plan for a larger study.*

We learned many things from the process evaluation of the dissemination pilot study that set the stage for a larger diffusion trial. First, we found that *interest* in a skin cancer prevention program at swimming pools is very high, especially in view of our limited promotional efforts. We also learned that, at present, many pools provide sun safety advice and support for their staff but fewer do so for the swimmers. Next, we found that the *decision to adopt* the program was apparently made at the time an application form was submitted, as there was less than 100 percent completion of the written pool reply form. We also learned a great deal about the operation of a dissemination project. We learned unequivocally that materials should be sent out before the beginning of the summer swim season, that a stronger training component was welcome, and that direct contact with pool managers should also occur if a district coordinator is the main liaison. We also learned that some materials that should be added to the materials package—all of which are feasible—are (1) a banner for each pool, (2) a training video, (3) larger sun safety signs, (4) more incentives, including some for lifeguards, (5) more discounts for sun safety products, (6) parent brochures, (7) special information about skin cancer risk for nonwhite children, (8) and materials that could be downloaded from the Web.

Conclusion

This chapter illustrates a process evaluation that was systematically designed alongside the outcome evaluation and provided substantial *value added* (that is, contributed to the overall study) and insights about the two phases of the study. The organizational setting for this cancer prevention program—swimming pools—is a novel setting for health promotion and one for which there was little preexisting guidance and information. Well-organized and carefully conducted process evaluation yielded great assets for Pool Cool. This information can be useful not only for this program's future diffusion efforts but also for other public health workers who conduct programs in partnership with recreation industry sites.

References

American Cancer Society. *Cancer Facts and Figures—2000.* Atlanta, Ga.: American Cancer Society, 2000.

Arthey, S., and Clarke, V. A. "Suntanning and Sun Protection: A Review of the Psychological Literature." *Social Science and Medicine,* 1995, *40,* 265–274.

Buller, D. B., and Borland, R. "Skin Cancer Prevention for Children: A Critical Review." *Health Education and Behavior,* 1999, *26,* 317–343.

Centers for Disease Control and Prevention. "Sun Protection Behaviors Used by Adults for Their Children: United States, 1997." *Journal of the American Medical Association,* 1998, *280,* 317–318.

Cohen, J. *Statistical Power Analysis for the Behavioral Sciences*. (2nd ed.) Hillsdale, N.J.: Erlbaum, 1988.

Diffey, B. L., Gibson, C. J., Haylock, R., and McKinlay, A. F. "Outdoor Ultraviolet Exposure of Children and Adolescents." *British Journal of Dermatology*, 1996, *134*, 1030–1034.

Geller, A. C., and others. "Impact of Skin Cancer Prevention on Outdoor Aquatics Staff: The Pool Cool Program in Hawaii and Massachusetts." *Preventive Medicine*, 2001, *33*, 155–161.

Gilchrest, B. A., Eller, M. S., Geller, A. C., and Yaar, M. "The Pathogenesis of Melanoma Induced by Ultraviolet Radiation." *New England Journal of Medicine*, 1999, *340*, 1341–1348.

Glanz, K., Carbone, E., and Song, V. "Formative Research for Developing Targeted Skin Cancer Prevention Programs for Children in Multiethnic Hawai'i." *Health Education Research*, 1999, *14*, 155–166.

Glanz, K., Lew, R. A., Song, V., and Murakami-Akatsuka, L. "Skin Cancer Prevention in Outdoor Recreation Settings: Effects of the Hawaii *SunSmart* Program." *Effective Clinical Practice*, 2000, *3*, 53–61.

Glanz, K., and others. "Skin Cancer Prevention for Children, Parents, and Caregivers: A Field Test of Hawaii's *SunSmart* Program." *Journal of the American Academy of Dermatology*, 1998, *38*, 413–417.

Glanz, K., and others. "A Randomized Trial of Skin Cancer Prevention in Aquatics Settings: The Pool Cool Program." *Health Psychology*, forthcoming.

Glasgow, R. E. "Evaluation Models for Theory-Based Interventions." In K. Glanz, B. K. Rimer, and F. M. Lewis (eds.), *Health Behavior and Health Education: Theory, Research, and Practice*. (3rd ed.) San Francisco: Jossey-Bass, 2002.

Glasgow, R. E., Vogt, T. M., and Boles, S. M. "Evaluating the Public Health Impact of Health Promotion Interventions: The RE-AIM Framework." *American Journal of Public Health*, 1999, *9*, 1322–1327.

Hill, L., and Ferrini, R. L. "Skin Cancer Prevention and Screening: Summary of the American College of Preventive Medicine's Practice Policy Statements." *CA: A Cancer Journal for Clinicians*, 1998, *48*, 232–235.

Howe, H. L., and others. "Annual Report to the Nation on the Status of Cancer (1973 Through 1998), Featuring Cancers with Recent Increasing Trends." *Journal of the National Cancer Institute*, 2001, *93*, 824–842.

Jemal, A., Devesa, S. S., Fears, T. R., and Hartge, P. "Cancer Surveillance Series: Changing Patterns of Cutaneous Malignant Melanoma Mortality Rates Among Whites in the United States." *Journal of the National Cancer Institute*, 2000, *92*, 811–818.

Koh, H. K., Bak, S. M., and Geller, A. C. "Sunbathing Habits and Sunscreen Use Among White Adults: Results of a National Survey." *American Journal of Public Health*, 1997, *87*, 1214–1217.

Lombard, D., Neubauer, T. E., Canfield, D., and Winett, R. A. "Behavioral Community Intervention to Reduce the Risk of Skin Cancer." *Journal of Applied Behavioral Analysis*, 1991, *24*, 677–686.

Mayer, J. A., and others. "Reducing Ultraviolet Exposure in Children." *Preventive Medicine*, 1997, *26*, 516–522.

National Cancer Institute. "SEER Cancer Incidence Public Uses Database, 1973–1996." Bethesda, Md.: National Cancer Institute, 1999. CD-ROM.

Newman, W. G., Agro, A. D., Woodruff, S. I., and Mayer, J. A. "A Survey of Recreational Sun Exposure of Residents of San Diego, California." *American Journal of Preventive Medicine*, 1996, *12*, 186–194.

Nunnally, J., and Bernstein, I. *Psychometric Theory.* (3rd ed.) New York: McGraw-Hill, 1994.

Preston, D. S., and Stern, R. S. "Nonmelanoma Cancers of the Skin." *New England Journal of Medicine,* 1992, *327,* 1649–1662.

Robinson, J. K., Rigel, D. S., and Amonette, M. D. "Sun Protection Behaviors Used by Adults for Their Children: United States, 1997." *Morbidity and Mortality Weekly Report,* 1998, *47,* 480–482.

Rogers, E. M. *Diffusion of Innovations.* (4th ed.) New York: Free Press, 1995.

Rosenberg, C., Mayer, J. A., and Eckhardt, L. "Skin Cancer Prevention Education: A National Survey of YMCAs." *Journal of Community Health,* 1997, *22,* 373–385.

U.S. Department of Health and Human Services. *Cancer Rates and Risks.* A. Harras (ed.). National Institutes of Health, Cancer Statistics Branch, Division of Cancer Prevention and Control. Washington, D.C.: Public Health Service, NIH Publ. No. 96–691, 1996.

Weinstock, M. A. "Assessment of Sun Sensitivity by Questionnaire: Validity of Items and Formulation of a Prediction Rule." *Journal of Clinical Epidemiology,* 1992, *44,* 547–552.

APPENDIX A: POOL COOL MONITORING FORM.

POOL COOL

Your Name _____

Your Pool _____

Pool Cool Monitoring Form
Lesson 1: Introducing Pool Cool Rules for Sun Safety

Marking Instructions		
Please use a pencil or blue or black ink.	Correct ●	Incorrect ⊘ ⊗ ⊖ ⊙

Date of the lesson: ☐ / ☐ / ☐
Month   Day   Year

Did you do the following?

A. Complete Lesson #1

     YES ○   NO ○

  If YES, how many minutes did this lesson take to complete?

  1 ○ 2 ○ 3 ○ 4 ○ 5 ○ 6 ○ 7 ○ 8 ○ 9 ○ 10 ○ >10 ○

B. Introduce the four Pool Cool Rules to the class YES ○ NO ○

C. Discuss the power of the sun YES ○ NO ○

D. How many children attended this lesson? ☐☐

E. How interested were the children in this lesson?

Not interested	A little interested	Somewhat interested	Interested	Very interested
○	○	○	○	○

F. Were any parents present for the lesson? YES ○ NO ○

If YES, how many? ☐☐

If YES, how interested were they in this lesson?

Not interested	A little interested	Somewhat interested	Interested	Very interested
○	○	○	○	○

For Office Use Only

1 2 3 4 5 6 7 8 9 0
☐ ○○○○○○○○○○
☐ ○○○○○○○○○○

APPENDIX B: SITE VISIT PROTOCOL AND FORMS.

Pool Cool Site Visit Protocol—*Highlight Sites,* Summer 2000
BEFORE VISIT

1. Schedule meeting with site (Plan on *at least* 1.5–2 hours)

2. Get directions to site

3. Checklist of material to bring

    ❍ Pool Cool shirt and hat for PC staff

    ❍ 20 Solartech cards

    ❍ Interview schedule/protocol

    ❍ Materials Use form

    ❍ Observation form

    ❍ Camera

    ❍ Pool info.—directions, travel arrangements, etc.

Site Visit Procedures

   ❑ Wear PC hat and shirt

   ❑ Introductions and purpose

   ❑ Interview (use attached form)

   ❑ Materials use (use attached form)

   ❑ Do Solartech card activity

   ❑ Watch lessons if possible

   ❑ Talk with other available involved persons

   ❑ Complete Observation form

   ❑ Sit back and watch pool (don't forget to take pictures)

Pool Cool Site Visit
Highlight Sites: Summer 2000
Interview {Open-Ended Questions}

Pool ID & Location: _____

Today's Date: _____

Names of Site Visitors: _____

Section A. General Background

1. Clarify liaison—person talking to—Are they the one who applied for Pool Cool? What is their title/position/role?

2. When did you receive the Pool Cool toolkit? _____

3. Did you complete, or are you planning, a training session for your lifeguards/aquatic instructor staff for Pool Cool?

○ Yes   ○ No

If *yes*, describe time, length, format:
-Group/individual
-Who led?
-How long?
-What was included?

Section B. ToolKit Use and Ratings

4. What components of the toolkit have you used, and which have you found to be the most helpful? Which have you found not to be useful? *(Ask "used" and "helpful" for each, mark if they state "NOT useful" but do not ask this question separately)*

	Used	Helpful/Very Helpful	Not Useful
a. Leader's Guide	❏	❏	❏
b. Lessons	❏	❏	❏
c. Decision Maker's Guide	❏	❏	❏
d. Resource Guide	❏	❏	❏
e. Mini Big Book	❏	❏	❏
f. Sun Signs	❏	❏	❏
g. Pool Cool Disk	❏	❏	❏

Comments:

5. Do you have suggestions about ways to make the Pool Cool toolkit easier to use?

Section C. Lessons and Support Use

6.   How often are the Pool Cool lessons taught at your pool?

7.   Do your lifeguards/staff members like to teach Pool Cool lessons?

8.   What kind of support have you used or are planning to use from Pool Cool? (ask each)

    a. Toll Free Hotline   ❑ Used   ❑ Plan to use

    b. E-mail   ❑ Used   ❑ Plan to use

    c. Fax   ❑ Used   ❑ Plan to use

    d. Other: _____ ❑ Used   ❑ Plan to use

Section D. Overall Opinion, Future Ideas, Suggestions

9.   Do the children and/or parents at your swimming pool enjoy Pool Cool?

10. Do you feel that Pool Cool is making a difference in the sun safety of the children at your pool?

11. Please help us plan for the future of Pool Cool. If they were available for Pool Cool, would you use . . . ?

    a. Training video   ◯ Yes   ◯ No

    b. Web site to download information and materials,
       and/or order brochures, incentives, and supplies   ◯ Yes   ◯ No

12. Other Suggestions:

**Thank you very much. Now, I have just a few
more specific questions to go over.**

Pool ID #: _____

Pool Location: _____

Date: _____

Site Visitors: _____

Pool Cool Site Visit
Highlight Sites, Summer 2000

Materials Use Questions	Yes	No
1. Leader's Guide		
a. Have you used or do you plan to use the **Leader's Guide?**	☐	☐
b. Did you make or do you plan to make copies of the **Leader's Guide?**	☐	☐
c. If yes, how many? _____		
2. Pool Cool Lessons		
a. Have you used or do you plan to use the **Pool Cool Lessons?**	☐	☐
b. Have you made or do you plan to make copies of the **Pool Cool Lessons?**	☐	☐
c. If yes, how many? _____		
3. Brochures/Pamphlets in the Leader's Guide		
a. Have you looked at the **brochures?**	☐	☐
b. Have your ordered or do you plan to order copies of brochures?	☐	☐
3. Decision Maker's Guide to Sun Safety		
a. Have you used or do you plan to use the **Decision Maker's Guide?**	☐	☐
b. Did you make or do you plan to make copies of the **Decision Maker's Guide?**	☐	☐
c. If yes, how many? _____		
4. Resource Guide		
a. Have you looked at the **Resource Guide?**	☐	☐
b. Do you plan to use the **Resource Guide?**	☐	☐
c. Did you order or do you plan to order items from the **Resource Guide?**	☐	☐
d. If yes, what are you planning to order?	☐	☐
5. Mini Big Book		
a. Have you used or do you plan to use the **Mini Big Book?**	☐	☐
6. Sun Signs		
a. Have you posted or do you plan to post the **Sun Signs?**	☐	☐
b. Where did you place the Sun Signs? _____	☐	☐

Materials Use Questions	Yes	No

7. **Pool Cool Disk**
   a. Have you used or do you plan to use the **Pool Cool Disk?**
   b. Have you used the Pool Cool Disk to make **Sun Signs?**
   c. Have you used the Pool Cool Disk to make a **Mini Big Book?**
   d. Have you used the Pool Cool Disk to make copies of **Lessons?**
   e. Have you used the Pool Cool Disk to make copies of the **Leader's Guide?**
   f. Have you used the Pool Cool Disk to make copies of the **Decision Maker's Guide?**

8. **Large Pump Bottle of Sunscreen**
   a. Have you used or do you plan to use the **Large Pump Bottle of Sunscreen?**
   b. Did you order or do you plan to order more **Large Pump Bottles of Sunscreen?**
   c. If yes, how much/how many? _____

Ask #9 only after July 22nd

9. **SunSafe Checklist, Evaluation Form, Surveys**
   a. Have you completed the **SunSafe Checklist?**
   b. Have you completed the **Pool Cool Evaluation Form?**
   c. Have your lifeguards/aquatic instructors completed the **Surveys?**
   d. If yes, how many? _____
   e. Have you distributed and collected the **Parent Surveys** at your pool?
   f. If yes, how many? _____

CHAPTER FOUR

Process Evaluation of the Adolescent Social Action Program in New Mexico

Deborah L. Helitzer and Soo-Jin Yoon

This chapter describes the process evaluation of a primary prevention program, the Adolescent Social Action Program (ASAP), which was aimed at reducing alcohol- and drug-related morbidity and mortality rates among New Mexico's youth. The program began in 1982 with supervised youth visits to the Emergency Room of the University of New Mexico (UNM) Hospital. During these visits, young people interviewed patients who had problems related to alcohol and drug use. Over the years since its inception, ASAP was successful in gaining various funding for its implementation and improvement. A curriculum was written around the core experience of the patient interviews, and, over time, ASAP broadened its focus to include tobacco, all types of drugs and substances, interpersonal violence, gangs, and other issues relevant to young people. With its evolution, the program's original name, Alcohol and Substance Abuse Prevention, was changed to Adolescent Social Action Program, to reflect its overall philosophy of empowering young people to become capable of promoting change in their communities.

In 1994, ASAP received a five-year research grant (mid-1994 to mid-1999) from the National Institute on Alcohol Abuse and Alcoholism (NIAAA). Although

The authors would like to acknowledge the contributions and assistance of Nina Wallerstein, Randall Starling, and Julie Griffin.

previous funding had produced extensive outcome evaluations for the program, the NIAAA grant provided ASAP with its first opportunity to conduct a systematic process evaluation. The process evaluation was designed at the beginning of the NIAAA grant period, along with the development of the outcome evaluation instruments, curriculum revision, and planning for program implementation. Because the quasi-experimental design of the NIAAA-funded outcome evaluation required ASAP to implement its intervention over a period of three and a half years (seven semesters between Spring 1995 and Spring 1998), the process evaluation was designed to capture information during this same period.

Process evaluation has been shown to (1) help determine if Type III error occurred (Steckler and others, 1992)—that is, if there was the belief that changes in program outcomes were due to the program when, in fact, there was an absence of intervention, and (2) enhance the understanding of program effects by linking exposure to outcome (McGraw and others, 1994). The purpose of this process evaluation was to document fidelity to the program (tracking students and documenting participation, attendance, and exposure), thereby enhancing the interpretation of the program's results. This check for *fidelity* (to ensure that the program was implemented as it was intended) was designed not only for the summative purpose of determining if Type III error had occurred but also for the formative purpose of reducing the possibility of such error through the program's constant monitoring of its implementation as well as appropriate activities to correct insufficient implementation. Evidence of program fidelity enhances investigators' ability to attribute changes in outcomes to the program's intervention. For the formative purpose of fine-tuning the program, this process evaluation was designed to provide immediate feedback to program personnel with data that would have to be, in a timely manner, analyzed, interpreted, and given back to the staff members who implemented the program.

The process evaluation design evolved slowly. The original design was based on literature available at the time, and subsequent modifications were made after the onset of the NIAAA grant. For example, focus groups consisting of young people were added to gain information about barriers and facilitators to participation. Observations of program sessions were added to check for the presence of theoretical constructs, which additionally enabled triangulation (Miles and Huberman, 1994) with other data sources. These modifications were based on a prior process evaluation study conducted by Deborah Helitzer for an obesity prevention program for Native American school children, in which twenty-seven sets of data collection instruments were developed, each set having between three and five instruments, from 1994 to 1999 (Helitzer and others, 1999).

A classic distinction in evaluation is whether the evaluator is internal or external to the program. External evaluators are assumed to be more objective, whereas internal evaluators are assumed to have better insight into program function and meaning (Weiss, 1998). The process evaluation of ASAP was conducted, for the most part, internally, which, in this case, involved the handling of design, instruments, data collection/documentation, and data management, as well as analysis of the process evaluation—functions considered to be part of the role of program implementers, which included two co-principal investigators, a full-time project director, a full-time program manager, and a small team of part-time staff members (site coordinators and research assistants). An external consultant was brought in for the process evaluation after the start of the grant, to increase the objectivity of the evaluation and to attempt to achieve some separation between program implementation and evaluation.

The Adolescent Social Action Program

Program Summary

The Adolescent Social Action Program had two primary long-term goals. The first was to prevent morbidity and mortality from risky behaviors—specifically tobacco and alcohol abuse—among low-income minority youth in high-risk communities. The second was to empower the young people to become leaders who were capable of promoting changes in their communities' behaviors, social values, and environmental policies and norms. The theoretical foundation of the program was based on protection motivation theory (Rogers, 1983) and Freire's empowerment dialogue method (Wallerstein and Bernstein, 1988). Over the course of sixteen years, ASAP operated in over thirty multiethnic (predominantly Hispanic and Native American) communities in New Mexico, served nearly sixteen hundred middle- and high school students, and trained over four hundred adult facilitators. The program was eventually expanded to serve twenty-seven hundred elementary school children through the program's peer education activities with younger students. ASAP attracted national and international attention and received an outstanding program award from the U.S. Department of Education's Safe and Drug-Free Schools Program for two consecutive years.

Participating Schools

In 1994, upon receipt of NIAAA funding, eight Albuquerque middle schools were invited to participate in the program and were informed that each of them would be randomly allocated to either the intervention or the comparison condition. Hence, four schools were randomly selected to receive the intervention during the research study period, whereas the other four schools received the delayed intervention (comparison condition). Before the onset of the research activities, ASAP gained Institutional Review Board approval from the Human Research Review Committee at UNM.

Youth Recruitment

Site coordinators, who were part-time paid personnel, had the responsibility of recruiting young people to participate in ASAP. The ASAP program manager and site coordinators consulted with the school administration to identify at each of the eight schools a seventh-grade teacher who facilitated access to his or her students and was willing to help in the recruitment process. These teachers were provided with a nominal stipend for their time spent on such tasks as arranging meeting spaces at the school for ASAP whenever needed, collecting consent forms, and reminding students of upcoming ASAP sessions. ASAP site coordinators entered the teachers' classrooms to recruit students, and ASAP research assistants accessed students for data collection (using questionnaires, forms, and saliva samples [for a cotinine assessment]). Those students who volunteered to participate were enrolled on a first-come, first-served basis. Between eighteen and twenty-one students were recruited each semester at each school. Site coordinators were responsible for orienting parents of the students and for coordinating transportation of the students to the program sites (either UNM hospital or Bernalillo County Detention Center).

ASAP Facilitators

An important part of the ASAP program was the group of adult facilitators who worked with the young people during the six-week hospital-detention center sessions (a more detailed explanation of the centers is given later in this chapter). Most facilitators were recruited through UNM classes and received university credit for their involvement, and some facilitators were community members who volunteered. (See the Results section for specific demographic information on facilitators.) All facilitators were required to attend a two-day training course at the beginning of the semester. During the semester, facilitators were required to attend a weekly seminar session, which included class readings of current literature on health issues related to young people and discussions about the progress of the hospital-detention center sessions. These sessions allowed the opportunity for facilitators to learn from each other's experiences and share lessons learned about how to keep the sessions on track.

The Core Curriculum: Hospital-Detention Center Sessions

Students who chose to participate in ASAP were assigned to a small group by school. ASAP attempted to recruit seven to nine students for each group. Due to attrition and the need to make up the numbers (for the appropriate sample size for the outcome evaluation), the number of students per group actually ranged from two to eleven. Each group of students was assigned two facilitators, who worked together to implement the core curriculum sessions held once a week for each group for six consecutive weeks.

The UNM hospital could handle only a moderate number of students without disrupting its normal operations, so the groups were staggered by day and by waves. In other words, the length of each semester allowed ASAP to schedule two waves of the six-week curriculum, and each group held a session one night a week (on a Monday, Tuesday, Wednesday, or Thursday). Hence, during a semester, between five and twelve groups of students went through the curriculum.

The first session of the six-week curriculum was a group-building session, followed by three supervised visits to the University-affiliated hospital and one visit to the county detention center. On these site visits, the students interviewed patients, their families, and jail residents who were affected by alcohol or substance abuse problems. After interviews, students and facilitators were debriefed on their experiences, using the SHOWED model (Helitzer, Yoon, Wallerstein, and Garcia-Velarde, 2000) to generate critical thinking and dialogue. This model was derived from ASAP's theoretical foundation. The acronym SHOWED stands for S—What did the students *see* and observe? H—What is *happening* in their stories? O—How do the stories relate to *our* lives? W—Why is this a problem? E—What would *empower* this person or us to change? and D—What can we *do* to improve our lives or the lives of others? A variety of other participatory learning exercises, designed to trigger topics relevant to young people, augmented each session. For example, for a media literacy activity, students constructed a mosaic of cigarette and alcohol advertisements from magazines and they discussed how advertisers target young people. The sixth session was a potluck dinner with family members, and it provided the opportunity for students to brainstorm about community projects in which they could further engage after the curriculum sessions.

Social Action Projects and Booster Sessions

After the core hospital-detention center experience, the site coordinators worked with the youth groups on social action projects. In alignment with the philosophy of the program of empowering young people, the student groups were encouraged to choose their own projects. These projects ranged from no project at all to establishing ASAP clubs at schools to painting murals on a school wall to creating educational music videos.

In addition, a booster session was conducted by ASAP site coordinators six months after the students received the core curriculum. This booster session consisted of a visit to a courtroom, where students witnessed live hearings and interviewed judges and lawyers to gain insight into the legal and financial ramifications of risky behaviors, such as drinking and driving drunk. As in the first six sessions, the booster included a thirty-minute debriefing that used the SHOWED model.

Outcome Evaluation

For the outcome evaluation, a questionnaire was developed to assess whether the program influenced students' attainment of constructs pertinent to protection motivation theory. The questionnaire appraised (1) *threat*—students' perception of their susceptibility and vulnerability to risky behaviors, (2) *coping*—students' perception of their self-efficacies and intentions to engage in self- or social protective behaviors, and (3) *empathy*—students' social relationships and their ability to experience vicariously the feelings and thoughts of others. Figure 4.1 illustrates the ASAP program theory model, which is explained in more detail in the Theoretical Framework section of this chapter (Wallerstein and Sanchez-Merki, 1994).

The outcome evaluation questionnaire was administered to each student in both the intervention and the comparison groups at pretest (immediately before they received the core curriculum), immediately posttest, and six weeks, eight months, and fifteen months posttest. In addition, a direct measure of tobacco use was collected in both groups through saliva samples at pretest and fifteen months posttest. During the course of seven school semesters, sixty-three groups of students participated in the project. Among the students who provided basic demographic information, 547 (63.2 percent) were female and 318 (36.8 percent) were male. Sixty four percent of the students self-identified as "Hispanic" (n = 557), 23.6 percent as "White/Anglo" (n = 204), 8.3 percent as "American Indian" (n = 72), 6.6 percent as "Black" (n = 57), 2.1 percent as "Asian American" (n = 18) and 7.2 percent as "Other" (n = 62). (These percentages add up to over 100 percent because nearly 10 percent of the students self-identified as belonging to more than one group. For example, forty-six students indicated that they were both Hispanic and white/Anglo). Follow-up rates at fifteen months were between 76 and 86 percent for both intervention and comparison students.

FIGURE 4.1. ASAP PROGRAM THEORY MODEL.

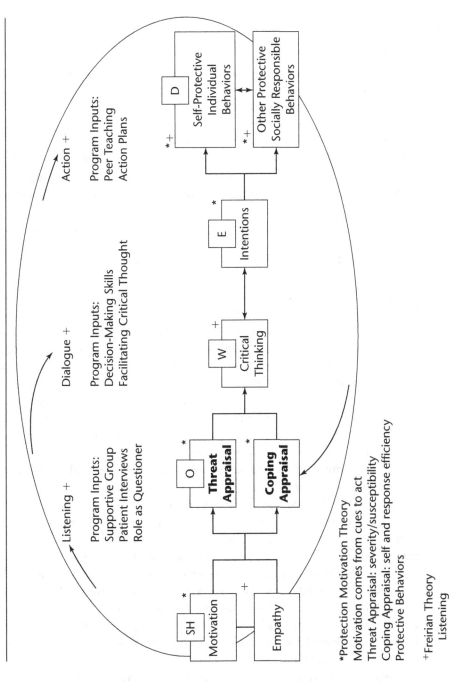

*Protection Motivation Theory
Motivation comes from cues to act
Threat Appraisal: severity/susceptibility
Coping Appraisal: self and response efficiency
Protective Behaviors

+Freirian Theory
  Listening
  Dialogue
  Action

Source: Wallerstein and Sanchez-Merki, 1994.

Theoretical Framework

The hypothesis of the ASAP program was that the experiential aspect of the program (for example, patient and inmate interviews), in combination with the facilitator-led dialogical method, would lead students to empathize with the patients and jail residents, in hearing their stories. Students were encouraged to talk about whether or how they identified with the issues raised in interviews and to critically analyze the influences that contributed to risky behaviors. For example, the specific targeting of young people by the liquor and tobacco industries is responsible for increasing levels of youth consumption of alcohol and cigarettes, and young people, being engaged in such risky behaviors, become negative role models for their friends and family members. The expectation was that the ability to analyze their own experiences would empower these young ASAP participants to take action.

The ASAP program focused on reducing risky behaviors and encouraging socially responsible behaviors that would protect others. The curriculum was based on two complementary theoretical perspectives that were woven together in the project curriculum: Freire's empowerment theory (Wallerstein and Bernstein, 1988; Wallerstein and Sanchez-Merki, 1994) and Rogers's protection motivation theory (Floyd, Prentice-Dunn, and Rogers, 2000; Rogers, 1983). Freire's approach was used in designing the structured dialogue component of the ASAP intervention. The theories used in ASAP were hypothesized to provide psychological empowerment, including personal efficacy, recognition of the need for group participation, critical consciousness, and the willingness to participate in collective action (Rissel and others, 1996). Figure 4.1 shows how the two theories and the SHOWED model were expected to move participants to empowerment.

The first theoretical framework was the Freirian dialogue method, which was used to foster critical thinking about adolescents' perception of alcohol, drug, or tobacco consumption and the meaning of such behavior to adolescents trying to achieve or maintain a certain self-image. For example, a teenage girl feels that smoking makes her look more grown up. The Freirian empowerment dialogue method is based on a continuous listening-dialogue-action cycle, in which program participants identify cues to action by listening to their own issues of emotional and social import, engaging in dialogues about these issues, and developing strategies for addressing them. The SHOWED model was derived from this theoretical foundation. This critical thinking process has been shown to influence youth engagement in such risky behaviors as drinking, smoking, and unexcused absence from school (Chassin, Presson, Sherman, and Steinberg, 1989; Jacobson, Atkins, and Hacker, 1983).

Rogers's protection motivation theory was a second theoretical foundation of the ASAP curriculum. Protection motivation theory hypothesizes that the decision to act is initiated through a range of informational sources and is mediated through a nonlinear cognitive perceptual process (Rogers, 1983; Rogers, Deckner, and Mewborn, 1978). A health-seeking response is expected when a health threat increases one's vulnerability and susceptibility, when self-efficacy and *response efficacy* (the belief that one's actions can have an effect and that one can respond correctly to a health threat) increase, and when the rewards for engaging in a maladaptive behavior decline (Rippetoe and Rogers, 1987; Rogers, 1983). The jail and hospital visits were expected to heighten the students' threat appraisal (or risk perception) of the seriousness of their own susceptibility to the consequences of substance abuse. The dialogue with patients and jail residents was expected to encourage the students to develop the ability to think through a situation and make an assessment that would lead to an appropriate behavioral response, as well as enhance their empathy, knowledge, and intention to change their own behaviors. It was anticipated that their coping skills and *self-efficacy* (personal responsibility) would be improved by their participation in peer resistance and decision-making exercises. For example, students were asked to enact scripted and improvised role-playing exercises in which they responded to common peer pressure situations.

Overall Program Results

Prior outcome evaluations demonstrated that the curriculum increased the students' social skills, competence, critical consciousness, knowledge, and self-efficacy for their own behaviors, as well as their social responsibility and prosocial behaviors, including their self-efficacy related to helping others, their recognition of the need for group participation, and their willingness to participate in collective action (Rissel and others, 1996).

However, the outcome results of the NIAAA-funded study of ASAP showed no significant differences in alcohol, tobacco, or other substance use among the young people—between the intervention groups and the comparison groups (Wallerstein and Woodall, 2000). In addition, no differences in other measures of threat appraisal or coping appraisal were found. The major pattern observed in the data was the regular increase over time in the proportion of students reporting ever having had an alcoholic drink. This percentage increased from 61.2 percent pretreatment to 64.0 percent posttreatment, to 66.3 percent at six months posttreatment, to 74.4 percent at the fifteen-month follow-up. In fact, compared with the outcomes of other published studies, the ASAP study participants reflected higher levels of alcohol initiation and exposure—higher than the national average for this age group. This was not surprising, given that the risk level of the study population was higher than the national average. All ethnic groups and both genders, in both the intervention and the control groups, showed, over the course of the study, an increased tendency to drink alcohol. The rate for females increased from 58.6 percent pretreatment to 75.7 percent at the fifteen-month follow-up.

Program Evaluation Design and Methods

The NIAAA-funded process evaluation of the ASAP program was designed to measure the following: (1) the fidelity of the implemented curriculum to the designed curriculum, (2) curriculum implementation consistency across groups of young people, (3) the level of exposure and participation of the students, (4) barriers and facilitators to participation, (5) competing or intervening influences on participation and exposure, (6) the existence of other health-related programs going on concurrently in both intervention and comparison populations, and (7) the characteristics of facilitators and students in the program. Figure 4.2 lists the actual evaluation questions.

The Role of Theory

The critical theoretical elements previously described were included in the design of several process evaluation instruments. Examples of theoretical constructs measured include the SHOWED model, social analysis, critical thinking, group process, facilitation style, cognitive dimensions, the continuous listening-dialogue-action cycle, cognitive appraisals of threat, and coping abilities.

Process Evaluation Design

The design of the process evaluation was an intervention/comparison group design with continuous measurement throughout the training and the seven semesters of intervention group implementation. Most of the data collection occurred

FIGURE 4.2. PROCESS EVALUATION QUESTIONS.

1. Was the curriculum implemented with fidelity to the original design?
2. Was the curriculum implemented similarly in each youth group?
3. What was the level of exposure/participation by students?
4. What were the barriers and facilitators to participation?
5. What were the competing or intervening influences on participation and exposure?
6. What were the characteristics of facilitators and students in the program?

at the intervention sites, as is appropriate for process evaluation. Some of the instruments were designed to contribute to a formative evaluation, some contributed to summative evaluation, and others were useful for both types of evaluation. Many of the instruments were designed to enable triangulation of data. Figure 4.3 shows the implementation model around which the process evaluation was designed.

Process Evaluation Resources

A small proportion of the grant funds were allocated to the process evaluation, from which the consultant was paid for 3 percent of her time for two years. A small percentage (~5 percent) of the salaries of all program staff members covered their data collection activities. In addition, one staff member conducted the process evaluation analyses, devoting to this function ~50 percent of her time for one year.

Data Collection, Sample, and Analyses

Fifteen instruments were used to collect both qualitative and quantitative information for the process evaluation data. Figure 4.3 shows the different types of information gathered and how they were related. The numbers next to each box correspond with the instruments listed in Table 4.1, which presents more details

FIGURE 4.3. IMPLEMENTATION MODEL.

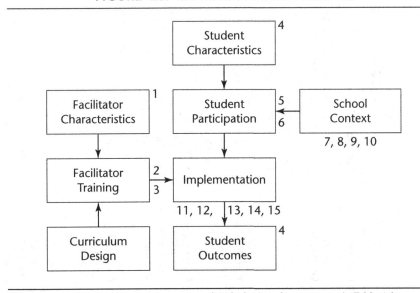

Note: The numbers in this model correspond with the list of instruments in Table 4.1.

TABLE 4.1. PROCESS EVALUATION INSTRUMENTS.

Instrument	Rationale/Purpose	Population/Sample	Analyses Method
1. Facilitator Questionnaire	• To assess facilitator characteristics, experience with drugs & alcohol, work with adolescents, self-efficacy [FORMATIVE & SUMMATIVE]	• Collected at pre- & postcurriculum	• Partially analyzed • Descriptive statistics performed on certain items [QUANTITATIVE & QUALITATIVE]
2. Facilitator Training Evaluation Form	• To assess facilitator perception of training & confidence in ability to implement curriculum [FORMATIVE]	• Forms administered in only 5 of 7 semesters • Total of 46 evaluation forms collected	• Reviewed by training director for immediate feedback • Scores for each item tallied [QUANTITATIVE & QUALITATIVE]
3. Facilitator Attendance Log of Weekly Class Sessions	• To assess participation/exposure to knowledge and skill enhancement sessions [FORMATIVE & SUMMATIVE]	• Collected weekly each of 7 semesters	• Monitored/tracked attendance of facilitator for the semester [QUANTITATIVE]
4. Student (Outcome) Questionnaire	• To assess student characteristics [SUMMATIVE]	• Collected at pre- & postcurriculum, 8-month & 15-month post [INTERVENTION & COMPARISON GROUPS]	• Descriptive statistics performed on certain items for process evaluation purposes [QUANTITATIVE]
5. 6-Session Curriculum Student Attendance Logs	• To assess participation (exposure) to curriculum • To assess whether there was a dose-response relationship [FORMATIVE & SUMMATIVE]	• One from each team of facilitators covering all 6 sessions • Total of 63 (100% response rate) [INTERVENTION GROUP]	• Attendance scores and percentages calculated by student and by group • Each student & group received a "Program Intensity" (dose) score [QUANTITATIVE]

	Purpose	Data Collection	Analysis
6. Master Attendance Log	• To assess participation (exposure) to curriculum, booster session, & social action projects • To assess whether there was a dose-response relationship [FORMATIVE & SUMMATIVE]	• One master attendance sheet for the entire program [INTERVENTION GROUP]	• Scores of attendance calculated [QUANTITATIVE]
7. Student Focus Group	• To assess barriers & facilitators to participation [FORMATIVE]	• One focus group conducted with ASAP participants from one school [INTERVENTION GROUP]	• Taped discussions were transcribed and coded for themes; themes were grouped into clusters [QUALITATIVE]
8. School Administrator & Teacher Focus Group	• To assess barriers & facilitators to participation	• School coordinators & administrators from each school [INTERVENTION SCHOOLS]	• Barriers and facilitators reviewed & summarized [QUALITATIVE]
9. Health-Related Program Inventory	• To assess competing programs in both intervention & comparison schools (school context) [SUMMATIVE]	• Collected yearly in January from each school, completed by administrator or teacher [INTERVENTION & COMPARISON SCHOOLS]	Not analyzed [QUANTITATIVE]
10. Health-Related Student Inventory	• To assess ASAP participants' involvement in other programs [SUMMATIVE]	• Collected at precurriculum at the same time as Student Outcome Questionnaire [INTERVENTION & COMPARISON GROUPS]	Not analyzed [QUANTITATIVE]
11. Facilitator Checkoff List	• To assess fidelity of curriculum implementation [FORMATIVE & SUMMATIVE]	• One from each team of facilitators covering all 6 sessions • Total of 63 (100% response rate) [INTERVENTION GROUP]	• Tally of scores by session, by content area, by group, & by semester • Reported in scores, percentages of coverage, & low, medium, or high scores of fidelity [QUANTITATIVE]

(continued)

TABLE 4.1. PROCESS EVALUATION INSTRUMENTS. (CONTINUED)

Instrument	Rationale/Purpose	Population/Sample	Analyses Method
12. Observation Checkoff List	• To assess fidelity of curriculum implementation • To assess group process • To assess student attainment of theoretical constructs [FORMATIVE & SUMMATIVE]	• 41 of 63 groups were observed during Session #5, but only 29 (46%) were done with the final version of the instrument [INTERVENTION GROUP]	• Partially analyzed • Fidelity score calculations were analyzed in the same manner as Facilitator Checkoff List & were compared with the scores reported by facilitators for the same sessions [QUANTITATIVE & QUALITATIVE]
13. Student Comment Sheet	• Check on fidelity of curriculum implementation • To assess student attainment of theoretical constructs [FORMATIVE & SUMMATIVE]	• All 6 sessions from all students • Total of 1,497 (91% response rate) [INTERVENTION GROUP]	Data quality was too poor to analyze (Students often did not answer questions or responded in only a few words) [QUALITATIVE]
14. Facilitator Log/Comment Sheet	• Check on fidelity of curriculum implementation • To provide feedback to training director on skill & confidence attainment [FORMATIVE & SUMMATIVE]	• All 6 sessions from all facilitators • Total of 548 (82% response rate) [INTERVENTION GROUP]	• Reviewed by training director for themes & areas to enhance in weekly class sessions [QUALITATIVE]
15. Participant Contact Documentation Sheet	• To document postcurriculum social action projects (extended exposure) [SUMMATIVE]	• Collected from Site Coordinators for each contact with each student [INTERVENTION GROUP]	Not analyzed [QUALITATIVE]

about the instruments—that is, the rationale and purpose of the instruments, the population sample from which the data were collected, and a brief description of the analysis methods used. The first three instruments (1, 2, and 3) were used to collect information on the facilitator characteristics and training, an outcome evaluation instrument (4) provided information on student characteristics, two instruments (5 and 6) examined student participation in and exposure to the program, four instruments (7, 8, 9, and 10) were used to examine school context, and five instruments (11, 12, 13, 14, and 15) measured the implementation of the program. As examples, the facilitator checkoff list and observation forms can be found in Appendixes A and B.

Student comment sheets and facilitator training evaluation forms were anonymous and coded by group or semester. The facilitator questionnaire, health-related student inventory, and student questionnaire did not include names but were coded to keep track of the individuals and to allow datasets to be merged by the code. This list of codes and names was maintained by ASAP research assistants and was not accessed by the outcome evaluation data analysts. The health-related program inventory and focus group were coded by school. Facilitator checkoff lists and log/comment sheets required the facilitators to include their names, as their class grade depended on their turning in these forms, and they were subsequently coded by group for analysis purposes. Student attendance information was initially tracked by student name, which program personnel used to boost attendance through follow-up, but it was eventually coded to be merged with other student-level data. Quantitative data were entered into an Excel spreadsheet (Microsoft Applications, 1995) as individual datasets by instrument and were later merged with the outcome dataset by student, group, or school code. Qualitative data were reviewed and analyzed for content where resources allowed. (Table 4.1 lists which data were collected by quantitative versus qualitative methods.)

Results

The information presented in this section describes only the results and use of data that were completely analyzed. As Table 4.1 shows, some data were found to be unreliable, whereas other data were not analyzed, because of resource constraints. Further discussion of issues related to the limitations of analyses and the use of results follows.

Facilitator Characteristics and Training

Because facilitators were so crucial to the program's success, we developed an extensive analysis of the facilitator characteristics, the training they received, their attendance at the weekly class sessions, and their ability to implement the program (Helitzer, Yoon, Wallerstein, and Garcia-Velarde, 2000). Facilitators were primarily undergraduate students (81 percent), Caucasian (60 percent), and Hispanic (30 percent), with varied experience working with teenagers (26 percent having less than a year, 33 percent having one to three years, and 13 percent having four years or more). These data were used only to create a profile of the facilitators for progress and final reports.

Data on training effectiveness were triangulated from several sources: facilitator training evaluation, facilitator checkoff list, observation checkoff list, student comment sheet, and facilitator log/comment sheet. Training evaluations revealed that 94 percent of the facilitators were confident that the preprogram two-day training workshop prepared them well for the program. However, the observation data and facilitator self-report data suggest that the facilitators were not competent to implement all of the facilitation methods used in the program and that they were inconsistent in their implementation of role-modeling behaviors. Findings revealed that facilitators showed inconsistent and lower than desirable implementation, especially by the later (fifth and sixth) sessions. When these data suggested that specific content or theoretical constructs were not fully grasped by the facilitators, the training director addressed these issues in the weekly class sessions for the benefit of other facilitators, whose sessions were not yet complete.

Exposure: Attendance and Implementation

Student attendance scores by group for the set of six sessions ranged from 43 to 100 percent. This was determined by calculating the total possible attendance for each group (the number of students in the group multiplied by six—the number of curriculum sessions) and then determining the mean attendance attained by all students in the group. Information on attendance was designed in such a way that program personnel had immediate access to the information for constant monitoring. This enabled program personnel to troubleshoot when attendance was declining and to ensure that efforts were being made to retain students for the six sessions.

Information about implementation of the curriculum was available from the facilitator checkoff list, the student comment sheet, the observation checkoff list, the participant contact documentation sheet, and the facilitator log. The data showed that implementation, as previously noted, was inconsistent. Implementation scores were calculated by session, by activity, and by group, based on the 0- to 3-point scoring system of the facilitator checkoff list (see Appendix A) and by totaling these scores. To check whether certain sessions were less implemented than others, actual scores from the checkoff list for each session were totaled across all sixty-three groups and checked against the total possible implementation score. There was a decline in implementation scores as sessions progressed over the six-week period, but this pattern was consistently repeated from semester to semester. Repeated elements like the interviews were highly implemented, but other, more difficult and less frequently implemented skills, such as role-playing, were often left out. Content/activity areas that received high implementation scores were those activities that were scripted versus improvised, repeated in several sessions, expected to be discussed in the seminars, and accompanied by visual materials. Poorly covered content areas (in which coverage was 50 percent or less) tended to be activities that were more abstract and more time-consuming, and which required more skill on the part of the facilitators. For example, though the patient/inmate interviews were well implemented, facilitators often failed to follow through with the next, more difficult and abstract, task of using the SHOWED model as a tool for engaging the young people in critical thinking and dialogue (Helitzer, Yoon, Wallerstein, and Garcia-Velarde, 2000).

Finally, a score for program exposure was calculated for each student. Exposure to each session was calculated by multiplying the student group's fidelity score for each session (1 = low, 2 = medium, 3 = high) by the student attendance score for that session (0 = not attended, 1 = attended). The program exposure score for the student was then calculated by totaling the exposure scores of six core sessions. Hence, the formula for program exposure was: Student Program Exposure = SUM[(Session Fidelity) × (attendance)]. The results revealed that there was inconsistent exposure to the curriculum across all of the students. With a possible score of 0 to 18, students' program exposure scores ranged from 2 to 17 ($\bar{x}$ = 10.6, n = 403).

Use of Process Evaluation Results

Some results from the process evaluation were used to inform ASAP about the process of program implementation, whereas other results were not available until after the completion of the implementation. For example, when initial data analyses suggested that the SHOWED model was being inconsistently implemented, quizzes were added to the weekly class sessions for facilitators. A final implementation score for each group (low, medium, or high) was calculated and could have been used for summative evaluation purposes for a dose response analysis, because one of the hypotheses was that there might be a positive dose-response relationship between exposure, participation, implementation, and outcome. Data on student participation (engagement) were not analyzed. The observation form was continually revised over two semesters in an attempt to improve low interrater reliability. Despite these efforts, when all of the data were analyzed, we found that observers who had previously been facilitators were more critical of student engagement than those who had never facilitated a session. As a result, it was difficult to aggregate data that was not comparable across groups.

Another hypothesis was that student characteristics might have influenced outcomes. For example, students' school performance or previous exposure to alcohol, drugs, or tobacco may have affected their future risk of negative outcomes. Outcome data suggested that the program had no overall effect on alcohol or tobacco consumption, and additional analyses were not conducted. Other information sources, such as the participant contact sheet, facilitator log, and student comment sheet, were not used, because of the lack of resources to embark on the labor-intensive qualitative analyses that these instruments required. Information on the school context (such as that provided by the barriers focus group, the health-related program inventory, and the health-related student inventory) was not used by the program, because the outcome data suggested that the program had not achieved its intended effect.

After the end of the grant period, Helitzer, Yoon, Wallerstein, and Garcia-Velarde (2000) described the relationship between training and implementation. At the time, a new grant submission was pending approval. It was thought that the new grant would be able to take advantage of this information. However, the grant was never awarded, which rendered the process evaluation results less useful than anticipated.

Lessons Learned About Process Evaluation

LESSON 1. *Get more out of less data.*

Our experience is that process evaluation data can easily become unmanageable. If an evaluator is highly detail-oriented, he or she will have the inclination to document every aspect of the project. However, it is unethical and a waste of resources to collect data that will not be used in some way. Unless an evaluator has a plan for data collection, analysis, and use, it is highly likely that he or she will collect more than is needed. It is a valuable exercise to find ways to overlap purposes for tools and for formative and summative applications. The most frequently asked or necessary questions, including both the *whether* and the *why* questions, can be formulated in advance. Early process evaluations, such as those for the CATCH and PATHWAYS projects (McGraw and others, 1994; Helitzer and others, 1999), had hundreds of instruments, but this is not realistic for most programs. Deciding what are the most important questions to answer will help the process evaluation be more efficient.

LESSON 2. *Use mixed methods and triangulate.*

In addition to being efficient with the collection of data, there is a need for data from different instruments, data sources, samples, and types of data. Qualitative methods, such as in-depth interviews and focus groups, are labor-intensive and perceived as subjective data because of the relationship between the data collector and the data. Furthermore, qualitative data tend to be seen as less valuable than quantitative data. Sometimes, this distinction is worded in terms of "soft" (qualitative) versus "hard" (quantitative) data. For these reasons, qualitative data can be seen as less desirable to include in evaluations than quantitative methods that are seen as more objective and less labor-intensive to collect and analyze (Helitzer and others, 1999). This debate and these biases have existed far too long in both primary and evaluation research. Using both qualitative and quantitative methods, we can better answer both the what and the why questions. Using mixed methods also provides more opportunities for triangulating data.

LESSON 3. *Use the information on time to improve the program.*

Process evaluation staff members should be included in project implementation discussions on a regular basis. In this way, these staff members can learn about the implementation process and can provide frequent feedback for midcourse corrections. This means that program staff people should expect implementation failure as a normal part of project implementation. If it is expected, then they can avoid being defensive about why it is happening, and as a result they can devote time and resources to fine-tuning and making changes based on feedback. We need to think about evaluation's purpose as program improvement rather than as a thumbs-up or thumbs-down judgment as to whether the program is effective. We need to create a culture of learning organizations as they relate to program implementation in public health.

LESSON 4. *Devote adequate attention and resources to process evaluation.*

Although evaluation has more recently been receiving a part of routine program funds, most of these funds and attention are still focused on outcome evaluation. The evidence suggests that most programs do not attain the outcomes they are designed to attain, and for this reason it is important that more attention be focused on process evaluation. Previously, process evaluation was thought of as "bean counting" because it routinely documented information on, for example, how many trainings were held, as well as how many trainees were trained. Process evaluation has the potential to provide much more information if it is properly planned and if sufficient resources are provided for it.

LESSON 5. *Use process evaluation to answer why, not just whether.*

Program implementation failure is to be expected and planned for. Also, programs under real-life conditions rarely show the same types of results that are published in research studies. This is the difference between program *efficacy* and program *effectiveness* (Green and Lewis, 1986). Because of this, it is more important to look at why programs do not demonstrate the same intensity of intended outcomes. Programs that are designed on paper and implemented in real life face challenges that often are not anticipated or planned for. For example, if teachers implement only parts of a curriculum, we could ask them why they chose the parts they did. However, it would be far more useful to have the original curriculum designers indicate which parts of the curriculum are linked to the theoretical framework of the program.

Some participants may benefit more from an intervention than others will. Process evaluation data can be used to examine whether a dose-response relationship exists between participation and outcome changes. If such a relationship exists, it may explain why some participants show increased changes as compared with others. In addition, other characteristics of the participants, such as age, sex, and ethnicity, can be examined for relationships.

Finally, programs may work better under certain conditions than others. A retrospective analysis can be conducted to examine participants for whom outcomes were favorable to see if individual, family, school, community, or program conditions were different for those participants whose outcomes were not as positive. A strength of process evaluation is its ability to provide more depth of information and the opportunity to build hypotheses for future research.

LESSON 6. *Theory, theory, theory.*

Both a strength and a weakness of the process evaluation described in this chapter was its evolving nature, reflecting new knowledge and expertise. The process evaluation of this study lacked a theoretical framework that might have examined in a comprehensive manner the assumptions upon which the program was based. However, we now know, in 2002, more about process evaluation, which enables us to be self-reflective. We recognize that a potential for process evaluation is the examination of both the implementation and the program theory, as described by Weiss (1998) as the program's "theories of change." Articulating a program's change theories helps us understand the assumptions on which the intervention is based, and it is essential for developing appropriate evaluation questions and evaluation design. Program theories of change help evaluators plan what data to collect and from whom, as well as what types of short- and long-term effects might be expected from the intervention. Using Weiss's theories of change approach, the process evaluation can focus on detailing and systematically documenting each step of the implementation. In this way, the process evaluation can be designed to examine some of the theoretical assumptions of the program.

Figures 4.4 and 4.5 illustrate how the theory of change model could have been used for the ASAP program. We inserted the instrument numbers into the figure to demonstrate the comprehensiveness of the original design in terms of program function but not in terms of theory. Process evaluation instruments were designed to measure *what* but not *why.* They were designed to document the implementation but not to look at the context and reasons behind the variable levels of

FIGURE 4.4. THEORY OF CHANGE MODEL FOR ASAP FACILITATORS.

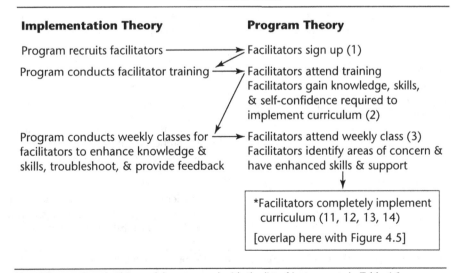

Note: The numbers in this model correspond with the list of instruments in Table 4.1.

FIGURE 4.5. THEORY OF CHANGE MODEL FOR ASAP CURRICULUM IMPLEMENTATION.

Implementation Theory

Program gains cooperation/support from school administration & teachers

Site coordinators recruit students from classrooms

Site coordinators make efforts to boost attendance with reminders, calls, transportation, etc.

*Facilitators completely implement curriculum (11, 12, 13, 14)

[overlap here with Figure 4.4]

Site coordinators provide support to student group for social action projects (6, 15)

Site coordinators provide booster session & contacts & invite students at 6-month postcurriculum; they also provide transportation & facilitate session (6, 15)

Program Theory

School teachers allow time in classrooms for recruitment; schools have low number of competing programs (8, 9, 10)

Students gain parental permission & sign up

Students attend 6-week curriculum sessions (5, 6, 7)

Patients/inmates are available for interviews (11, 12, 13, 14)

Students participate fully (12)

Students determine a social action project at the end of 6-week curriculum

Students attend, participate in, & complete social action project (6, 15)

Students attend & participate in booster session (6, 15)

Students attain/increase & maintain theoretical elements (e.g., self-efficacy & coping skills) for at least 15 months (4)

Students decrease in risky behaviors (e.g., smoking, alcohol, & drug consumption) for at least 15 months (4)

Note: The numbers in this model correspond with the list of instruments in Table 4.1.

implementation. Many of the instruments measured the same component, and triangulation was desirable, but given limited resources, it would have been more effective to have more instruments or sections of instruments to measure a greater proportion of theoretical components.

Using Weiss's theoretical framework (1998) has been helpful to us in our process evaluation efforts. We recently developed a methodology for working closely with investigators and program designers in the early stages of planning and program design. We use implementation and program theory logic models, such as those shown in Figures 4.4 and 4.5, as a framework to

- Articulate the program and implementation theory
- Identify where the theory components can be found in the implementation
- Identify which components are critical to program success
- Articulate what assumptions are held about the relationship between theory and outcome
- Identify which program components require tracking

In this way, we can be more efficient about collecting data. Included in this planning process are schedules for pilot testing and feedback, as well as discussions about timing for feedback, in order to make the feedback most useful for mid-course corrections.

In summary, the lessons learned from this study are important for the future practice of process evaluation. First, evaluators need to gain from investigators and program staff members *support for* and *interest in* the process evaluation. Their support helps ensure the timely and accurate collection of process evaluation measures and it helps ensure that the evaluation continues despite preliminary outcome data findings. Second, evaluators working with staff members and investigators need to build their *capacity for understanding* the value of process evaluation. Such a process might include discussions early on in the evaluation and implementation process to help everyone involved in the project understand the important and interconnected role that all phases of evaluation—formative, process, and outcome—have in a full and insightful understanding of interventions. Evaluations are often broken into the familiar parts of formative, process, and outcome, but for evaluation to be most effective, greater emphasis must be placed on the fact that these parts are an integrated whole evaluation. Such an understanding will go a long way toward resolving the often inadequate resources that are directed toward the design, collection, and analysis of process as well as formative evaluation data. Finally, *planning* is essential in successful evaluations, including the process component, and in our experience it is extremely helpful for program designers and evaluators alike.

Conclusions

The process evaluation described in this chapter represents an ambitious undertaking for the amount of resources it was allotted, and it reflects the state of knowledge and experience about process evaluation that existed in the mid-1990s. It is through these types of projects that we can be self-reflective and take away lessons that can improve the knowledge base from which future process evaluations will be designed.

What follows in this concluding section is a list and discussion of (1) the strengths of this process evaluation and (2) the limitations and opportunities for learning.

Strengths

The existence of a process evaluation. It is significant, given the level of knowledge about process evaluation at the time, that some funding for process evaluation was provided by the NIAAA and that the principal investigators had the wisdom to plan for and allocate these resources to hire a process evaluation consultant. In addition, the design represented a praiseworthy attempt to be conceptually thorough. Program personnel did an excellent and thorough job of collecting and managing the voluminous amount of data. Response rates were extremely high (see Table 4.1) for most instruments. Data were organized and easy to access for analysis.

The multipurpose design of instruments. A second strength of this process evaluation is that instruments were designed to provide both formative and summative data. For example, the attendance logs were intended to be used to provide information on participation for formative purposes, allowing quick response to improve poor attendance by site coordinators. Attendance data also could have been used to calculate the dose response rate for each student, correlating this rate with the alcohol use behavior outcome measures.

Triangulation. A third strength of this process evaluation is the ability to triangulate data from different instruments, data sources, samples, and types of data. Some of the triangulation was accomplished by using both qualitative and quantitative data. Other triangulation was undertaken by using two or more types of informants. For example, the observation checklist was designed to estimate the fidelity of facilitators to the curriculum by an independent observer during one session. Facilitator checklist data and student comment sheets for the same session were compared with observer data to determine whether facilitators were accurately representing their coverage of curriculum components. It was the ability to triangulate the data from the checklists, comment sheets, and observations that enabled facilitators to determine that midcourse corrections were needed.

Limitations and Opportunities for Learning

Insufficient planning for the analysis process. Despite the ambitious design and allocation of some resources to process evaluation, the program did not dedicate sufficient attention to planning for the analysis process so that it would provide useful and timely feedback to the program. This could have been because human resources were mainly focused on the collection and implementation of outcome data. For example, the process evaluation consultant was not brought on board until well into the grant period. When the consultant was brought on, data were already being collected without a plan for the management and analysis of the data. No one anticipated how much data there would be, how long the data analysis would take, or how labor-intensive it would be. Therefore, much of the process evaluation data were not analyzed and synthesized in a time frame that would have enabled the program to make corrective changes to improve the program's implementation. For example, if the data regarding facilitator implementation had been analyzed throughout the project rather than just at the end, the training process could have been improved to increase fidelity to the curriculum (Helitzer, Yoon, Wallerstein, and Garcia-Velarde, 2000).

Insufficient understanding, interest, and appreciation. Although the process evaluation design was thoughtful, there was only partial appreciation for the value of process evaluation and the contribution that its results could make. This lack of knowledge about the various ways the process evaluation could be used resulted in insufficient attention being paid to it during the course of the project. For example, weekly meetings of the project staff often did not include discussions of process evaluation data, and rarely were requests made for data to be analyzed for a specific purpose. Also, the process evaluation expert was paid only 3 percent of her salary to work on the project, which provided insufficient time for the thoughtful incorporation of process evaluation results.

Process evaluation data were not being used to answer the question Why? When the outcome data suggested that there were no intervention effects, process evaluation data could have been used to understand whether or *why* there was program failure and whether or *why* the theoretical assumptions about the curriculum were not sound. For example, once we realized that the facilitators were implementing some parts of the curriculum more consistently than other parts, we could have used the qualitative data from facilitator logs to try to understand why the facilitators seemed to have more difficulty with components requiring role-playing behavior than with those involving the introduction and review of content areas.

Limited use of qualitative data. Most of the qualitative data were not analyzed. These data were a rich source of information (for example, participant contact documentation sheets were the logs of site coordinators working on social action projects) and could have provided insight into unintended outcomes. However, the reality of qualitative data is that it can be unwieldy and that it requires a long time to analyze properly. Qualitative analysis requires not only adequate time and human resources devoted to it but also personnel who possess the appropriate research skills. In the case of ASAP, the human resources devoted to research were not adequate to be extended to most of the qualitative analyses.

References

Chassin, L., Presson, C. C., Sherman, S. J., and Steinberg, L. "Adolescent Smokeless Tobacco Use: Future Research Needs." *NCI Monograph*, 1989, *8*, 101–105.

Floyd, D. L., Prentice-Dunn, S., and Rogers, R. W. "A Meta-Analysis of Research on Protection Motivation Theory." *Journal of Applied Social Psychology*, 2000, *30*(2), 407–429.

Green, L. W., and Lewis, F. M. *Measurement and Evaluation in Health Education and Health Promotion*. Mountain View, Calif.: Mayfield, 1986.

Helitzer, D. L., Yoon, S., Wallerstein, N., and Garcia-Velarde, L. "The Role of Process Evaluation in the Training of Facilitators for an Adolescent Health Education Program." *Journal of School Health*, 2000, *7*(4), 141–147.

Helitzer, D. L., and others. "Process Evaluation in a Multisite, Primary Obesity-Prevention Trial in American Indian Schoolchildren." *American Journal of Clinical Nutrition*, 1999, *69* (supp.), 816S–824S.

Jacobson, M., Atkins, R., and Hacker, G. *The Booze Merchants: The Inebriating of America*. Washington, D.C.: Center for Science in the Public Interest, 1983.

McGraw, S. A., and others. "Design of Process Evaluation Within the Child and Adolescent Trial for Cardiovascular Health (CATCH)." *Health Education Quarterly*, 1994, *2* (supp.), S5–26.

Microsoft Applications, *Microsoft Excel*, 1995. Software.

Miles, M. B., and Huberman, A. M. *Qualitative Data Analysis: An Expanded Sourcebook*. (2nd ed.). Thousand Oaks, Calif.: Sage, 1994.

Rippetoe, P. A., and Rogers, R. W. "Effects of Components of Protection-Motivation Theory on Adaptive and Maladaptive Coping with a Health Threat." *Journal of Personality and Social Psychology*, 1987, *52*(3), 596–604.

Rissel, C. E., and others. "Empowerment, Alcohol, Eighth-Grade Students and Health Promotion." *Journal of Alcohol and Drug Education*, 1996, *41*(2), 105–119.

Rogers, R. W. "Cognitive and Physiological Processes in Attitudinal Change: A Revised Theory of Protection-Motivation." In J. Cacioppo and R. Petty (eds.), *Social Psychophysiology*. New York: Guilford Press, 1983.

Rogers, R. W. "Changing Health-Related Attitudes and Behavior: The Role of Preventive Health Psychology." In R. McGlyn, J. Maddox, C. Stoltenbery, and R. J. Harvey (eds.), *Interfaces in Psychology*. Lubbock: Texas Tech University Press, 1994.

Rogers, R. W., Deckner, C. W., and Mewborn, C. R. "An Expectancy-Value Theory Approach to the Long-Term Modification of Smoking Behavior." *Journal of Clinical Psychology*, 1978, *34*, 562–566.

Steckler, A., and others. "Toward Integrating Qualitative and Quantitative Methods: An Introduction." *Health Education Quarterly,* 1992, *19,* 1–9.

Wallerstein, N., and Bernstein, E. "Empowerment Education: Freire's Ideas Adapted to Health Education." *Health Education Quarterly,* 1988, *15*(4), 379–394.

Wallerstein, N., and Sanchez-Merki, V. "Freirian Praxis in Health Education: Research Results from an Adolescent Prevention Program." *Health Education Research,* 1994, *9*(1), 105–118.

Wallerstein, N., and Woodall, G. *ASAP Project Final Report for NIAAA.* Albuquerque: University of New Mexico, 2000.

Weiss, C. H. *Evaluation.* Englewood Cliffs, N.J.: Prentice Hall, 1998.

APPENDIX A: FACILITATOR CHECKOFF LIST.

School _____

Facilitators _____

_____

Date _____

NIAAA Facilitator's H/DC Checkoff List

As part of the NIAAA Evaluation Process, the ASAP program requests that you track the activities during your H/DC experience. Please indicate by degree all of the activities that you and your cofacilitator completed for each session and return it to our office at the completion of session six. Please use the following scale: **0 = didn't cover; 1 = touched on briefly; 2 = mostly covered; 3 = completely covered**

Introductory Session I

__1. Group Introduction
__2. Brainstorm Norms with Students
__3. Who I Am/Tree of Life
__4. Culture and Stereotyping—Wood Plank Activity
__5. Norm Perception Questionnaire
__6. Choose a Theme! Wildside Video
__7. Student Comment Sheet

Hospital Session Two: Hospital Introduction

__1. Review Group Norms & Hospital Guidelines
__2. Participant Expectation
__3. Definitions
__4. Communication Interview Skills
__5. Interview Patients
__6. Discussion of Patients
__7. Role-Play on Coping Skills
__8. Interview Home Assignment
__9. Student Comment Sheets

Hospital Session Three

__1. Icebreaker
__2. Communication
__3. Patient Interview
__4. Dealing with Problems "Right or Wrong"
__5. ABC's of Smoking Chart
__6. Preparing for Session Four
__7. Student Comment Sheets

Jail Session Four

__1. Introductions
__2. Interview Residents
__3. 8:00 PM Interview Debrief at a Local Restaurant
__4. Student Comment Sheets
__5. Collage Activity in Session Five

Hospital Session Five

__1. Advertising Activity
__2. Discussion of Students' Communities
__3. Patient Interviews
__4. The "But Why?" Root Cause Analysis of Problems
__5. Student Comment Sheets
__6. Preparation for Session Six

Session Six

Social Action Project Development Student Group

__1. Shaping Your Community Activity
__2. Brainstorm a Social Action Project
__3. Resources
__4. Action Steps

Parents and School Site Representative Group

__1. South Valley Pride
__2. Discussion of ASAP
__3. Prepare to Rejoin Students

Parents and Students Back Together

__1. Presentation of Project
__2. Wrap-Up and Public Commitment

APPENDIX B: ASAP SESSION V OBSERVATION FORM.

ASAP OBSERVATION CHECKLIST (Session V)

School _____   Facilitators A) _____   Date _____

Number of Students _____   B) _____

_____ Females

_____ Males   Observed by _____

****

DK = Don't Know   NA = Not Applicable

****

STUDENT BEHAVIOR

For questions pertaining to student groups, high majority (at least 5/7, 4/6, 4/5, 3/4, 2/3, 2/2) of students should exhibit the behavior. (Circle appropriate one.)

1. At least one student articulates a belief in group action.	Yes	No	DK
2. Students articulate belief in group action.	Yes	No	DK
3. Students demonstrate a sense of belonging to the ASAP group.	Yes	No	DK
4. At least one student articulates self-efficacy toward doing group action. (e.g., "I feel that I can . . . because . . .).	Yes	No	DK
5. Students articulate self-efficacy toward doing group action (e.g., "I feel that I can . . . because . . .).	Yes	No	DK
6. At least one student articulates a sense of responsibility to take social action (e.g., "It's my job to . . .).	Yes	No	DK
7. Students articulate a sense of responsibility to take social action (e.g., "It's my job to . . .).	Yes	No	DK
8. At least one student articulates the social context.	Yes	No	DK
9. Students articulate the social context.	Yes	No	DK
10. At least one student discussed his or her own risky behavior.	Yes	No	DK
11. At least one student discussed the risky behavior of his or her family or friends.	Yes	No	DK

For the following question, use this rating scale:

3	2	1	0	DK
All of the model	Most of the model	Some of the model	None of the model	Don't know

12. Students use the SHOWED model in analyzing problems.   3 2 1 0 DK

For the remaining questions in this section, use the following rating scale:

3	2	1	0	DK	{ NA }
All of the time	Most of the time	Some of the time	None of the time	Don't know	{ Not Applicable }

13. The group process encourages participation.   3 2 1 0 DK

14. The students as a group are attentive to the issues being discussed. 3 2 1 0 DK

15. The students as a group are attentive to each other.   3 2 1 0 DK

(Continued)

APPENDIX B: ASAP SESSION V OBSERVATION FORM. (CONTINUED)

STUDENT BEHAVIOR

16. The students as a group are attentive to the facilitators.	3 2 1 0 DK
17. Students are quiet or uncomfortable during discussion.	3 2 1 0 DK
18. Students are respectful of each other.	3 2 1 0 DK
19. The students as a whole appear to be bored or impatient.	3 2 1 0 DK
20. Hostility or group division among the students is apparent.	3 2 1 0 DK
21. Teasing and unacceptable behavior is taking place among the students.	3 2 1 0 DK
22. There is an appropriate amount of humor in the session.	3 2 1 0 DK
23. There is an inappropriate amount of humor in the session.	3 2 1 0 DK
24. The students as a group are attentive to the patients.	3 2 1 0 DK NA
25. Students pose open-ended questions to patients.	3 2 1 0 DK NA
26. Debriefing occurred as a result of _____ and _____.	Yes No DK
27. The group discussions are superficial.	3 2 1 0 DK
28. Topics are addressed in group discussions in depth.	3 2 1 0 DK
29. Topics discussed elicit student stories about their lives, social analysis, and critical thinking.	3 2 1 0 DK
30. Group discussions have a prevention orientation.	3 2 1 0 DK
31. The students articulate alternative actions/strategies to problems presented to them.	3 2 1 0 DK
32. The concept of "community" is discussed (e.g., a sense of belonging/responsibility to larger group).	Yes No DK
33. The concept of "culture" is discussed (e.g., religion, foods, beliefs, language, ethnicity).	Yes No DK
34. The concept of "stereotype" is discussed.	Yes No DK

FACILITATORS

35. Facilitator A places him- or herself among the students.	Yes No DK
36. Facilitator B places him- or herself among the students.	Yes No DK
37. Facilitator A ensures that students are okay after seeing patients.	Yes No DK NA
38. Facilitator B ensures that students are okay after seeing patients.	Yes No DK NA
39. Facilitator A allowed time for debriefing and dialogue.	Yes No DK
40. Facilitator B allowed time for debriefing and dialogue.	Yes No DK
41. Facilitator A leads a dialogue based on the SHOWED model.	Yes No DK
42. Facilitator B leads a dialogue based on the SHOWED model.	Yes No DK
43. Facilitator A uses the patients as triggers for dialogue.	Yes No DK NA
44. Facilitator B uses the patients as triggers for dialogue.	Yes No DK NA
45. Facilitator A recalls specific incidents to support and obtain more reactions and ideas from the students.	Yes No DK
46. Facilitator B recalls specific incidents to support and obtain more reactions and ideas from the students.	Yes No DK

APPENDIX B: (CONTINUED)

FACILITATORS

For the next section, use the following rating scale:

3	2	1	0	DK
All of the time	Most of the time	Some of the time	None of the time	Don't know

47. Facilitator A encourages students to ask questions of each other.	3 2 1 0 DK
48. Facilitator B encourages students to ask questions of each other.	3 2 1 0 DK
49. Facilitator A lectures on what students should or shouldn't do.	3 2 1 0 DK
50. Facilitator B lectures on what students should or shouldn't do.	3 2 1 0 DK
51. Facilitator A works well with and reinforces the other facilitator.	3 2 1 0 DK
52. Facilitator B works well with and reinforces the other facilitator.	3 2 1 0 DK
53. Facilitator A dominates.	3 2 1 0 DK
54. Facilitator B dominates.	3 2 1 0 DK
55. Facilitator A is respectful of students.	3 2 1 0 DK
56. Facilitator B is respectful of students.	3 2 1 0 DK
57. Facilitator A is impatient.	3 2 1 0 DK
58. Facilitator B is impatient.	3 2 1 0 DK
59. Facilitator A follows up on issues raised by the students.	3 2 1 0 DK
60. Facilitator B follows up on issues raised by the students.	3 2 1 0 DK
61. Facilitator A offers explanations to students' questions and concerns.	3 2 1 0 DK
62. Facilitator B offers explanations to students' questions and concerns.	3 2 1 0 DK
63. Facilitator A leads dialogue about healthy behaviors.	3 2 1 0 DK
64. Facilitator B leads dialogue about healthy behaviors.	3 2 1 0 DK
65. The discussion promotes student ability to handle situations such as peer pressure.	3 2 1 0 DK

For this section, please use the scale:

0 = didn't cover   1 = touched on briefly   2 = mostly covered   3 = completely covered

66. _____	Advertising activity	Comments:
67. _____	Discussion of students' communities	Comments:
68. _____	Patient interviews	Comments:
69. _____	Debrief SHOWED model	Comments:
70. _____	The "but why?" root cause analysis of problems	Comments:
71. _____	Preparing for session six	Comments:
72. _____	Student Comment Sheets	Comments:

WHAT ISSUES WERE TALKED ABOUT DURING THIS SESSION?

COMMENTS (Please use back of this page):

CHAPTER FIVE

Process Evaluation of the Church-Based PRAISE! Project

Partnership to Reach African Americans to Increase Smart Eating

Alice Ammerman

This chapter describes the design, implementation, and findings of the process evaluation of Partnership to Reach African Americans to Increase Smart Eating (PRAISE!), a five-year faith-based intervention (1996–2001) funded by the National Cancer Institute and designed to reduce cancer risk through dietary change. This study was funded in response to a program announcement requesting studies designed to reach high-risk minority populations through culturally sensitive intervention strategies.

It is well known that African Americans suffer from disproportionately high rates of many types of cancers for which diet is a risk factor (American Cancer Society, 2001). However, clinical trials and intervention studies aimed at cancer prevention have often failed to reach this priority population effectively (Brawley and Tejeda, 1995; Millon-Underwood, Sanders, and Davis, 1993; Swanson and Ward, 1995; Kaluzny and others, 1993). Explanations for past failures to reach African Americans through cancer prevention clinical trials include their historical mistrust of research and medical institutions, the lack of culturally relevant lifestyle change interventions, and a failure on the part of researchers to design and implement interventions that continue to give back to the community through long-term sustainability and broader diffusion (Corbie-Smith, Thomas, Williams, and Moody-Ayers, 1999; Paskett, DeGraffinreid, Tatum, and Margitic, 1996; Harris, Gorelick, Samuels, and Bempong, 1996). We designed the PRAISE! project to more effectively reach a high-risk population by identifying and overcoming these common barriers. The process evaluation provides information to assess the degree to which we were successful in this effort.

PRAISE! Project Description

Study Design

The PRAISE! study was designed as a multisite, randomized controlled trial to assess the effectiveness of a twelve-month intervention to increase fruit, vegetable, and fiber intake and to decrease fat consumption (see Figure 5.1). After the collection of baseline data, sixty churches were randomized to receive either an immediate nutrition intervention (Group I) or a delayed nutrition intervention (Group II) with an interim nonnutrition intervention. Follow-up outcome data were collected at twelve months and Group II then received the delayed nutrition intervention.

Recruitment of Churches and Participants

Churches. African American churches were recruited from eight counties (urban and rural) in the central and coastal regions of North Carolina, with a recruitment goal of ten churches per county. At the outset, a list was compiled of all African American churches in these counties. Churches were eligible if they had a hundred active members or more, were 90 percent African American, and had not participated in significant nutrition education activities in the last ten years. Churches with congregations of fewer than a hundred members were given the option of pairing with a sister church in order to meet the hundred-member eligibility requirement. Once churches officially joined the project, the pastor appointed a church liaison to act as a link between the church and the project staff and to act as the Health Action Team (HAT) leader. The HAT took primary responsibility for implementing the intervention at each participating church.

Participants. To assess the impact of the church-based intervention, a convenience sample from each church was recruited to serve as the measurement group. Pastors made an announcement about the program during a worship service and HAT members recruited church members individually. Initial enrollment occurred immediately after the service during which the program was announced. The recruitment goal for each church or church pair was to enroll thirty volunteers, with the allowable range being ten to forty-five. To be included in the measurement group, participants had to be at least eighteen years old and no older than seventy-five, they had to attend church services at least once a month, they could not be either pregnant or breast feeding, and they had to be able to make dietary

FIGURE 5.1. PARTNERSHIP DEVELOPMENT AND RECRUITMENT.

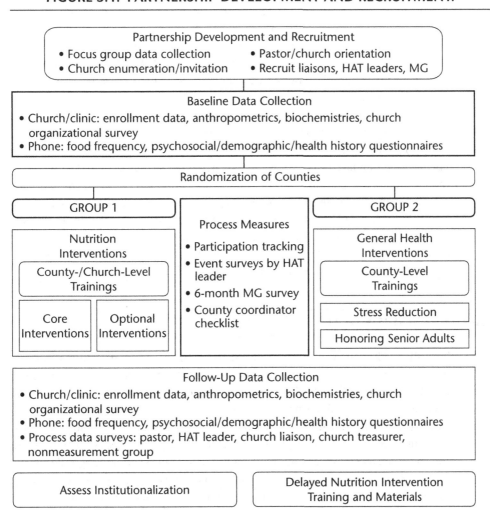

Partnership Development and Recruitment
- Focus group data collection
- Church enumeration/invitation
- Pastor/church orientation
- Recruit liaisons, HAT leaders, MG

Baseline Data Collection
- Church/clinic: enrollment data, anthropometrics, biochemistries, church organizational survey
- Phone: food frequency, psychosocial/demographic/health history questionnaires

Randomization of Counties

GROUP 1

Nutrition Interventions

County-/Church-Level Trainings

Core Interventions | Optional Interventions

Process Measures
- Participation tracking
- Event surveys by HAT leader
- 6-month MG survey
- County coordinator checklist

GROUP 2

General Health Interventions

County-Level Trainings

Stress Reduction

Honoring Senior Adults

Follow-Up Data Collection
- Church/clinic: enrollment data, anthropometrics, biochemistries, church organizational survey
- Phone: food frequency, psychosocial/demographic/health history questionnaires
- Process data surveys: pastor, HAT leader, church liaison, church treasurer, nonmeasurement group

Assess Institutionalization

Delayed Nutrition Intervention Training and Materials

changes. Although study measures were collected primarily on the measurement group, the PRAISE! intervention was designed to reach the entire church, and all church members were encouraged to participate.

Randomization and Data Collection

To avoid contamination between the Group I and Group II interventions, randomization occurred at the county level rather than by church. In some cases, two smaller (less populated) counties were combined into one *county unit*. Before recruitment of churches began, the six county units were matched into three pairs, according to county population and region within the state. For logistical reasons, baseline data collection, randomization, and intervention implementation were performed sequentially, by county unit pair (Waves I–III). Within each Wave, churches were randomized by county to either Group I (nutrition intervention) or Group II (delayed intervention control). After follow-up data collection, Group II health action teams were trained in the implementation of the PRAISE! intervention and provided with all of the necessary materials.

Weight and height, along with fasting blood measures, were collected at baseline by using standard protocols. A baseline psychosocial, health, and demographic questionnaire was administered by trained telephone interviewers, who also assessed dietary intake, using a food frequency instrument modified to reflect the Southern diet. All of these measures were repeated at the twelve-month follow-up. Process measures, including participation tracking, event surveys, county coordinator checklists, pastor surveys, and HAT leader surveys, were collected both during and following the intervention (see Figure 5.1).

Theoretical Basis of the Intervention

The PRAISE! intervention was multilevel, with components addressing the intrapersonal, interpersonal, organizational, and community levels of the social ecological framework (McLeroy, Bibeau, Steckler, and Glanz, 1988). It was designed with particular attention given to cultural appropriateness, long-term institutionalization within the church environment, and the potential for dissemination/diffusion to other interested church organizations. At the intra- and interpersonal levels, social cognitive theory guided intervention design (Bandura, 1986), whereas organizational theory and community organization models were used at the more "upstream" levels of the social ecological framework.

Organizational theory has been used to describe the processes of institutionalization and diffusion. Many different terms and models have been put forth in an attempt to understand how innovations are adopted and sustained in community organizations (Barab, Redman, and Froman, 1998; Basch, Eveland, and Portnoy, 1986; Ford, Kaluzny, and Sondik, 1990; McMichael, Smith, and Corvalan, 2000; O'Loughlin and others, 1998). In the PRAISE! project, *institutionalization* refers to the long-term integration of the intervention into an individual church. *Sustainability* refers to the perpetuation of the program in the surrounding community as well as in the church. The potential for *diffusion* has to do with the components of the intervention design that make possible the dissemination of the program to other interested churches by those churches where it had become institutionalized.

Institutionalization and Sustainability

Early work in this area was guided by Katz and Kahn (1978), who describe a series of steps or stages experienced by an organization in order for an innovation to be successfully introduced, adopted, and sustained. Goodman and Steckler (1989) have looked more specifically at institutionalization of change within organizations, particularly at schools and worksites (see also Goodman, McLeroy, Steckler, and Hoyle, 1993; Steckler and others, 1992). The terms *institutionalization* and *sustainability* have often been used interchangeably to describe the integration of a program into its host organization and the attainment of long-term viability.

More recently, Shediac-Rizkallah and Bone (1998) offer a conceptual framework for sustainable community-based health programs that gives the term *sustainability* a broader application with regard to program continuation, with the term referring to elements of the community as well as organizational capacity. These authors are among the first to advocate *planning* for sustainability in the design of the intervention. A community-based model such as this did not exist when we designed the PRAISE! intervention, but we believe it captures the essence of our approach, which was largely guided by organizational theory adapted to reflect the guidance of our community-based church partners. Table 5.1 illustrates how PRAISE! intervention components match the Shediac framework for conceptualizing program sustainability.

Shediac-Rizkallah and Bone (1998) argue that key groups of factors behind the potential for sustainability include (1) project design and implementation factors, (2) factors within the organizational setting, and (3) factors in the broader community environment. Therefore, planning for sustainability must focus on program design and implementation that considers the barriers to implementation while building on the strengths of the organization and community. Because positive dietary behaviors must be sustained in order to maintain good health over a lifetime, interventions that influence these behaviors must be sustainable.

Diffusion

Diffusion theory attempts to identify predictable program adoption patterns across a variety of innovations and populations. Oldenburg, Hardcastle, and Kok (1997), basing their findings on the work of Rogers (1983) and Zaltman and

TABLE 5.1.   FRAMEWORK FOR CONCEPTUALIZING PROGRAM SUSTAINABILITY.

Sustainability Planning Guideline	Elements of the PRAISE! Intervention Designed to Foster Sustainability
Project Design and Implementation	
Project negotiation process	Whereas the funding source (National Cancer Institute) determined the health focus, interventions were designed with extensive input from church leadership/members and with flexibility to address broader concerns associated with chronic disease prevention.
Project effectiveness	Information regarding the effect of diet on chronic disease and the effectiveness of similar intervention on dietary change was presented to church members. Diet and health outcome measures will be shared with study participants. Formative data suggests that members believe dietary change will have many positive secondary effects.
Project duration	The PRAISE! team worked with study participants to establish a church infrastructure/health ministry during a five-year funding period that could sustain the program over the long term.
Project financing	Interventions were designed to require minimal external funding support or draw on community resources. Research-related study costs were covered by the PRAISE! project.
Project type	The focus of the project is preventative vs. curative, which necessitates a long-term approach to foster sustainability.
Training	Pastor training included CE credits and developed capacity among the pastors to address lifestyle modification as a part of their role as spiritual leaders of the church. HAT and HAT leader training focused on a train-the-trainer model, providing skill-building and educational resources to church members who carry out the interventions directly. Sharing sessions among church HATs were designed to help build networking and support among the churches.
Factors Within the Organizational Setting	
Institutionalization strength	Black churches were selected to implement the intervention, based on their historic strength and central role in the African American community.
Integration with existing programs/service	Some churches have existing "Health Ministries" or have started them as a result of participating in the PRAISE! project. PRAISE! activities are integrated into the existing church calendar and functions and can be adapted to the needs of the individual church. Churches are encouraged to draw on local health resources and professionals.
Program champion/leadership	In most cases, the pastors play a very strong and critical leadership/champion role at the spiritual/inspirational/motivational level. HAT leaders and the HAT provide the day-to-day leadership for program implementation.

TABLE 5.1. (CONTINUED)

Factors in the Broader Community Environment

Socioeconomic and political considerations	Although churches have not traditionally been involved in health promotion, pastors seem to be embracing this as an important new direction that fits well within the spiritual priorities of the church. The black church plays a critical role in the lives of African Americans across socioeconomic strata.
Community participation	Many PRAISE! churches took the initiative to invite the broader community to PRAISE! events. There appears to be a strong sense of local ownership of the program, and many churches have indicated an interest in sharing the program with other nearby churches or through their larger denominational affiliations.

Duncan (1977), identified twelve key determinants of the speed and extent of diffusion. Table 5.2 lists these key determinants and how the PRAISE! intervention is designed to address these factors. We recommend an additional determinant for church-based interventions: concordance with the organizational mission.

Process Evaluation Context, Design, and Methods

In keeping with our efforts to design an intervention approach that was culturally sensitive, was sustainable within the study churches, and could be feasibly disseminated to other churches—*and* to test this intervention within a true research partnership between the university and faith-based communities, we designed our process evaluation to focus on three areas:

1. *Intervention implementation*—the *fidelity* of the intervention (how well the intervention was carried out as it was intended), the perceived "fit" in the church, and organizational/leadership factors that facilitated or inhibited implementation

2. *Research partnership*—the degree to which church members and leaders were comfortable with the research process and felt that they were research partners rather than "research subjects"

3. *Potential for sustainability and diffusion*—the degree to which intervention implementers at the church level perceived the intervention as sustainable at each church and whether they thought it could be shared with other churches

TABLE 5.2. KEY DETERMINANTS OF DIFFUSION'S SPEED AND EXTENT: A GUIDE TO DESIGNING THE PRAISE! INTERVENTION.

Key Determinant	PRAISE! Intervention Characteristic
Relative advantage Better than what it will replace?	Most churches/pastors reported that they are interested in health issues but currently have no health ministry and limited other activities in this area. PRAISE! offers training and educational resources to implement a program that would fill this gap.
Compatibility Fit the intended audience?	Focus group data facilitated an intervention designed to blend with existing church program and culture, such as food events associated with homecoming and pastor's anniversary celebrations. Recommended dietary changes focus on strengths of the Southern diet (greens, dry peas and beans, vegetables) and modifications to culturally valued foods that reduce the fat content or increase fruit, vegetable, and fiber intake.
Trialability Can the innovation be subjected to trial?	Optional interventions gave churches the chance to try the interventions they felt would work best for them. Taste testing allowed congregants to experience healthier food choices before making a major commitment to changes in food preparation for church events.
Observability Are results observable/ easily measurable?	Cancer risk reduction is NOT readily detected; however, process data suggest that congregants notice a difference in the types of meals served at church functions. Others report feeling better and losing weight as a result of the intervention.
Impact on social relations Disruptive effect on social environment?	Interventions were designed to build on social support and bring church members together. Many churches invited members of other churches and the community at large to their PRAISE! events. Given implementation flexibility, many HATs found creative ways to introduce healthier foods without disrupting social norms (like putting smaller pieces of fried chicken at the END of the buffet line).
Reversibility Discontinued easily?	In the case of dietary change, this is a detrimental component of higher diffusabilty. It is all too easy to reverse healthier dietary behaviors. PRAISE! project influence on evolving social norms toward healthier eating, along with role modeling of church leaders, can help prevent reversal of positive dietary trends.
Communicability Understood clearly and easily?	The PRAISE! intervention was delivered entirely through trained church leaders and members who could tailor the educational messages to the interest and understanding of the church membership. This assured that messages were understood.
Time required Adopted with minimal investment of time?	The interventions were designed to blend with existing church activities vs. adding extra programming; therefore, the time demanded of an individual (outside the data collection requirements) was quite minimal.
Risk and uncertainty level Adopted with minimal risk/uncertainty?	Dietary change is very low-risk except for fears of unpalatability and high cost. Intervention materials and strategies were specifically designed to address both of these barriers.

TABLE 5.2. (CONTINUED)

Commitment required Used effectively with modest commitment?	The interventions were designed to blend with existing church activities versus adding extra programming; however, significant time was required of the HAT. By having a large enough team that can rotate membership, it is hoped that the time requirements will be shared among members.
Modifiability Able to be updated and modified over time?	Training materials for HATs offer suggestions rather than a set curriculum that can be adapted over time. PRAISE! packets mailed on a quarterly basis allowed seasonal modification and intervention updates.
Concordance with organizational mission Fits with goals/objectives of organization	Formative focus group data suggested that although most churches did not have active health ministries, the notion of physical health blended very well with the church's primary emphasis on spiritual health, and this idea was well supported by scripture.

Research Questions

Multiple data collection instruments and methods were used to collect data from church leaders and participants many times during the study. Figure 5.1 shows how process data collection interfaced with the overall study design and other data collection elements. Table 5.3 provides more detail about individual data collection instruments, the types of questions included, and which of the three major foci of our process evaluation—*intervention implementation, research partnership,* and *potential for sustainability/diffusion*—were addressed. Because the intent was to design an intervention that was not only sufficiently structured to guide the church implementers but also flexible enough to permit tailoring to each church environment, many process measures included questions to elicit the details of intervention content and delivery. Table 5.4 provides detailed information about specific intervention components and the degree to which they were implemented by the churches.

Research questions addressed in the area of *intervention implementation* include

- To what degree were the core (required) and optional interventions implemented by participating churches?
- To what extent did both measurement group and general congregation members participate in core and optional interventions?
- From the perspective of church leaders and HAT members, what were some of the church-related resources and organizational and leadership factors that facilitated or inhibited both *specific* and *overall* intervention delivery and participation?

TABLE 5.3. PROCESS EVALUATION INSTRUMENTS: ADMINISTRATION, CONTENT, AND APPLICATION.

Instrument Sample and Measurement Period	Intervention Implementation	Research Partnership	Potential for Sustainability/ Diffusion	Instrument Content and Purpose	Application/Analysis
Pastor Survey —Baseline (Groups I & II)	*	*	*	—church organization, resources, and facilities —pastor demographics and training —pastor health concerns for self and congregation —interest in research partnership—decision to participate	*Formative data for intervention design *Quantitative data for church and pastor demographics
Pastor Survey —Follow-Up (Groups I & II)	*	*	*	—enthusiasm for and participation in intervention —personal efforts at lifestyle change —perceived participation of other church leaders —acceptability and dynamics of research partnership —steps toward and interest in sustainability and diffusion	*Role of pastor in intervention implementation and institutionalization *Association between pastor characteristics and attitudes and intervention success.
Health Action Team (HAT) *Leader* Surveys —Interim and —Follow-Up (Group I)	*	*	*	—specific/detailed feedback on each intervention re attendance, activities included, overall success, challenges in planning, use of church and community resources, perceived likelihood of sustainability, perceived ease of dissemination —demographics and past/current church leadership —personal level of involvement with intervention —perceived effectiveness of HAT and church leadership in implementing programs —major challenges and adequacy of support —confidence in leadership ability	*Role of HAT and HAT leader in intervention implementation *Association between HAT involvement and intervention success

Health Action Team (HAT) *Member* Survey —Follow-Up (Group I)	—dynamics of HAT in terms of leadership and teamwork in carrying out the interventions —past and current leadership roles —relevance of PRAISE! to church mission —church attendance —reasons for PRAISE! involvement —length and extent of service on HAT —perceived role in HAT and level of satisfaction	*Role of Health Action Team and in intervention implementation *Association between HAT involvement and intervention success
Non-measurement Group Survey (General church congregation) —Follow-Up (Group I)	—familiarity with project and goals —relevance of PRAISE! to church mission —decision not to participate in MG —involvement in PRAISE! activities —perception of inclusion —impact on church and on own dietary behavior	*Reasons for nonparticipation in measurement group and impact on overall level of involvement and satisfaction with PRAISE!
HAT Leader Follow-Up Evaluation for Specific Intervention "events" and ongoing activities —Events: immediately following —Ongoing: at 12-month survey	**Follow-up evaluation for specific intervention "events"** —4 food events —1 food festival —music fest (optional) —gleaning (optional) **Ongoing interventions ("non-events")** —personal health bulletin —communication center —PRAISE! packets —New Leaf and PRAISE! partners —congregation skills and treasures —inspirational booklets and tapes **Content for both "event" and ongoing interventions** —overall satisfaction —challenges of planning and implementing intervention —perceived enthusiasm of participants —assistance from HAT in planning/conducting intervention —use of resources outside church —receptivity of church members —perceived likelihood of institutionalization in the church —perceived ease of dissemination to other churches	*Acceptability and institutional-ization/dissemination potential for specific intervention components

TABLE 5.3. PROCESS EVALUATION INSTRUMENTS: ADMINISTRATION, CONTENT, AND APPLICATION. (CONTINUED)

Instrument Sample and Measurement Period	Intervention Implementation	Research Partnership	Potential for Sustainability/ Diffusion	Instrument Content and Purpose	Application/Analysis
Church Liaison Survey —Follow-Up (Group 1)	*	*	*	—demographics and past/current church leadership —personal level of involvement with intervention —perceived effectiveness of HAT and church leadership in implementing programs —major challenges and adequacy of support —confidence in leadership ability —satisfaction with research partnership	*Role of church liaison in intervention implementation and research components of partnership *Association between church liaison and data collection success
County Coordinator Checklist— Completed at 3, 6, 9, and 12 months	*		*	**Assistance provided to churches (quantified)** —phone calls to and from church HAT leader and church liaison —church and office **Church involvement and need for assistance (relative ranking among churches)** —assistance needed/requested in implementing PRAISE! project —leadership/participation/communication —evidence of institutionalization of PRAISE! **Evidence of outreach and potential for dissemination to other churches**	*Role of county coordinator in intervention implementation and research components *Association between county coordinator role and church level of satisfaction/success
Church Treasurer Survey —Follow-Up (Group 1)	*		*	—other leadership roles in church —adequacy of training —acceptability of role in terms of time demands and required activities —level of comfort with approach to financial transactions —perceived challenges of treasurer role	*Role of church treasurer in running the financial component of the project—feasibility and acceptability

PRAISE!
Partner Survey

*

*

—decision to participate
—adequacy of training and comfort in role
—level of involvement with PRAISE! partner activities
—interest from church members
—use of New Leaf educational materials
—acceptability of role in terms of time and required activities
—other involvement in church activities

*Role of PRAISE! partner in intervention implementation
*Association between PRAISE! partner role and church level satisfaction/success

Measurement
Group
Acceptability
Survey
—Follow-Up
(Group I and II)

*

*

Group I
—importance of church in program implementation
—assessment of relative impact, importance, and acceptability of different intervention components
—likelihood of sustainability of behavior change
—interest in institutionalizing program at the church
—interest in dissemination role
—acceptability of research partnership (e.g., blood draws, surveys)
—helpfulness of specific church level and PRAISE! field staff

Group II
—satisfaction with disappointment in involvement in Group II vs. Group I
—involvement in Group II interim interventions and perceived impact
—participation in nutrition counseling or programming outside of PRAISE! (potential contamination)

*Satisfaction of Measurement Group participants with PRAISE! program, relative acceptability to Group I vs. Group II

TABLE 5.4. PRAISE! CORE INTERVENTION ELEMENTS.

Intervention Element	Description CORE interventions were expected of all churches; OPTIONAL were offered as opportunities for those who were interested.	Expected Implemen-tation
Pastors' Health Promotion Workshops CORE	Developed and supported the role of the pastor as health promotion leader and change agent by providing biblically based nutrition information to help them promote goals of the project. Pastors learned the basics of good nutrition and developed strategies to reinforce positive changes in their church. Continuing education credits offered. (All 30 Group I churches implemented at least one, averaging 1.6 per church.)	3 per church
PRAISE! Communication Center CORE	A table and/or bulletin board displaying health educational materials, information regarding PRAISE! activities, and making available fruits and vegetables from gleaning trips. Maintained by the HAT, who often used materials provided in the PRAISE! packets (described below) related to seasonal or spiritual themes. (All 30 Group I churches implemented.)	1 per church
PRAISE! Quarterly Packets CORE	Included bulletin board kits, activity ideas, camera-ready church bulletin inserts, nutrition resources and games, clip art, and certificates. First packet distributed during the individual HAT training sessions and subsequent packets mailed to HAT leaders quarterly. Theme of each packet based on the target dietary goals and included scripture-based messages. HATs used materials from the packets and/or developed their own ideas related to the theme. (All 30 Group I churches implemented.)	4 delivered/ mailed to each church
Tailored Health Bulletin CORE	Computer-tailored health bulletin developed for all measurement group (MG) participants and produced using information from baseline surveys regarding personal health practices, knowledge, and beliefs. Provided participants with suggestions and tips relevant to their own personal health practices. A general (nontailored) bulletin was developed for church members who were not part of the MG. (All 30 Group I churches implemented.)	1 newsletter mailed to each Group 1 MG participant
Food Festival CORE	At the food fair, similar to what happens at a health fair, church and community members participated in taste testing, label reading, and cook-offs. Local physicians, public health professionals, and community leaders provided additional services, such as health screenings and information booths. Designed to be a fun way for people to learn more about eating smarter for a positive impact on their own health as well as on the health of their loved ones. (All 30 Group I churches implemented.)	1 per church
Food Events CORE	Usually conducted in conjunction with other church activities, such as anniversaries, homecomings, and other services. At food events, smaller in scale than a food festival, church members sampled recipes from project cookbooks, tested new preparation techniques, and shared ways to make smarter food choices. Members were often surprised that the very palatable foods they were eating were considered "smart" foods. (Twenty-seven churches implemented 4 food events, 3 churches implemented 3.)	4 per church

TABLE 5.4.   (CONTINUED)

Intervention Element	Description CORE interventions were expected of all churches; OPTIONAL were offered as opportunities for those who were interested.	Expected Implemen- tation
PRAISE! Partners (New Leaf) CORE	New Leaf, Choices for Healthy Living is a structured assessment and educational package designed to help participants review their eating habits, identify practices they would like to change, and make choices to help them reach their goal. PRAISE! partners are church members who completed a one-day workshop on how to serve as peer counselors using the New Leaf. Church members were given the option of working with New Leaf on their own, with a friend or in a group. (All 30 Group I churches implemented.)	Aim of training 4–6 PRAISE! Partners per church
Congregation Skills and Treasures CORE	A checklist designed to tap hidden congregation talents related to food and nutrition. Based on the assets mapping model (McKnight and Kretzman, 1992) identified members in each congregation who had skills and "treasures" of knowledge to help other members make smart food choices, such as seasoning greens without fatback, modifying recipes to increase fiber, and growing and "putting up" tomatoes. Survey results (including names, phone numbers, and skills/treasures) were used to create directories for each church and were made available to the respective pastor and church leaders. (All 30 Group I churches implemented.)	Intended for all churches
Inspirational Booklets CORE	Pocket-sized booklets containing inspirational Bible verses and testimonials from PRAISE! participants who had attempted to make dietary changes in the past. The booklets were based on the stage theory of change and gave practical tips for making dietary changes based on the self-determined stage of the participant. (Implemented in 20 of the 30 Group I churches.)	Intended for all churches
Gleaning OPTIONAL	Gleaning is a practice dating back to biblical times. Because modern mechanical agricultural harvesters often leave a significant portion behind in the field, some farmers open their fields to others to pick from the crops that were left behind. Gleaning trips were arranged by the county coordinator, who contacted a philanthropic organization to arrange gleaning opportunities with local farmers. PRAISE! participants gleaned sweet potatoes and collard greens, taking back car- and truckloads of the vegetables to share with their churches and communities. (Implemented in 8 churches.)	OPTIONAL
Music Festival OPTIONAL	Music is an important part of the African American worship experience, and thus it is a good channel to promote positive messages in church. PRAISE! music festivals were a way to promote smart eating through song and various types of music. For example, in one church, PRAISE! kids made up the song "Broccoli Rap." Music festivals provided the congregation with an opportunity to be creative and used the talents of different people in the congregation to promote smart eating. (Implemented in 4 churches.)	OPTIONAL

- From the perspective of the PRAISE! staff (locally based county coordinators), what were some of the church-related resources and organizational and leadership factors that facilitated or inhibited the overall intervention delivery and participation?
- To what extent did the implementers feel that they had adequate support and direction from the research team for each intervention?

Research questions addressed in the area of *research partnership* include

- What do church leaders and members consider to be critical factors in a successful church-university partnership?
- To what extent do church leaders and members feel that UNC met their expectations for a successful partnership during the implementation of the PRAISE! project?
- To what extent do church leaders and members believe that their participation in both the research and the intervention components of the project was "worth the time and effort"?

Research questions addressed in the area of *potential for sustainability and diffusion* include

- What is the evidence for short-term institutionalization of the interventions within the church (was the project mentioned from the pulpit, mentioned at board meetings, or included in the church bulletin or newsletter)?
- To what extent do church leaders believe that the intervention components (individually, collectively, and in principle) are likely to be continued at the church after the project is over?
- To what extent do church leaders believe that the intervention components (individually, collectively, and in principle) could be disseminated to other churches with minimal or no help from UNC other than the training materials?

Process Data Design, Sample, and Data Collection

Table 5.3 provides a detailed description of the process data we collected at different points in the study. Data were collected from four primary sources: (1) church leader and church-based intervention implementers, (2) church member participants either in the measurement group or not, (3) PRAISE! staff county coordinators who were based in the counties where the project was implemented, and (4) testimonials by church members and leaders at the "Share, Tell, and Look

Forward Session" that took place in each Wave after follow-up data collection. As noted in Figure 5.1, process measures were primarily collected at baseline and follow-up, with intervention tracking and acceptability assessment conducted throughout the intervention period. During the entire study, frequent informal contact with church leaders and members, either directly or through the county coordinators (described later), was key to fine-tuning our measurement and intervention strategies.

Church Leaders and Church-Based Intervention Implementers

To determine existing organizational resources and health promotion programming that could support PRAISE! interventions, as well as to assess the pastor's role in the introduction of innovations to church programming, pastors in both Group I and Group II were interviewed at baseline. At follow-up, Group I pastors were asked about their perceptions of program implementation (they were asked who the primary implementers were and to what degree church members attended and embraced the program). They were also queried extensively about their expectations regarding a research partnership and the degree to which these expectations were met. Finally, the pastors were asked whether they felt the PRAISE! intervention would be maintained in their church after the formal research period had ended and whether they felt the program could be easily disseminated to other churches. Group I HAT leaders and church liaisons were asked very similar questions regarding intervention implementation, the research partnership, and the potential for institutionalization and dissemination.

Extensive data regarding the implementation of specific interventions were also collected during the course of the intervention period (see Appendixes A and B). HAT leaders and church liaisons were asked to complete brief data collection forms after each intervention event (such as a food event, food festival, gleaning trip, or music festival), documenting the number of attendees from both the measurement group and the general church membership. Additional data collection forms were used to elicit information about the specific intervention components delivered, acceptability to participants, and the challenges involved in delivering the intervention. For intervention components that were delivered over time rather than at a single event (referred to as "nonevent interventions"), similar data forms were completed at six months and again at twelve months.

Church Member Participants

All Group I and Group II church members included in the measurement group (MG) completed a telephone survey at baseline and follow-up that included some data relative to our process evaluation, such as their perception of innovation adoption by both their pastor and the church as a whole and the level of satisfaction of participants in a research project. MG participants also completed a six- and twelve-month survey regarding the acceptability of specific intervention components and the perceived impact of each on their dietary knowledge, attitudes, and practices. For intervention events, similar data were collected on-site from both MG and non-MG members immediately following the program. As part of the twelve-month survey, MG participants were asked about their interest in helping to keep the program going (institutionalization) at their own church, and the degree to which they would like to participate in helping to share the PRAISE! program (dissemination) with other churches. Finally, a brief survey was distributed through church bulletins at the end of the intervention period in Group I to assess the degree to which non-MG church members felt they were included in the program and were able to benefit from it.

PRAISE! Staff County Coordinators

To assist with data collection and support intervention implementation efforts at the church level, county coordinators (CCs) were hired from each of the participating counties. They were asked to play a "backseat" role in intervention delivery so as to test an intervention implementation strategy that could be replicated without them. At the third, sixth, ninth, and twelfth month of the intervention, the CCs were asked to complete a grid (see Appendix C) to document for each Group I church (relative to other participating churches) (1) the magnitude of assistance needed by the church in terms of HAT recruitment, leadership development, technical assistance, and intervention implementation and (2) the degree of success experienced by the church in terms of pastor and HAT leadership, HAT team communication and functioning, the general level of church member enthusiasm and commitment to the project, and the involvement of resources and agencies outside the church who could support the intervention efforts.

At twelve months, CCs were asked to assess current and predicted institutionalization at each church, indicating the degree to which PRAISE! principles were becoming a regular part of all food events and the extent to which informal policies related to PRAISE! goals and objectives had been implemented, as well as answering the question "How likely is this church to continue PRAISE! activities after the formal intervention period is over?" At twelve months, CCs were also asked to document current and predicted dissemination efforts by each church, the degree to which the church had already involved other community members in PRAISE!, the pastor's interest in sharing the PRAISE! intervention with other churches, the likelihood that the church would take an active role in disseminating PRAISE!, and the HAT's readiness to train others with minimal assistance.

Testimonials at the "Share, Tell, and Look Forward" Session

Although we wanted to celebrate the completion of the research phase of the project with our church partners, we made every effort to avoid sending the message that the intervention had come to an end as well. In the spirit of "passing the baton" to church members to continue PRAISE! long after the research team was gone, we held three separate "Share Tell and Look Forward" sessions at the end of each Wave. At each of these three sessions, up to ten church leaders and PRAISE! participants from each of the ten Group I churches were invited to share a healthy meal (prepared with our assistance by local caterers) and to share (by whatever creative means they chose) something about what they got out of their involvement in the project as well as their plans to "keep PRAISE! going" at their church. The audio- and videotapes of these sessions are a rich source of qualitative process data on how the interventions were implemented as well as what plans have been made for sustainability and dissemination.

Results

Overall Study Participation

A total of 1,309 participants recruited from sixty churches met eligibility criteria and completed baseline measures and were randomized to either Group I or Group II. Seventy-six percent completed follow-up blood work and the two telephone surveys. None of the sixty churches dropped from the study. Of the participants, three quarters were women, the mean age was forty-seven, and 62 percent had belonged to their church for more than ten years. Chronic disease and related risk factor rates were high, with 40 percent reporting that they had smoked (21 percent reporting that they still smoked), 13 percent reporting having diabetes, and 42 percent reporting having hypertension.

Implementation

The various process data collection strategies previously described have resulted in an immense amount of process data. Some of the results regarding implementation of the core and optional interventions are presented in Table 5.4. All thirty Group I churches completed each of the nine core intervention elements, including four food events. Other core intervention elements included pastors' health promotion workshops, a PRAISE! communication center, quarterly packets, tailored health bulletins, a food festival, PRAISE Partners (peer counselors), inspirational booklets, and the "Congregation Skills and Treasures" directory. Optional interventions that were conducted by a number of churches included gleaning (harvesting crops left by mechanical pickers) and music fests featuring nutrition/health-related music and sharing. Much of the information collected regarding implementation is church-specific and thus does not lend itself to summary data but will instead be used to form indices to predict church- and individual-level effects of the intervention, as discussed later in this chapter.

Research Partnership

Regarding the research partnership, both pastors and HAT leaders appeared quite satisfied with their experience. Of the thirty pastors participating in Group I, twenty-three completed follow-up surveys. Twenty of the thirty participating HAT leaders in Group I completed a follow-up survey.

Table 5.5 provides some insight into the experience of Group I pastors and HAT leaders.

TABLE 5.5.   RESEARCH PARTNERSHIP.

Question	Strongly Disagree > Neutral, DK		Agree		Strongly Agree	
	Pastor	HAT L	Pastor	HAT L	Pastor	HAT L
Participating in the *research* component of PRAISE! was worth the time and effort required by *me*	0	DK 5%	31%	50%	69%	45%
Participating in the *nutrition* component of PRAISE! was worth the time and effort required by *me*	0	0	22%	40%	78%	60%
Participating in the *research* component of PRAISE! was worth the time and effort required by *members of the congregation*	0	DK 5%	35%	50%	61%	45%
Participating in the *nutrition* component of PRAISE! was worth the time and effort required by *members of the congregation*		DK 5%	22%	40%	78%	60%

When asked to rate the importance of twelve characteristics of research partnerships, pastors, and HAT leaders, at least 50 percent of the pastors and HAT leaders ranked the following as extremely important:

- An honest and complete description of the purpose and requirement of the research project
- Minimal paperwork
- The churches' receipt of results when the study is complete
- The university's interaction with church participants as partners rather than as "research subjects"
- Sufficient financial resources to cover costs associated with the research project

Potential Sustainability and Dissemination

In the area of potential sustainability and dissemination, many of the process data collected are either intervention- or church-specific and will be used to help refine interventions for future work to enhance the likelihood that intervention programs will become institutionalized at an individual church and perhaps shared with other churches as well. At a more general level, the pastor and HAT leader follow-up surveys provide some useful information regarding current and potential sustainability of the program as a whole (see Tables 5.6 and 5.7).

Strengths of the PRAISE! Project Process Evaluation

Comprehensive Process Evaluation

Several members of our research team had been involved in prior research projects that took place in African American churches. Community-based projects implemented in multiple sites some distance from the research institution are difficult to monitor. In the prior studies, those involved found themselves wishing they had collected more process data, as they were trying to analyze and interpret the results. Because each participating site has its own "personality" and cast of characters, intervention implementation can vary widely and this will be largely unknown to the researcher unless good process data are collected. Without this information, it is impossible to determine what factors might be responsible for the fact that the intervention was more successful in some sites than in others. Having learned from our prior experience with inadequate process data collection, we decided, during our grant application phase, that good process data collection would be a priority.

TABLE 5.6.   SUSTAINABILITY AND DISSEMINATION: HAT LEADER FOLLOW-UP SURVEY.

Please answer some questions about how often the following things have happened at your church	Missing, Never, NA, DK	Rarely	Some-times	Often	Very often
How often is PRAISE! part of the agenda for church business meetings?	20%	10%	35%	15%	15%
How often are comments or announce-ments made from the pulpit supporting the project?	15%	15%	30%	15%	25%
How often does the church bulletin include updates about PRAISE!?	20%	10%	20%	20%	30%
How often is food that is served at the church noticeably more healthy?	10%	5%	10%	35%	40%
How often has the church budget included money for PRAISE! activities beyond what is provided by UNC?	40%	5%	25%	10%	20%
How often do menu planners use PRAISE! goals to plan meals for church functions?	10%	5%	25%	35%	25%

For these statements, we are interested in your opinion about whether or not PRAISE! activities should continue at your church	Strongly Disagree or Missing	Disagree	Agree	Strongly Agree
Some members of my church have expressed an interest in continuing to plan and implement healthy eating activities at church.	5% SD 5% M	25%	40%	25%
Continuation of PRAISE! activities would be strongly supported by church members.	0 SD 5% M	20%	40%	30%
With a little extra training, our HAT would be ready to work with other churches to implement activities similar to those of PRAISE!	5% M	20%	45%	30%
Our HAT has been talking about the idea of sharing PRAISE! activities with other churches.	0	40%	40%	10%

Documentation of a Complex Intervention Implementation

Inadequate process data can severely compromise the ability to fully analyze and interpret research findings. Like many community-based lifestyle interventions, PRAISE! was based on a menu of different intervention strategies, some of which were core (required) and others of which were optional. Because the churches were given some flexibility with regard to which interventions would be implemented and how, we decided that it was important to obtain adequate

TABLE 5.7. SUSTAINABILITY AND DISSEMINATION: PASTOR FOLLOW-UP SURVEY.

Now, I'm going to ask your thoughts about continuing PRAISE! activities at your church	Strongly Disagree, Disagree, DK	Neutral	Agree	Strongly Agree
PRAISE! is high on the list of the church's priorities	9%	0	52%	39%
PRAISE! is high on the list of pastoral priorities	9%	4%	39%	48%
I would like to continue PRAISE! activities after the research component ends	0	0	43%	57%
I believe the majority of my congregation is interested in continuing PRAISE! activities	0	0	70%	30%
I will work with my church treasurer and/or those responsible for the church finances to find continuing support for PRAISE! activities	4% DK	0	61%	30%
I believe that healthier lifestyles, including eating smarter, should be a part of the church's mission	4% SD	4%	31%	61%
I believe that it is feasible to make eating smarter a part of the church's mission	0	0	43%	57%
I believe that as a result of this project, people in my congregation want to eat smarter on a regular basis	0	0	52%	48%
If my members are interested in continuing a smart eating program at this church, I will support them	0	0	35%	65%
Thinking about the project as a whole, I believe that other churches can and would do this project if given the opportunity	9% DK	0	39%	52%
I would be willing to assist other pastors in developing the PRAISE! project at their churches			Yes 91%	No 9%

How would you assist other pastors in developing PRAISE! at their churches?
   78% Pass information on to other pastors orally
   90% Pass on written materials about PRAISE! to other pastors
   83% Identify someone in the church to pass the information on to the pastors

process data to allow us to describe the *dose* (that is, the amount delivered) of the intervention later. This included strategies for intervention delivery, the rates of participation, and the level of satisfaction with different interventions—on the part of both the participants and the church-based implementers. Because the study was implemented in three Waves, process data collected during Wave 1 allowed us to fine-tune and improve our implementation approach for Waves II and III.

Assessment of Initial and Potential Sustainability and Dissemination

Our desire to design a sustainable intervention prompted us to seek a fuller understanding of the factors that impeded or facilitated implementation at the church level. An important rationale for collecting process data was our intention to give the churches significant autonomy in how they implemented the intervention while retaining our ability to describe what happened. As previously discussed, our intent was to evaluate an intervention that could be implemented primarily by members of the church in order to increase the likelihood of long-term sustainability and, ultimately, dissemination to other churches. We developed extensive curriculum materials and trained the church-based HATs regarding each intervention, but we gave them sufficient latitude to implement the interventions in a way that would befit their church culture and environment. Although we feel that this is a strong approach to community-based interventions, it raises specific challenges regarding the use of process measures to determine the fidelity of the intervention. It may be more appropriate to describe it as the spirit and intent of the intervention.

Evaluation of the Research Partnership

Because the PRAISE! project researchers were faced with challenges that so many prior researchers had been confronted with—in terms of reaching, recruiting, and retaining members of the African American community in a cancer prevention research effort, we felt it would be very useful to fully document the research partnership process. Most of the process evaluation data for this effort were collected at follow-up. Although, ideally, we would have collected measures early in the partnership process as well, it was our belief that until the partnership and a level of trust were firmly established, it would be difficult for our church partners to communicate to us their reservations about working with a university and participating in a research project. However, we believe that by the end of the project, church leaders were able to be quite honest with us about what worked for them and about where there were problems.

Lessons Learned About Process Evaluation

LESSON 1. *Apply theory prospectively when possible.*

At the time of implementing the PRAISE! project intervention and measures, we did not have anyone on the research team who could be considered an expert in process measures. Theoretical frameworks well suited to guide development of a sustainable intervention in the church environment were also limited. However, we did have a field staff that was very experienced in community-based research and with African American churches. Investigators with expertise in nutrition-related behavior change interventions worked closely with the field staff to determine what process variables should be measured and how they could be implemented to minimize the burden of both participants and church leaders. Later, when Shediac-Rizkallah and Bone's article (1998) about their model of sustainability was published, we were able to match many of our approaches with components of the model. Clearly, it would have been preferable to use a specified theory from the beginning in designing our process evaluation.

LESSON 2. *Design a comprehensive process evaluation plan early and pilot test it if possible.*

Although we were committed to the importance of a comprehensive process evaluation from the beginning, we found ourselves assembling the components in a more piecemeal fashion than desirable. This made it difficult to carry themes throughout different process evaluation instruments or to assure that, for example, the questions asked of one church leader were phrased the same way for another. In retrospect, we would recommend that those projects that have the benefit of beginning with a pilot phase use this opportunity to carefully map out and test the process evaluation design.

LESSON 3. *Be parsimonious so as to avoid excess respondent burden.*

Given the demanding nature of implementing a large community-based intervention, researchers are often racing to keep up with the design of appropriate process evaluation measures for each stage of the program. This can result in the inclusion of too many instruments that have too many questions, in an effort to make sure that nothing is overlooked or forgotten. Some potential consequences of this are that (1) the measures will interfere with intervention delivery, (2) participants will be overwhelmed and may develop the impression that the measures are more important than the intervention, and (3) the response rate may be lowered. It is our hope that a comprehensive analysis of our evaluation data for PRAISE! will provide us with a better understanding of which process measures were most useful and which could be dropped in future studies.

Summary

Lessons learned from the PRAISE! project process evaluation will be useful in guiding future efforts. The effort expended by both the research team and our church partners has greatly enabled our understanding of the effects of this intervention and how it could be refined for future application. In addition to the more standard measures related to intervention fidelity and dose, we encourage researchers to selectively address process issues that can be of great benefit to the larger research community. In the case of PRAISE!, we included process evaluation measures related to the sustainability and dissemination potential of the intervention as well as an assessment of the research partnership in what has traditionally been an environment of suspicion and mistrust. Having collected these data, it is now our obligation to ensure that both the researchers and the study participants benefit from what we have learned.

References

American Cancer Society. *Cancer Facts and Figures.* American Cancer Society, 2001.

Bandura, A. *Social Foundations of Thought and Action: A Social Cognitive Theory.* Englewood Cliffs, N.J., Prentice-Hall, 1986.

Barab, S. A., Redman, B. K., and Froman, R. D. "Measurement Characteristics of the Levels of Institutionalization Scales: Examining Reliability and Validity." *Journal of Nursing Measures,* 1998, *6*(1), 19–33.

Basch, C. E., Eveland, J. D., and Portnoy, B. "Diffusion Systems for Education and Learning About Health." *Family and Community Health,* 1986, *9*(2), 1–26.

Brawley, O. W., and Tejeda, H. "Minority Inclusion in Clinical Trials Issues and Potential Strategies." *Journal of the National Cancer Institute. Monographs,* 1995, *17,* 55–57.

Corbie-Smith, G., Thomas, S. B., Williams, M. V., and Moody-Ayers, S. "Attitudes and Beliefs of African Americans Toward Participation in Medical Research." *Journal of General Internal Medicine,* 1999, *14*(9), 537–546.

Ford, L., Kaluzny, A. D., and Sondik, E. "Diffusion and Adoption of State-of-the-Art Therapy." *Seminar on Oncology,* 1990, *17*(4), 485–494.

Goodman, R. M., and Steckler, A. "A Framework for Assessing Program Institutionalization." *International Journal of Knowledge Transfer,* 1989, *2,* 55–71.

Goodman, R. M., McLeroy, K. R., Steckler, A. B., and Hoyle, R. H. "Development of Level of Institutionalization Scales for Health Promotion Programs." *Health Education Quarterly,* 1993, *20*(2), 161–178.

Harris, Y., Gorelick, P. B., Samuels, P., and Bempong, I. "Why African Americans May Not Be Participating in Clinical Trials." *Journal of the National Medical Association,* 1996, *88*(10), 630–634.

Kaluzny, A., and others. "Assuring Access to State-of-the-Art Care for U.S. Minority Populations: The First Two Years of the Minority-Based Community Clinical Oncology Program." *Journal of the National Cancer Institute,* 1993, *85*(23), 1945–1950.

Katz, D., and Kahn, R. L. *The Social Psychology of Organizations.* New York: Wiley, 1978.

Kretzman, J. P., and McKnight, J. L. *Building Communities from the Inside and Out: A Path Toward Finding and Mobilizing a Community's Assets.* Evanston, Ill.: Northwestern University Center for Urban Affairs and Policy Research, 1993.

McLeroy, K. R., Bibeau, D., Steckler, A., and Glanz, K. "An Ecological Perspective on Health Promotion Programs." *Health Education Quarterly,* 1988, *15,* 351–377.

McMichael, A. J., Smith, K. R., and Corvalan, C. F. "The Sustainability Transition: A New Challenge." *Bulletin of World Health Organization,* 2000, *78*(9), 1067.

Millon-Underwood, S., Sanders, E., and Davis, M. "Determinants of Participation in State-of-the-Art Cancer Prevention, Early Detection/Screening, and Treatment Trials Among African Americans." *Cancer Nursing,* 1993, *16*(1), 25–33.

Oldenburg, B., Hardcastle, D. M., and Kok, G. "Diffusion of Innovations." In K. Glanz, F. Lewis, and B. Rimer (eds.), *Health Behavior and Health Education, Theory, Research, and Practice.* (2nd ed.) San Francisco: Jossey-Bass, 1997.

O'Loughlin, J., and others. "Correlates of the Sustainability of Community-Based Heart Health Promotion Interventions." *Preventive Medicine,* 1998, *27*(5, Pt. 1), 702–712.

Paskett, E. D., DeGraffinreid, C., Tatum, C. M., and Margitic, S. E. "The Recruitment of African Americans to Cancer Prevention and Control Studies." *Preventive Medicine,* 1996, *25*(5), 547–553.

Rogers, E. M. *Diffusion of Innovations.* (3rd ed.) New York: Free Press, 1983.

Shediac-Rizkallah, M. C., and Bone, L. R. "Planning for the Sustainability of Community-Based Health Programs: Conceptual Frameworks and Future Directions for Research, Practice and Policy." *Health Education Research,* 1998, *13*(1), 87–108.

Steckler, A., and others. "Measuring the Diffusion of Innovative Health Promotion Programs." *American Journal of Health Promotion,* 1992, *6*(3), 214–224.

Swanson, G. M., and Ward, A. J. "Recruiting Minorities into Clinical Trials: Toward a Participant-Friendly System." *Journal of the National Cancer Institute,* 1995, *87*(23), 1747–1759.

Zaltman, G., and Duncan, R. *Strategies for Planned Change.* New York: Wiley, 1977.

APPENDIX A: PRAISE! PROJECT INTERVENTION FOLLOW-UP FORM
FOR HAT LEADER: FOOD EVENT.

Please provide the following information about the Food Event that you planned for the members of your church. What you tell us about your experience with planning and conducting the event is vital to our understanding of how to help others carry out similar activities.

Church name: _____

County name: _____

Activity name: _____

Person completing form: _____

Date of activity: ☐☐ ☐☐ ☐☐☐☐

How many people (including measurement group) attended the event? ☐☐☐

About how many of all participants were adult men (age 18 and over)? ☐☐☐

About how many of all participants were adult women (age 18 and over)? ☐☐☐

About how many of all participants were children? ☐☐☐

Overall, how pleased are you with the way this activity turned out?

Displeased	☐ somewhat displeased	☐ very displeased
Pleased	☐ somewhat pleased	☐ very pleased

Did this activity turn out the way you planned it?   ☐ yes   ☐ no

If you have any comments about why this did not turn out as you planned, please write them in below.

Planning and organizing a new activity can bring challenges or problems. For each of the following statements, please mark "yes" if this was a challenge for you or "no" if this was not a challenge for you in organizing this Food Event.

☐ yes   ☐ no   I did not know exactly where to start.

☐ yes   ☐ no   I did not have enough help.

☐ yes   ☐ no   It took too much time.

☐ yes   ☐ no   There were too many activities to coordinate.

☐ yes   ☐ no   It was hard to offer so many different kinds of food.

☐ yes   ☐ no   This event cost too much.

Was this Food Event part of another church program?   ☐ yes   ☐ no

APPENDIX A: (CONTINUED)

If this Food Event was part of another church program, please "X" which one.

□ Homecoming
□ Pastor's Anniversary
□ Choir Anniversary
□ Revival Service

If this Food Event was part of a church program other than these, write below.

How many of these activities were included in this Food Event? You may "X" more than one.

□ Taste testing.
□ Cooking demonstration.
□ Participants brought healthy food from home.
□ Educational materials were handed out.
□ Special speaker on nutrition/health issues.

If this Food Event included other activities, please list those activities below.

Overall, how would you rate the level of enthusiasm of
your church members regarding this Food Event?

□ very high   □ high medium   □ low   □ very low

How easy or difficult was it for you to plan and implement this activity in your church?

Difficult   □ somewhat difficult   □ very difficult
Easy   □ somewhat easy   □ very easy

How much cooperation did you get from church members
in planning and conducting this Food Event?

□ a great deal   □ quite a bit   □ some   □ not much   □ none

Did you use resources outside your church to conduct this Food Event?   □ yes   □ no

If yes, please "X" any of these resources that were used:

□ food from a farmer's market
□ food from a gleaning trip
□ help from health professionals in the community
□ help from community businesses (such as donated food)
□ help from the PRAISE! staff

(Continued)

APPENDIX A: PRAISE! PROJECT INTERVENTION FOLLOW-UP FORM
FOR HAT LEADER: FOOD EVENT. (CONTINUED)

Overall, how receptive were church members to trying foods prepared a different way?

Unreceptive	☐ somewhat unreceptive	☐ very unreceptive
Receptive	☐ somewhat receptive	☐ very receptive
Does not apply	☐ didn't prepare foods differently	

Do you think that other churches like yours could plan and carry
out a Food Event using only the training and intervention manual   ☐ yes   ☐ no
you received from PRAISE!? *Please write any comments about
your answer in the box below.*

Do you think your church will continue
this activity after the project is over?   ☐ yes   ☐ no

List comments made to you (both good and bad) by people who participated in
this Food Event.

If you have other comments or suggestions about the Food Event,
please write them below.

APPENDIX B: PRAISE! FOOD EVENT: MEASUREMENT GROUP ONLY.

Please answer the following questions about the PRAISE! Food Event you have just attended. What you tell us will help the PRAISE! staff improve programs like this in the future. Please feel free to disagree! Your honest answers will help us the most. To choose your answer, please mark an "X" in the box.

Please write your name here.

Please write the date you attended the food event in the boxes.
(For example, if it was held on September 6, you would write 09-06-1998.) ☐☐- ☐☐- ☐☐☐☐

Did this food event include any information or activities related to   ☐ yes ☐ no
eating less fat?

Did this food event include any information or activities related   ☐ yes ☐ no
to eating more fruits and vegetables?

Did this food event include any information or activities related   ☐ yes ☐ no
to eating more fiber (roughage)?

For the next statements, please think about what you learned from this Food Event. Decide whether you agree or disagree with the statement and then "X" the box beside how strongly you feel. Please mark only one box for each statement.

I learned something new to help me "eat smarter"

| *Disagree* | ☐ Disagree a little | ☐ Disagree quite a bit | ☐ Disagree a lot |
| *Agree* | ☐ Agree a little | ☐ Agree quite a bit | ☐ Agree a lot |

This Food Event helped me feel that others are supporting my efforts to eat smarter.

| *Disagree* | ☐ Disagree a little | ☐ Disagree quite a bit | ☐ Disagree a lot |
| *Agree* | ☐ Agree a little | ☐ Agree quite a bit | ☐ Agree a lot |

This activity gave me the confidence that I can eat smarter.

| *Disagree* | ☐ Disagree a little | ☐ Disagree quite a bit | ☐ Disagree a lot |
| *Agree* | ☐ Agree a little | ☐ Agree quite a bit | ☐ Agree a lot |

This Food Event caused me to think more seriously about changing my eating habits.

| *Disagree* | ☐ Disagree a little | ☐ Disagree quite a bit | ☐ Disagree a lot |
| *Agree* | ☐ Agree a little | ☐ Agree quite a bit | ☐ Agree a lot |

(Continued)

APPENDIX B: PRAISE! FOOD EVENT: MEASUREMENT GROUP ONLY. (CONTINUED)

I learned some new ways to deal with things that make it hard to eat smart.

Disagree	☐ Disagree a little	☐ Disagree quite a bit	☐ Disagree a lot
Agree	☐ Agree a little	☐ Agree quite a bit	☐ Agree a lot

This Food Event helped me recognize more of the benefits of eating smart.

Disagree	☐ Disagree a little	☐ Disagree quite a bit	☐ Disagree a lot
Agree	☐ Agree a little	☐ Agree quite a bit	☐ Agree a lot

This activity inspired me to eat smarter.

Disagree	☐ Disagree a little	☐ Disagree quite a bit	☐ Disagree a lot
Agree	☐ Agree a little	☐ Agree quite a bit	☐ Agree a lot

It was easy to fit this Food Event into my schedule.

Disagree	☐ Disagree a little	☐ Disagree quite a bit	☐ Disagree a lot
Agree	☐ Agree a little	☐ Agree quite a bit	☐ Agree a lot

This activity was fun.

Disagree	☐ Disagree a little	☐ Disagree quite a bit	☐ Disagree a lot
Agree	☐ Agree a little	☐ Agree quite a bit	☐ Agree a lot

I plan to put into practice what I learned from this Food Event.

Disagree	☐ Disagree a little	☐ Disagree quite a bit	☐ Disagree a lot
Agree	☐ Agree a little	☐ Agree quite a bit	☐ Agree a lot

If you have any other comments about this Food Event, please write them below:

APPENDIX C: COUNTY COORDINATOR CHECKLIST.

County Coordinator: _____ **Date:** _____ **Time Period: (3, 6, 9, or 12 months)** **County:** _____

Thinking about the AVERAGE church during this time period, please give a rough number estimate for the following (please use a single number rather than a range):

1. Number of *phone calls* per week made **by you** to the church liaison _____

2. Number of *phone calls* per week made **by you** to the HAT leader _____

3. Number of *phone calls* made by the church liaison **to you** _____

4. Number of *phone calls* made by the HAT leader **to you** _____

5. Number of *visits* made **by you** to the church for PRAISE! intervention events _____

6. Number of *visits* made **by you** to the church for anything other than PRAISE! intervention events _____ (such as planning meetings, providing assistance, etc.)

7. Number of times HAT leader or church liaison stopped by the office to request assistance _____

KEY FOR CHARTS ON THE *FOLLOWING PAGES*
1 = much less than most churches
2 = somewhat less than most churches
3 = about average relative to most churches
4 = somewhat more than other churches
5 = much more than other churches
NA = Not Applicable for time period or otherwise   **DK** = Don't know (not enough info.)

APPENDIX C: COUNTY COORDINATOR CHECKLIST. (CONTINUED)

FOR LAST TIME PERIOD (12 months) ONLY

Church Name

For the following items, please describe each church (using numbering key on the front page), relative to the other churches in the same county

INSTITUTIONALIZATION

Item							
PRAISE! principles are becoming a regular part of all food events at the church							
Church members have implemented informal policies related to PRAISE! goals and objectives (such as serving water at all meals)							
Church members are discussing the continuation of PRAISE! activities							
Church members are actively planning activities beyond the end of the intervention period							
The pastor is likely to continue promoting PRAISE! objectives							
The HAT is likely to remain an active team							
Some of the HAT members are likely to change							
The HAT leadership is likely to change							
In your opinion, how likely is this church to continue PRAISE! activities after the formal intervention period is over?							

DISSEMINATION

Item							
The church has already involved other community members in PRAISE! activities							
The pastor appears interested in outreach to other churches re PRAISE!							
In your opinion, how likely is this church to take an active role in spreading the word about PRAISE! objectives to other churches?							
In your opinion, how ready is the HAT (from this church) to train others about PRAISE! Interventions with minimal assistance?							

Notes:

County Coordinator: _____ Date: _____ Time Period: _____

Church Name												
For the following items, please describe each church (using numbering key on the front page), relative to the other churches in the same county												
ASSISTANCE NEEDED/REQUESTED												
Needed help with HAT recruitment												
Hat leader needed leadership development assistance												
Church liaison needed leadership development assistance												
The HAT leader or liaison stopped by the office for assistance												
Phone calls from me to the church liaison												
Phone calls from me to the HAT leader												
Phone calls from the HAT leader to me												
Phone calls from the church liaison to me												
Needed technical support for PRAISE! intervention implementation												
Needed help/encouragement to complete paperwork												
Needed assistance with the budget												
Needed assistance with implementation of PRAISE! in general												
The HAT requested my attendance at planning meetings												
The HAT requested my attendance at PRAISE! intervention events												
Notes:												

(Continued)

APPENDIX C: COUNTY COORDINATOR CHECKLIST. (CONTINUED)

County Coordinator: _____ Date: _____ Time Period: _____

Church Name

For the following items, please describe each church (using numbering key on front page), relative to the other churches in the same county

LEADERSHIP/PARTICIPATION/COMMUNICATION												
Overall HAT member energy and enthusiasm												
Degree to which work was spread evenly among HAT members												
HAT members communicate well with each other												
HAT members work well together as a team												
HAT manages conflict effectively												
HAT is effective as a group in getting the work done												
HAT members "get the word out" about activities												
Church liaison is a confident leader												
Church liaison is an effective leader												
HAT leader is a confident leader												
HAT leader is an effective leader												
HAT leader and church liaison work well together												
Pastor support of PRAISE! activities												
Pastor involvement with PRAISE! activities												
General level of measurement group participation												
General level of church membership (non-MG) participation												
Participation in PRAISE! events by people from broader community												
Involvement of county agencies/resources from outside the church												

Notes:

PART TWO

Worksite-Related Process Evaluation Efforts

More than 60 percent of U.S. adults are employed and spend a large percentage of their waking hours at work. The worksite has been recognized as an important setting for reaching large numbers of individuals with public health interventions. The two chapters in this section that focus on worksite-based process evaluation efforts represent important efforts, with great variation in size, scope, and focus.

In Chapter Six, Linnan, Thompson, and Kobetz describe selected process evaluation results from the national Working Well Trial (WWT). Working Well was the largest federally funded, worksite-based, cancer prevention trial, as it covered 114 worksites in sixteen states, reaching more than twenty-eight thousand employees. This study was conducted from 1989 to 1994, a period of growth in process evaluation skills, expertise, and conceptual thinking. The purpose of the WWT was to test whether a comprehensive, sustained cancer prevention intervention aimed at individuals and organizations could significantly improve selected health behavior outcomes in smoking and nutrition over outcomes produced by minimal intervention in the comparison worksites. Study investigators designed the intervention protocol with a strong theoretical foundation based on the transtheoretical model of behavior change, social cognitive theory, and community organizing principles. A common intervention protocol was developed and delivered by all study centers over a two-and-a-half-year intervention period (Chapter Six, Table 6.2). The experimental intervention included both individual and environmental intervention strategies.

The process evaluation was designed to measure the extent to which the intervention was delivered as intended and to measure the cost of the intervention. Results reported by Linnan and colleagues focus on (1) *implementation*—a measure of the extent to which the intervention was delivered as intended (for example, the percentage of process objectives in the standardized intervention that were delivered and recorded within the Working Well Intervention Tracking System [WWITS]), (2) *awareness*—a measure or indicator of the receipt of the intervention as employees self-report that they were "aware of" specific types of health promotion programs being offered at their worksite, as recorded on the final employee survey, (3) *resources*—a measure or indicator of the receipt of the intervention by way of materials used, as recorded in WWITS on the Materials Tracking Form, and (4) *dose*—a measure or indicator of the proportion of workers in an entire worksite who participated in the intervention. Results from the larger trial revealed both modest and significant trial-wide effects on nutrition outcomes. But no significant trial-wide effects on smoking cessation were demonstrated, despite clear evidence through reported process evaluation results that the intervention was delivered as intended and that the dose delivered (and received) was fairly good among program participants. The authors use process evaluation results to help shed light on plausible explanations for trial-wide results.

The WWT process evaluation effort was comprehensive and systematic, and it represents one of the earliest studies to undertake such an effort. The WWT process evaluation effort demonstrated a true commitment to developing a systematic approach to process evaluation that was linked to the study intervention protocol by specific, measurable process objectives. This represented a true advance on a number of previous process evaluation efforts. Yet evaluators had few models to go on, and they created a complex tracking system that was burdensome to the staff in ways that may have limited getting complete and accurate data. Despite this, the WWT process evaluation has been the foundation for generating new, improved worksite and other community-based tracking systems over time.

In Chapter Seven, the second worksite-based chapter in this section, Tessaro, Campbell, and Benedict describe selected process evaluation efforts associated with Health Works for Women (HWW), a five-year Centers for Disease Control and Prevention-funded study that took place in nine rural, manufacturing worksites in eastern North Carolina. The project used a randomized two-group experimental design to test the effect of the two intervention components—tailored health messages and the Natural Helper program—on changes in the multiple behaviors of physical inactivity, unhealthy eating (high fat and low fruit and vegetable intake), smoking, and failing to get breast and cervical cancer screening. Results showed that at the eighteen-month follow-up, the intervention group had increased fruit and vegetable consumption by 0.7 daily servings, compared with no change in the delayed group. Significant differences in fat intake were observed at six months but not at eighteen months. The intervention group also demonstrated improvements in strengthening and flexibility exercise, compared with the delayed group. The rates of smoking cessation and cancer screening did not differ between the study groups.

The process evaluation for HWW was important for formative assessment to design the intervention, monitor progress, and make midcourse corrections, and it was important for understanding the study outcomes. Process evaluation of one component of the HWW intervention—the Natural Helper program—was designed to answer the question How would a natural helper intervention best be adapted to a worksite setting? For HWW, formative evaluation was done through focus groups and field notes, as well as through personal interviews and process questions in the study survey that were designed to help explain exposure related to the Natural Helper program and the tailored health messages, as well as explain how they each functioned to effect change. Several of the process evaluation results are based on qualitative data, which tends to offer rich detail not available through other data sources.

Unique to this chapter is the investigators' ability to trace the way in which process evaluation results, especially those done formatively, were used to help create and shape the natural helper intervention to the expressed needs and interests of the study participants—rural, blue-collar women. This population represents an underserved, high-risk group that warrants the detailed, thoughtful process undertaken in this study. The authors also mention the need for flexibility in study planning and implementation efforts, so as to accommodate information gained in the formative stages. This has implications both for the funders, in terms of how much time and resources are made available to conduct formative research with underserved populations, and for the project staff, in terms of how much time is needed to work with these populations to ensure intervention success. As a result, this study makes a unique and important contribution to the book.

These two worksite-based chapters underscore the importance of designing comprehensive process evaluation efforts to support worksite-based health promotion interventions. The worksite will continue to be an important channel for reaching large numbers of adults with health promotion programs and services. In addition, new efforts to reach dependents and other family members by delivering both worksite and family interventions makes this setting a mainstay for future generations of applied public health interventions. Process evaluation efforts are a key component of understanding what interventions work best, under what conditions they are most effective, and for whom they are most beneficial.

CHAPTER SIX

The Working Well Trial

Selected Process Evaluation Results

Laura Linnan, Beti Thompson, and Erin N. Kobetz

Most of the U.S. adult population are employed and spend a large percentage of their waking hours at work (U.S. Bureau of Labor Statistics, 2001). Work has both direct and indirect influences on the U.S. public's health. Worksite health promotion programs have demonstrated an ability to improve worker health (Heaney and Goetzel, 1996; Sorensen, Emmons, Hunt, and Johnston, 1998) and to control health care costs (Yen and others, 2001).

The National Cancer Institute (NCI) funded a large-scale project—the Working Well Trial (WWT) (1989–1994)—to investigate whether a worksite health promotion program, aimed at both individual employees and the work environment, could reduce for employees the health risks associated with cancer. The two primary objectives of the overall intervention were to promote smoking cessation and low-fat, high-fiber eating, in response to estimates that 50 to 70 percent of cancer deaths can be prevented through selected lifestyle behavior changes. Teams of investigators at four study centers (The University of Texas's M. D. Anderson Cancer Center, the Dana Farber Cancer Institute of Harvard's School of Public Health, the University of Florida (which did not target smoking as a risk factor),

This study was funded by the National Cancer Institute, grant P01CA50087. The authors want to thank members of the Working Well Process Evaluation Working Group, Gloria Sorenson (chair); intervention staff at all study centers who collected the data; members of the study coordinating center; and all participating workplaces.

155

and Brown University's Miriam Hospital) recruited worksites to participate in the national trial. A study coordinating center for the national trial was located at the Fred Hutchinson Cancer Center in Seattle. Principal investigators from each study center, the study coordinating center, and the NCI made up a steering committee for the national trial. Investigators from each of the study centers and the study coordinating center were organized into national working groups to address the following key measurement and intervention issues: smoking, nutrition, participatory strategies, cost-effectiveness, evaluation, publications/presentations, organizational variables, and process evaluation (see Appendix A for a roster of national working group members).

Working Well investigators developed an extensive process tracking system—the Working Well Intervention Tracking System (WWITS)—to monitor the extent to which the intervention was delivered as intended on a trial-wide basis. This chapter focuses on a description of the WWT intervention, explains how the intervention and the WWITS process evaluation effort were linked through a series of trial-wide process objectives, describes selected results that give additional insight to enhance our understanding of the larger study results already published, and shares lessons learned from the process evaluation effort.

Description of the Working Well Trial

The Working Well Trial included 114 worksites and more than twenty-eight thousand employees in a five-year randomized controlled trial, with the worksite as the unit of randomization, intervention, and analysis (Abrams and others, 1994). Each study center team was responsible for recruiting worksites into the study. The study centers used specific eligibility requirements and recruitment methods, as described in Table 6.1. After worksite recruitment, employees in each participating worksite were invited to complete written baseline surveys, and another survey was conducted of worksite employees at the study's conclusion (approximately thirty months later) to assess targeted primary health behavior outcomes (Abrams and others, 1994; Heimendinger and others, 1995; Sorensen and others, 1996). As part of baseline data collection, structured interviews were conducted with the CEOs, the human resource directors, the benefits managers, union representatives (if appropriate), and other key informants of the worksites to assess environmental and organizational factors, hypothesized to influence targeted individual health behaviors (Abrams and others, 1994). These surveys were also repeated at the midpoint of the intervention period (twelve months), and at the study's conclusion (approximately thirty months).

The purpose of the WWT was to test whether a comprehensive, sustained, multilevel cancer prevention intervention could significantly improve selected health behavior outcomes—relative to smoking and nutrition—over outcomes produced

TABLE 6.1. WORKSITE ELIGIBILITY REQUIREMENTS AND RECRUITMENT METHODS BY STUDY CENTER.

Study Center	Worksite Eligibility	Recruitment Method
Brown University	• Employed 200–1,000 workers, the majority of whom (80%) can read and write English • Located within 60 miles of Providence, RI • Allowed smoking within workplace or failed to adequately enforce smoking ban	• Identified eligible worksites using a Dunn & Bradstreet database • Promoted study in trade magazines • Contacted company CEO and human resource director by phone and mail • Visited worksite to facilitate enrollment and ensure eligibility
University of Florida	• Designated as GTE South Telephone Operations unit • Located near Gainesville • Included on-site cafeteria • Employed more than 100 workers	• Collaborated with GTE to identify eligible worksites
Dana Farber Cancer Institute	• Employed between 200 and 2,500 workers, the majority of whom (80%) can read and write English • Located within central or eastern Massachusetts • Have a turnover rate of less than 20% annually • Use a known or suspected carcinogen	• Identified eligible worksites using an on-line Dunn & Bradstreet database • Searched database using SIC codes to identify companies likely to use carcinogenic substances
M. D. Anderson Cancer Center	• Worksites were either electric companies included as part of the National Rural Electric Cooperative Association (NRECA), with 100 full-time employees or a large gas pipeline district for various local and multinational corporations	• Engaged support of NRECA to generate interest among and enlistment of independent rural electric companies • Relied on existing relationships with regional gas pipeline industry leaders to facilitate worksite recruitment

by a minimal intervention in the comparison worksites. Study investigators designed the intervention protocol with a strong theoretical foundation based on the transtheoretical model of behavior change, social cognitive theory, and community organizing principles (Abrams and others, 1994). A common intervention protocol was developed and delivered by all the study centers over a two-and-a-half-year intervention period (see Table 6.2). The intervention protocol was designed to allow commonality of intervention activities, with enough flexibility that individual worksites could tailor the activities to meet their specific needs. Within experimental worksites, at the individual level, the intervention protocol included a worksite-wide kickoff event with interactive activities and, for each risk factor addressed, a series of educational brochures and videos, as well as self-assessment materials with feedback, self-help materials, contests or campaigns, and educational groups. Interventions aimed to influence the worksite environment by promoting smoke-free workplace policies and instituting healthy food access within catering policies, as well as improving employee access to healthy food choices in the cafeteria and at vending machines. Within comparison worksites, three of the four study centers received a minimal intervention that was limited to the distribution of commonly available printed materials at the worksite (Abrams and others, 1994).

Based on a community organizing approach, all the study centers used participatory strategies as a means of implementing the standardized intervention protocol at the experimental worksites. An employee advisory board (EAB) made up of eight to twelve employees representing a diverse group of employees—for example, management and labor, as well as representation from all the key departments and shifts—was organized at each experimental worksite to assist with planning, implementation, and promotion of the intervention activities. In addition, the EAB members helped tailor the standardized intervention to the needs and interests of a particular worksite.

The Working Well study overview (Abrams and others, 1994), baseline results (Heimendinger and others, 1995), and final study results (Sorensen and others, 1996) have been published elsewhere. In brief, there were significant changes in targeted nutrition outcomes at the individual employee level, from baseline to final at the experimental worksites (versus control worksites). There were no significant outcomes (although change did occur in the intended direction) on individual smoking cessation outcomes (Sorensen and others, 1996). Individual changes in nutrition outcomes within the experimental worksites were associated with significant changes in the worksite environment that supported increasing awareness of and access to healthy food choices (Biener and others, 1999). Similarly, the nonsignificant trial-wide smoking cessation changes at the individual employee level were associated with the fact that there were no significant smoking policy changes at either the experimental worksites or the comparison worksites at the time of the final survey (Biener and others, 1999). Thus, the WWT is among the first studies to provide

TABLE 6.2. WORKING WELL TRIAL CORE INDIVIDUAL
INTERVENTION ELEMENTS.

Core Intervention Elements— for Smoking and Nutrition Outcomes	Description	By Intervention Midpoint	By Intervention Conclusion	Total # Delivered per RF
Interactive kickoff activity	Multiactivity, multiple risk factor, interactive event to initiate Working Well intervention within the worksite	1	1	1
Posters	Print posters placed at key, visible locations throughout worksite, conveying an educational message	2	4	4
Video/single-session presentation	Either video presentation or single-session presentation made by professional or trained lay individual, with an educational message	1	3	3
Self-assessment + feedback	Individuals assess smoking or nutrition status (through quizzes, health risk assessments, self-tests, etc.) and receive individualized feedback based on the assessment results	1	2	2
Self-help programs	Materials used by individuals to initiate or maintain health behavior change on their own	1	2	2
Multisession direct education	Small- or moderate-sized groups with a minimum of two sessions and at least 30 minutes of educational information provided	1	2	2
Campaign/Contests	Multiactivity, single risk factor focus with a theme, educational messages, and incentives	0	1	1

evidence of a positive association between the individual employee and organizational and environmental change in the workplace (Biener and others, 1999).

Process Evaluation

Overview. A process evaluation working group (see Appendix A for a roster of national working group members) was responsible for developing a method of assessing the extent of the intervention's implementation as well as its cost. For each component of the intervention protocol (see Table 6.2), a measurable process objective was written so that the intervention's implementation could be monitored over the course of the intervention period. The extent of the intervention's implementation was assessed by the degree to which process objectives and participation goals were met. The process objectives defined a targeted number of specific activities to be offered within a specified period of time.

The WWITS was a dynamic, computerized intervention tracking system based in FoxPro, a relational database program that was designed to be user-friendly and to require only basic computer skills, so as to avoid overburdening project staff members who collected the data in the field or the data managers at each site who managed both the paper trail and the local data entry efforts. The system permitted staff members to input information based on the risk factor targeted, the type of intervention activity, the number of activities, the types of materials used, the duration of activity, and the number of participants. Dates and costs were also entered. A staff member at the study coordinating center reviewed the WWITS databases from each study center on a monthly basis.

Standardized tracking forms were developed and pretested over a six- to eight-month period. Once pretesting was complete, all intervention staff members in the national trial attended a two-day orientation/training workshop covering the purpose of the tracking system, the use of the tracking system forms, and quality control procedures. Staff members who later joined the study completed a training/certification process to ensure standardization of the data collection and form-completion procedures. The study coordinating center initiated quality control procedures for the process evaluation effort, which included monthly conference calls between the study coordinating center, data managers, and representative intervention coordinators at each study center to answer questions and solve coding problems. In addition, periodic reports that summarized questions from the study coordinating center focused on missing data requests, coding questions, and feedback on completed forms.

Procedures. As part of the intervention protocol, one intervention coordinator (IC) was assigned to work with each participating worksite and each full-time IC was typically responsible for between four and ten experimental worksites. The

IC also worked with the EAB to make sure all activities in the intervention protocol were delivered (for example, all process objectives related to those activities were achieved). Each IC worked with experimental worksites to develop an intervention plan that included a schedule of how and when activities would be offered during the intervention period. The WWITS was used to monitor the extent to which the intervention was delivered as intended by tracking where and when each process objective in the standardized intervention protocol was delivered. Figure 6.1 depicts a simplified overview of WWITS.

When the EAB planned a particular activity, the IC initiated a Planned Activity Tracking Form (Appendix B), providing detail on the risk factor addressed, the method of intervention (such as groups, self-help, self-assessment and feedback, and mailings), and the duration of the intervention (number of sessions or number of minutes). This form was submitted to the tracking coordinator (TC) at each study center for data entry into the WWITS relational database.

Once the data were entered into a Planned Activity Tracking Form, a sequential code was assigned to the activity. Simultaneously, a Materials Tracking Form and a Personnel Tracking Form (for ICs, EAB members, and nonproject personnel) were generated and linked to the same activity code.

The Materials Tracking Form was a means of tracking resources used in the study, ensuring some quality control of materials used, and estimating costs of the intervention. Early in the trial, potential intervention materials for each risk factor were reviewed and an inventory of "approved" intervention materials was constructed. The approved materials met the overall theoretical underpinnings of behavior change adopted by the trial; specifically, the materials were designed to raise employee awareness of risk factors and health, motivate employees to make a behavior change, provide employees with skills required for behavior change, or encourage environmental changes to support employee behavior change. Material types included audiovisual materials, brochures, pamphlets, kits to facilitate behavior change (such as smoking quit kits and fat counters), posters and banners posted

FIGURE 6.1. WORKING WELL INTERVENTION TRACKING SYSTEM.

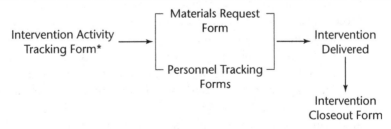

*The intervention is assigned a sequential code number that clarifies risk factor, study center, and worksite and is used to track the activity over the course of the study

throughout the worksite, slides and software for behavior change, recipes that followed the fat and fiber recommendations of the trial, incentives materials, and demonstration equipment. These approved materials were entered into WWITS to facilitate the ordering of materials. In addition to the approved materials, study center staff members could input recommended materials for consideration for use by other sites; these were called "recommended materials."

The Personnel Tracking Form (for ICs, EAB members, and nonproject personnel) tracked personnel costs associated with each activity. Each IC would track the amount of time he or she spent on each activity (for both planning and implementation) and would turn the forms in monthly. Each IC would bring to the EAB a personalized sheet that listed activities that were under way at that site. For the monthly EAB meetings, each member would estimate the number of minutes (if any) he or she had spent on a particular activity in the past month. Each EAB member could also report time spent that was not necessarily linked to a particular activity. The IC would then collect the EAB members' information and submit it to the TC at each study center for local data entry.

The IC was also responsible for making sure that all planning and implementation efforts related to each activity were recorded. After implementation of the activity, an activity-specific Closeout Form (Appendix C) was used for recording what actually transpired in the field, compared with what was planned (as some activities changed over time). Actual or estimated participation, materials used, and personnel involved were recorded and linked by the original activity code on the Closeout Form.

The data collected for this national trial was voluminous; therefore, only selected process evaluation results are provided here. Specifically, we report results associated with (1) *implementation*—a measure of the extent to which the intervention was delivered as intended (such as the percentage of process objectives in the standardized intervention that were delivered and recorded within the WWITS), (2) *awareness*—a measure or indicator of the receipt of the intervention as employees report that they were "aware of" specific types of health promotion programs being offered at their worksite, as recorded on the final employee survey, (3) *resources*—a measure or indicator of the receipt of the intervention by way of materials used, as recorded in WWITS on the Materials Tracking Form, and (4) *dose*—a measure or indicator of the proportion of workers at a worksite who participated in the intervention. Only smoking dose calculations are presented in this chapter. (Dose related to nutrition outcomes can be found in Patterson and others, 1997.)

As noted previously, the worksite was the unit of randomization, intervention, and analysis in this study. Worksites were embedded in study centers and participants/employees were embedded in worksites. Whenever possible, we report worksite data, using aggregated employee data or study center-level findings, as well as aggregated worksite data. In this manner, we attempt to shed additional light on the larger study findings and then we report lessons learned from this process evaluation effort.

Results

Implementation

The process objectives that were achieved trial-wide and at each study center are reported in Table 6.3, and they were also reported previously (Sorensen and others, 1996). Overall, 74 percent of the smoking process objectives and 82 percent of the nutrition process objectives were achieved. For smoking, the percentage process objectives achieved varied from 56 percent for M. D. Anderson to 92 percent for Brown. Self-assessment programs (85 percent) and self-help programs (81 percent) were the objectives most likely to be achieved, whereas group education programs (58 percent) and video/single-session presentations (67 percent) were achieved less often. For nutrition, the range of process objectives achieved varied from 57 percent for M. D. Anderson to 100 percent for Brown, followed closely by Florida (98 percent) and Dana Farber (93 percent). Nutritional interactive activities in the kickoff event (96 percent), self-assessment (88 percent), videos (84 percent), and posters (82 percent) were most likely to be achieved, whereas self-help programs (69 percent) were the least likely to be achieved.

Despite the fact that the Working Well intervention staff generally appears to have delivered the intervention as planned, the outcomes achieved were fairly modest. A few plausible explanations for these results, as well as remaining questions to be answered, are offered here. First, although process objectives were met, the intervention may not have been powerful enough to motivate behavior change among employees, or it may not have lasted long enough to promote change. Second, there may have been larger social or environmental factors influencing employee health behaviors that overwhelmed the effect of the individually focused intervention activities. In fact, Biener and others (1999) demonstrated that there was an association between individual and environmental change in nutrition. Future studies should explore these relationships more fully. Third, practical and logistical issues at certain study centers—such as M. D. Anderson, whose sites were spread across sixteen states and involved difficult-to-reach pipeline workers—may have precluded them from offering certain types of interventions, such as multi-session classes, whereas other study centers may have had worksites where special arrangements to facilitate implementation—such as requiring employee attendance at classes—could be negotiated. Fourth, measuring only the extent

TABLE 6.3. IMPLEMENTATION OF THE WORKING WELL TRIAL
INTERVENTION: PERCENTAGE OF PROCESS OBJECTIVES
ACHIEVED BY SMOKING AND NUTRITION TARGETS.

Process Objectives Achieved[1]	Brown	Dana Farber	Florida[2]	M. D. Anderson	All Centers Combined
Kickoff Participation (goal = 50% of employees/worksite)	48%	60%	69%	84%	68%
Nutrition[3]					
Interactive activity held at kickoff (1)	100	92	100	95	96
Posters (4)	100	98	100	51	82
Video/Single session presentation (3)	97	83	100	68	84
Self-assessment + feedback (2)	100	100	100	68	88
Self-help program (2)	100	96	96	45	78
Multisession direct education	100	92	100	20	69
Campaign/Contests	100	92	92	50	78
Total % of Nutrition	100	93	98	57	82
Smoking[3]					
Interactive activity held at kickoff (1)	100	92	NA	45	72
Posters (4)	98	92	NA	66	81
Video/Single session presentation (3)	91	56	NA	62	67
Self-assessment + feedback (2)	91	96	NA	75	85
Self-help program (2)	100	100	NA	60	81
Multisession direct education	100	58	NA	35	58
Campaign/Contests	100	83	NA	56	74
Total % of Smoking	97	82	NA	56	74

[1]Excludes process objectives directed toward environmental change; numbers in parentheses indicate the number of times an activity was to be done.

[2]Not applicable, as Florida had no smoking intervention.

[3]Conducted at each worksite.

Source: Sorensen and others, 1996, p. 943.

to which the intervention objectives were met—such as implementation—does not indicate whether employees participated in the activities or show the quality of the intervention delivered. This points to the importance of having other process evaluation measures—such as dose, fidelity, and participation—as a means of comparing or making sense of these results.

Awareness

Awareness is often an initial indicator that participants have "received" an intervention. In the case of Working Well, an intervention aimed at influencing the behaviors of all employees within a worksite, including making them aware of the availability of health promotion programs at work, is a key process variable. Awareness was captured by using data aggregated from the employees' final health survey responses. An awareness index was calculated by asking employees about their knowledge of a list of available smoking and nutrition activities being offered at the worksite. Responses to the questions were scored as "0" (no) or "1" (yes), summed, and divided by the number of activities in the list. Chronbach's alpha for the awareness index ranged between 0.75 and 0.85. Bootstrap regression estimates depict the extent to which the awareness index was associated with intervention outcomes (calculated as the difference between experimental and control worksites on smoking and nutrition outcomes) (see Table 6.4). For both sets of

TABLE 6.4. AWARENESS INDEX BY STUDY CENTER FOR SMOKING AND NUTRITION.

Awareness Index	Intervention-Control Difference	SE	p	95% CI
Smoking Awareness[1]				
Brown	0.15	0.09	0.15	−0.05, 0.36
Dana-Farber	0.09	0.06	0.15	−0.02, 0.28
M. D. Anderson	0.16	0.04	0.00	0.08, 0.27
All centers combined	0.14	0.03	0.00	0.08, 0.22
Nutrition Awareness				
Brown	0.22	0.07	0.02	0.05, 0.40
Dana-Farber	0.22	0.05	0.00	0.10, 0.33
Florida	0.14	0.03	0.01	0.09, 0.24
M. D. Anderson	0.15	0.04	0.00	0.07, 0.24
All centers combined	0.17	0.02	0.00	0.13, 0.22

Note: SE = standard error, CI = confidential interval.

Source: Sorensen and others, 1996, p. 944.

[1]Florida did not address smoking.

outcomes, difference scores were significant (p < .001), and provide evidence that employees at experimental worksites were more aware of the health promotion materials available at their workplace than were employees at the comparison worksites. Some variation in the magnitude of the difference existed among study centers, yet no significant center-by-treatment interactions were observed (Sorensen and others, 1996).

Thus, employee awareness about nutrition and smoking resources was generally high, and it was significantly higher at the experimental worksites than at the control worksites—as expected. And people paid more attention to the availability of nutrition information and programs than they did to smoking-related activities—probably because some people smoke but everyone eats. In addition, it may mean that more nutrition-related activities than smoking-related activities were offered at the Working Well experimental worksites (see Table 6.3), so it is possible that the level of awareness was linked to the number of interventions sponsored, whereas awareness alone did not translate into behavior change. However, measuring awareness and verifying that it was in the expected direction allows investigators to rule out the possibility that employees' lack of awareness of the availability of these programs at the experimental worksites explains nonsignificant findings.

Resources Used

WWT investigators conducted an extensive review of educational materials—such as print materials, videotapes, and slides—and created an inventory of approved materials and resources for the national trial. Table 6.5 indicates the intervention materials approved or recommended for the trial by risk factor and the number of approved or recommended materials used by the study centers. As can be seen from Table 6.5, there were considerable differences between study centers in the use of approved or recommended materials. For the category of brochures, pamphlets, and other written materials, the difference was most pronounced, with M. D. Anderson using the fewest materials for both smoking and nutrition. In turn, Brown used more materials for smoking than did Dana Farber. However, with regard to nutrition, Dana Farber reported using many more materials than were approved or recommended, but it is not clear if this refers to multiple uses of the same materials.

Although the number of approved or recommended intervention materials used varied substantially from one study center to the next, it is not clear whether such differences were related to the number of trial process objectives achieved or to differences in study outcomes across study centers. Process objectives achieved have been reported in detail elsewhere (see Table 6.3). For smoking, however,

TABLE 6.5. INTERVENTION MATERIALS APPROVED AND RECOMMENDED BY RISK FACTOR AND NUMBER OF MATERIALS USED BY STUDY CENTER IN THE WORKING WELL TRIAL.

Risk Factor and Material	Number of materials approved	Number of materials recommended	Number of materials used			
			Brown	Dana Farber	MD Anderson	U of Florida[1]
Smoking						
Audiovisual	14	2	9	3	6	N/A
Brochures and pamphlets	61	17	57	37	16	N/A
Kits	8	2	3	7	2	N/A
Posters/Banners	1	0	8	12	2	N/A
Other[2]	0	0	6	5	2	N/A
Nutrition						
Audiovisual	17	3	8	16	6	2
Brochures and pamphlets	26	21	41	119	16	33
Kits	12	7	3	12	6	0
Slides and software	5	1	0	4	0	1
Recipes	0	0	9	1	0	0
Posters/Banners	3	0	5	7	5	1
Other[3]	0	7	16	20	3	14

[1]N/A = Not applicable, as Florida did not have a smoking intervention.

[2]Includes equipment, general supplies, and incentives.

[3]Includes equipment, food, general supplies, and incentives.

the percentage process objectives achieved varied from a low of 56 percent for M. D. Anderson to a high of 92 percent for Brown. This finding may be compared with the fact that M. D. Anderson had the lowest usage of trial approved or recommended materials and Brown had the highest usage. For nutrition, the percentage of process objectives achieved varied from a low of 57 percent for M. D. Anderson to a high of 100 percent for Brown. Again, this is consistent with M. D. Anderson having the lowest usage of materials for nutrition. Although Brown had the highest percentage of process objectives met, Dana Farber followed closely with 93 percent, which is congruent with its usage of materials. However, Florida met 98 percent of its nutrition process objectives but was only third in the usage of trial approved and recommended materials.

There is little consistency between the usage of trial materials and trial outcomes. M. D. Anderson used fewer smoking cessation materials than either Brown or Dana Farber yet still showed a decrease in the six-month smoking abstinence rate (Sorensen and others, 1996). However, only Dana Faber (not Brown) showed a significant increase in the six-month smoking abstinence rate at study conclusion (Sorensen and others, 1996). With regard to nutrition outcomes, Florida showed a significant increase in dietary fiber and a percentage increase in fruits and vegetables consumed, despite using relatively few of the study-wide approved or recommended intervention materials. Similarly, M. D. Anderson achieved a significant percentage increase in fruits and vegetables consumed, even though the use of approved or recommended materials was low compared with that of other study centers (Sorensen and others, 1996).

The materials inventory was an ambitious effort to ensure that intervention materials met selected quality control characteristics, but the actual implementation of this aspect of WWITS proved even more challenging. First, the inventory list was established approximately six months after the intervention was under way; therefore, planning for a number of interventions had already occurred. Second, when doing retrospective tracking, ICs were able to simply list any new materials used in the intervention. When the data was entered in this manner, widespread adoption of excellent materials used in one study center may have been delayed or prevented because others never learned that these materials existed. Third, using participatory approaches made it difficult for ICs to use only materials from the approved materials inventory. Members of the EAB, or experienced ICs, often suggested materials not included in the materials inventory. Finally, the actual tracking of materials used was time-consuming. Intervention staff had to count (or estimate) materials used at the numerous interventions occurring at each worksite. This was not a favorite task of the intervention staff, and it may have contributed to either the underreporting or the overreporting of actual materials used.

Dose

In this chapter, we focus only on dose as it relates to the smoking outcome. Defining *dose* for a comprehensive intervention study is a complex undertaking. Substantial differences existed in the type of activities offered as part of the national trial, making it difficult to add a quantity of one activity with another. For example, the participation of smokers in a series of smoking cessation classes could not realistically be thought to equate in any way with the receipt, through company mail, of a smoking cessation flyer. Quantitative weighting of variables was also not considered appropriate, as it would be unrealistic to rationalize that one activity would be worth two of another activity. Conversely, however, entering each of the different activity types into a model with a behavior as a dependent variable was not feasible, given the diversity of activity types. Thus, the first step in calculating worksite level was to reduce the number of activity types.

From the overall standardized intervention protocol, six key smoking-related activities were identified: (1) attendance at a kickoff event, (2) direct educational activities that included lectures or presentations, such as classes on smoking cessation, (3) demonstration activities, such as pulmonary lung function tests and expired CO tests, (4) contests and campaigns, such as incentives for quitting, (5) information opportunities, such as a table or pamphlet holder where employees could take information at will, and (6) company-wide material distribution, such as putting flyers in every worker's mailbox or sending messages to workers' homes. Data from WWITS also tracked the number of materials distributed in each activity type or the total number of employees who participated in the activity type, though the participation of each individual worker was not tracked (except at Brown). This was not viewed as problematic, since, to obtain a meaningful level of intervention dose within the entire worksite, the proportion of total worksite employees receiving an intervention activity was considered more important than participation by any individual. The key criterion for dose, therefore, was the proportion of workers who participated in the intervention activities.

Most smoking cessation activities attempted to involve smokers at each worksite. According to the baseline survey, the trial-wide prevalence of smoking was approximately 25 percent (Heimendinger and others, 1995), though as many as 31 percent of employees failed to report smoking status, suggesting that the actual proportion of smokers may be higher. Evidence demonstrates that nonrespondents to surveys are more likely to be smokers (Heimendinger and others, 1995). Therefore, intervention dose was calculated both for the total number of employees per worksite and for the number of smokers as reported in the baseline survey. To calculate the worksite-wide level of exposure for each activity, all participants at an event (such as at a lecture or presentation) were summed and were then divided by the total number of employees at the worksite. For materials distribution, the total number of materials distributed was divided by the total number of employees. To calculate the rate for smokers only, the denominator was the total number of smokers at the worksite at baseline. Both methods produced rates with no upper bounds, since employees could participate more than once in an activity. Indeed, the higher the number, the greater the dose that was delivered.

The WWT emphasized the importance of changing the smoking environment as well as individual behavior. Specifically, the protocol required that worksites engage in activities to increase the restrictiveness of smoking policies. Since worksites varied considerably in their attempts to change the environment, dose of intervention at the environmental level was also calculated. Every three months, worksite representatives completed a form stating whether or not they had worked on developing or instituting a more restrictive smoking policy. Baseline policies were recorded and rated on a scale of 1 to 4: 1 = smoking is allowed everywhere,

2 = smoking is allowed everywhere except in designated "no smoking" areas, 3 = smoking is allowed only in a few designated smoking areas, and 4 = smoking is not allowed. Any action toward a more restrictive smoking policy was considered part of the intervention dose. To assess the level of change, the baseline policy strength is subtracted from the policy strength at study conclusion. A negative number reflecting change to a less restrictive policy was not included (this occurred at only one worksite). Thus, for all worksites that included a smoking intervention, dose was assessed by examining the six individual intervention activities and the one environmental activity (see Table 6.6).

There was substantial variation among the three study centers that addressed smoking in the dose variables (data not shown). Two study centers had participation rates in the kickoff that were considerably higher than the third. One study center had virtually no participation in contests and campaigns, compared with the others. One study center had a threefold higher rate of material distribution than the other two but had a lower rate of information picked up by employees through information opportunities.

Table 6.7 summarizes the median and range of the seven smoking dose variables at the forty-three experimental worksites that addressed smoking. Kickoff activities included all components of the intervention, not just smoking cessation,

TABLE 6.6.   REGRESSION OF WORKSITE-LEVEL SIX-MONTH QUIT RATE AGAINST BASELINE PREVALENCE AND DOSE FOR ALL EMPLOYEES AT THE WORKSITE AND FOR SMOKERS ONLY ADJUSTED FOR EDUCATION, GENDER, AND AGE AT FORTY-THREE WORKSITES IN WORKING WELL.

Variables	All Employees in the Worksite			Smokers Only in the Worksite		
	Relative Change in Quit Rate	S.E.	p value	Relative Change in Quit Rate	S.E.	p value
Baseline Prevalence	0.48	0.23	.04	0.27	0.22	.23
Dose Activities						
Kickoff	0.10	0.04	.03	0.09	0.04	.03
Direct education	−0.01	0.01	.50	−.001	0.003	.62
Demonstrations	−0.04	0.03	.14	−0.009	0.006	.13
Contests	−0.14	0.12	.26	−0.04	0.03	.20
Informational pickup	−0.01	0.01	.25	−0.001	0.001	.41
Material distribution	−0.003	0.005	.59	−0.001	0.001	.54
More restrictive policy	−0.01	0.01	.38	−0.009	0.009	.34

TABLE 6.7. VARIABLES OF SMOKING CESSATION DOSE BY MEDIAN AND RANGE OF PARTICIPATION AMONG SMOKERS AT FORTY-THREE WORKSITES IN THE WORKING WELL TRIAL.

Dose Element	Median	Range
Individual Activities		
Kickoff (percentage of smokers attending)	72.0	21 to 100
Direct education (number of sessions per smoker)	1.2	0.0 to 32.1
Demonstration activities (number of activities per smoker)	2.6	0.0 to 10.1
Contests (number of smokers per contest)	0.0	0.0 to 2.4
Information opportunity (number of materials taken per employee)	4.5	0.6 to 33.5
Material distribution (number of materials distributed per smoker)	0.0	0.0 to 52.3
Environmental Activity		
More restrictive smoking policy (number of steps increased)	1.0	0.0 to 4.0

and involved the majority of employees at most worksites. Three worksites did not have direct educational activities, contests and campaigns were conducted by only eight of the forty-three worksites, and employee-wide information distribution was done at eleven worksites. More restrictive smoking policies were enacted at twenty-four worksites. Of those that increased restrictiveness, eight increased one level of restrictiveness, ten increased two levels, and three worksites each increased three and four levels. The range for all of the dose measures indicates that substantial variation existed between worksites.

Some of the dose variables were correlated: kickoff participation was significantly correlated with both direct education ($r = .55$, $p < .01$) and demonstrations ($r = .43$, $p < .01$); informational pickup opportunities were correlated with contests ($r = .39$, $p < .01$). None of the other variables was significantly correlated. Regressions of six-month smoking cessation against baseline prevalence, dose variables using the entire worksite population as the denominator, and smokers only as the denominator are given in Table 6.8. All of the dose variables were entered into the model as predictor variables, with smoking cessation being the response variable. Regressions were adjusted for gender, education level, and age. No relationships were found between dose and program awareness when all the worksite respondents were used as the denominator. For smokers only, awareness of contests and campaigns was inversely related to six-month cessation.

TABLE 6.8.   REGRESSION OF AWARENESS RECEIPT INDICES AGAINST
DOSE VARIABLES FOR ALL EMPLOYEES AT THE WORKSITE AND
FOR SMOKERS AND QUITTERS ONLY, ADJUSTED FOR BASELINE
PREVALENCE, EDUCATION LEVEL, GENDER, AND AGE AT
FORTY-THREE WORKSITES IN THE WORKING WELL TRIAL.

| | Awareness Index | | | | | |
| | All Employees ($N = 7188$) | | | Smokers and Quitters Only ($N = 1840$) | | |
Dose Variable	Relative Change in Awareness Rate	S.E.	p value	Relative Change in Awareness Rate	S.E.	p value
Kickoff	0.03	0.07	.71	0.05	0.06	.46
Direct education	−0.004	0.004	.38	−0.004	0.004	.31
Demonstrations	0.01	0.01	.20	0.01	0.01	.23
Contests	−0.08	0.05	.11	−0.11	0.04	.02
Information opportunities	0.002	0.002	.35	0.002	0.002	.29
Material distribution	−0.0002	0.02	.93	−0.001	0.002	.79
Policy change	0.02	0.02	.28	0.02	0.01	.28

Strengths and Limitations

The WWT process evaluation effort had a number of important strengths and
has served as a model for the development of process evaluation efforts in several
subsequent worksite- and community-based intervention studies. A highly qualified and experienced team of investigators from the study centers and the study
coordinating center collaborated to develop the process evaluation effort for this
study. The steering committee made a commitment of personnel time and resources to develop a comprehensive process evaluation effort, despite the fact that
budget was not allocated up front for local data entry or coding. Another strength
of this study was the development of a standardized national training of ICs and
data managers. Each study center staff member involved in the process evaluation effort was required to take a written exam and complete a certification process.
An extensive pretest was done of the forms, as well as of the database, prior to
full-scale implementation of the process tracking system.

Despite these strengths, several limitations are also noteworthy. A major limitation was that the pretest of WWITS was done during the actual intervention

period rather than prior to the intervention; thus, retrospective data collection and entry occurred. This frustrated the project staff and reduced the overall time available to do process tracking (and intervention). Another limitation was the complexity of WWITS itself. Unlike some current paperless systems, WWITS involved myriad supplementary forms that branched out from the Planned Activity and Closeout Form to track all aspects of the comprehensive and evolving intervention effort. Each time a new form was introduced, staff members were required to become familiar with it, adopt it, and retrospectively "correct" interventions that had been tracked without the "new" form. This placed great demands on project staff members at all levels of the tracking effort. Third, the commitment to process tracking was not consistent over time or across study centers. In addition to incomplete record keeping from the field staff, by the time available data were entered, cleaned, and ready for analysis, investigators who might have published manuscripts on these results had moved on to other projects. Thus, the sheer volume of data collected in the process evaluation served to limit this study. However, it would have been useful to collect *more* data on the comparison intervention. For example, smoking-specific study results revealed that both the experimental worksites and the comparison worksites had achieved positive smoking cessation results, and thus there was no overall treatment effect. It would have been desirable to have more detail about the amount and type of intervention, as well as employee participation, in the comparison sites. Lack of comparison site process data is a limitation of Working Well, as it is of many other community-based studies that include process evaluation components.

Lessons Learned About Process Evaluation

Process evaluation efforts undertaken as part of the WWT were among the most comprehensive carried out, compared with other community-based studies during that time period. A national process evaluation working group that included representation from all of the study centers, as well as from the study coordinating center, was formed specifically to focus on this issue. Several important lessons were learned in the development, implementation, and evaluation of the Working Well process evaluation effort.

LESSON 1. *It is often feasible to tailor and improve existing forms and tools that other studies have created.*

Several investigators, including several steering committee members and working group chairs, had previous experience with process evaluation efforts as part of the community cardiovascular disease intervention studies in the state of Minnesota and in Pawtucket, Rhode Island, as well as experience with the Community Intervention Trial for Smoking Cessation (COMMIT). When developing community-based interventions, we often fail to make use of lessons learned from others who have faced similar challenges. The chapters in this book give many examples and sample forms that should be exceedingly useful to build upon when developing tools for future trials.

LESSON 2. *Clearly articulate the purpose of the process evaluation.*

In the WWT, clear objectives for the process evaluation were stated up front when the national process evaluation working group was organized. If the purpose is clear, then the data one needs to collect will reflect this clarity. If expectations for the process evaluation are not clear in advance, investigators (especially in a large complex trial) may believe that the process tracking system is collecting something it is not designed to collect. Alternatively, investigators may ask to have a process evaluation system collect far more data than will ever be examined. Clear expectations and regular progress reports should be featured in future process evaluation efforts.

LESSON 3. *Pretest the overall system and its component parts prior to intervention implementation.*

The WWITS computerized system was "pretested" as a paper system for nearly eight months. This pretest gave study investigators an opportunity to develop and troubleshoot use of all the forms prior to doing the final computer programming to make the system operational. By having the pretest, study investigators avoided huge programming expenses for the multiple changes and iterations that were required, based on problems identified in the field. However, another lesson we learned about the pretest is that it should be take place much earlier, so that it is completed prior to the start of the intervention. ICs were already in the field and had completed several months of activities before the WWITS system became fully operational. Though ICs were filling out the "paper system," it is likely that the retrospective tracking of time and materials introduced a recall bias in the data collected prior to when the system was fully operational. It is important to recognize, however, that the process evaluation planning often occurs after a project is under way. As the intervention progresses, a process evaluation system must be flexible enough to accommodate changes as the project evolves, thereby minimizing staff burden.

LESSON 4. *Use the best technology available, making sure that it is easy to use and that staff members are trained appropriately.*

At the time that this project occurred, several guiding principles in the development of the process tracking system were adopted trial-wide. A few examples of principles that guided the development of the process evaluation are (1) "in recording data for WWITS, whenever possible intervention staff will be asked to document, and computations will be done by the system"; (2) "minimizing the documentation burden on project staff and companies is a high priority"; and (3) "the impact on programming is an important consideration." Taking these guiding principles into consideration, the WWT created a comprehensive process tracking system that used state-of-the-art software, including a relational database that could link multiple sources of data while managing a large volume of data.

Unfortunately, at the local study centers, ICs were required to complete paper forms, as they did not have access to computers, which would have allowed them to enter data immediately into the database. This paper system proved both time-consuming and unwieldy. Now that laptops and other portable data collection devices are available at a reasonable cost, these barriers are not likely to persist. However, finding a match between the practical use of technology and facilitating timely data entry, increasing the quality control of data entry, and reducing the overall time costs for data entry remains an important consideration when planning for process evaluation efforts. Initial and ongoing staff training in the use of selected technology is an important key to success as well.

LESSON 5. *Be sensitive to the staff and participant data collection burden.*

An important lesson learned in the Working Well process tracking experience suggests that the study investigators planning the effort should focus clearly on the objectives of the process evaluation and should collect only the data necessary to answer those questions. The Working Well intervention protocol was ambitious, and ICs worked long hours to ensure that the protocol was met. In addition, they were asked to manage a very challenging documentation task for WWITS—one that involved several changes over the first several months while the pretest occurred. Then, when the final version of WWITS was available, and ICs received extensive training on the system, several months of documentation effort had to be redone on the "new, final" forms. It is possible that the amount of time spent documenting the intervention effort in WWITS took time away from intervention.

In addition to minimizing the burden on project staff, it is critical to keep to a minimum the efforts that study participants are asked to make in assisting with data collection and monitoring. At one Working Well study center (Brown), an attempt was made to collect individual employee-level participation at all study events and activities. This placed an added burden on employees to complete sign-ins or some other checklist at each event, since it required additional steps to guard against the loss of privacy, it increased the annoyance factor of requiring the filling out of more forms, and it took time away from participating in the intervention. Adjustments were made at mid-study to limit employee participation records at selected events, and a streamlining of the forms was accomplished, but it is clear that future studies should evaluate the amount of information gained against the extra burden on staff members and participants to accomplish this level of record keeping.

The tracking burden might have been minimized further by the following strategies:

- Complete a pilot test of the entire system before the intervention began to ensure that no "extra" documentation was required.
- Work more closely with ICs to develop the pilot test of the data collection process and the various forms used.
- Consider a paperless system by issuing laptops so that project staff members can do immediate data entry while in the field.
- Give employees "swipe" cards (versus paper forms) to record participation.
- Talk with the worksite contacts to determine if they might be able to maintain some forms/database files (such as EAB member files) that the study center could send electronically or by diskette (versus tracking by paper at each EAB meeting).
- Hire nonintervention personnel to enter the paper form data into a computerized system.

With advance planning and more dialogue between end users (ICs, project staff members, and worksite contacts), creative solutions could have been devised for overcoming the burden of various process tracking forms on respondents. This was especially true of participant tracking forms, which required extra effort on the part of staff members. A swipe card for employees to use when attending Working Well-sponsored events would have greatly facilitated the tracking of individual participants in the study. Minimizing the data collection burden for project staff members and end users is key to long-term practicality and the success of process evaluation efforts.

LESSON 6. *Create brief and clear feedback reports and disseminate them early and often.*

One of the strengths of a comprehensive process tracking system is the ability to create timely, informative reports. In Working Well, the reports most often generated were those from the study coordinating center to the project staff, informing individuals of where problems in the dataset, or missing data, should be addressed. Although study centers could generate their own reports, it was seldom done. At Brown, monthly reports were generated to inform the project director of how many process objectives were met at monthly intervals. Reports were generated by worksite, risk factor, or IC, so that strategies could be employed to facilitate completion of the intervention protocol by the end of the study period. Reports were also generated that compared participation across experimental worksites. ICs could "show" a particular EAB where it was located on a chart that compared all experimental worksites in the study (identified only by a unique code). Thus, EAB members could set realistic expectations about increasing participation, meeting process objectives, responding to surveys, and so on. Creating useful reports helped stimulate interest in and commitment to the process evaluation effort—for both the project staff and the participants. Management at the participating worksites responded favorably when reports were shared that highlighted progress toward meeting the study objectives and showed the participation rates and outcomes of a particular intervention activity.

Conclusion

Theoretically, to achieve behavior change, a comprehensive intervention program needs to be built on interventions that have demonstrated previous success in a variety of settings, can be implemented as intended, reach the intended target population, reduce barriers to participation, and ensure that participants use the intervention. As some other large group-randomized trials have discovered, however, the links between the various parts of an intervention and individual behavior change are tenuous and not guaranteed (Glasgow and others, 1996; Sorensen, Emmons, Hunt, and Johnston, 1998; Sorensen and others, 1999). In Working Well, the association between awareness, the use of approved and recommended materials, the number of process objectives achieved, and final trial outcomes was not at all clear. The trial was certainly built on sound theoretical foundations (Abrams and others, 1994). Both intervention strategies and intervention materials were designed to be congruent with successful interventions in other settings and studies. Overall, the intervention appeared to be implemented as intended. Reports by employees indicated that they were both aware of and participated in some of the intervention activities (Sorensen and others, 1996). Despite all this, overall, the trial saw no change in smoking cessation, and it saw only a modest decrease in dietary fat intake (-0.35) as well as a modest increase in servings of fruits and vegetables per day (0.18).

Process evaluation can be key to understanding why an intervention program did not produce the desired result. It can help identify failures in intervention, assess the linkages between various levels of evaluation, and provide valuable insight into research that is needed. In Working Well, for example, process evaluation results indicated that few individual health behavior changes were made, despite awareness of and participation in the intervention. Plausible explanations for these findings include important, unmeasured, and possibly multilevel contextual influences that occurred during the time of the intervention period. For example, a number of worksites in one study center closed during the course of the study, and several other sites experienced severe economic downturns. It is possible that employees at those worksites faced serious concerns—health and stress-related threats that overwhelmed intervention effects. Moreover, there were important changes in the larger social environment that supported changes in norms about smoking, as well as in the carcinogenic risks of environmental tobacco smoke, that may have motivated all worksites (including comparison worksites) to adopt smoking policy changes, thus wiping out any possible differences between the experimental sites and the control sites with regard to smoking policy change. The fact that Biener and others (1999) reported an association between individual and environmental change suggests that testing the independent and combined effects of an environmental and individual intervention may be warranted. Moreover, careful documentation of the contextual influences occurring during a study is also needed in a thorough process evaluation effort.

Puzzling results from the process and outcome evaluations also suggest that more research is needed to identify strategies that transfer employee participation in an intervention to actual behavior change—that is, the process evaluation component called "initial use" (Baranowski and Stables, 2000). Certain intervention strategies—such as self-assessment plus feedback—present opportunities for employees to assess a particular health status indicator—such as the results of a strength test, the level of carbon monoxide shown in their expired air, or an index of their body mass—and get immediate feedback about the result and what it means relative to their personal health. We need to investigate why certain intervention methods stimulate greater behavior change, and under what conditions this change is most likely to occur. Process evaluation data can be particularly helpful when answering these questions in future studies.

Alternatively, these results may suggest a fresh look at the theory underlying the trial. For example, Linnan and others (2001) have considered macrosocial theories—such as political economy of health—that identify potential social drivers of participation in worksite health promotion programs and ultimately act as important determinants of health behavior. Using ecological approaches, future studies may need to move beyond the intrapersonal and organizational theories that informed the WWT intervention and integrate theories that address inter-personal, community, or society levels. Measurement and analytic strategies will need to keep pace with these advances in theory.

More time and effort is needed to understand the linkages between specific types and amounts of intervention delivered within the context of a comprehensive worksite health promotion program. For example, there may be certain interventions that, when employees participate in them, will stimulate an increase in health behavior change. Or perhaps certain changes in health, such as increasing physical activity, may lead an individual to attempt other health behavior changes—such as ceasing to smoke. The notion of "gateway" behaviors for making health changes can be investigated with process and outcome evaluations (French, Hennrikus, and Jeffrey, 1996; Gomel and others, 1997). Process evaluation efforts can help unravel the "black box" of intervention strategies that are more or less likely to produce and sustain desired health changes among individuals and within the work environment.

References

Abrams, D. B., and others. "Cancer Control at the Workplace: The Working Well Trial." *Preventive Medicine,* 1994, *23,* 15–27.

Baranowski, T., and Stables, G. "Process Evaluations of the 5-a-Day Projects." *Health Education and Behavior,* 2000, *27*(2), 157–166.

Biener, L., and others. "Impact of the Working Well Trial on the Worksite Smoking and Nutrition Environment." *Health Education and Behavior,* 1999, *26*(4), 478–494.

French, S. A., Hennrikus, D. J., and Jeffrey, R. W. "Smoking Status, Dietary Intake, and Physical Activity in a Sample of Working Adults." *Health Psychology,* 1996, *15*(6), 448–454.

Glasgow, R. E., and others. "Promoting Worksite Smoking Control Policies and Actions: The Community Intervention Trial for Smoking Cessation (COMMIT) Experience. The COMMIT Research Group." *Preventive Medicine,* 1996, *25*(2), 186–194.

Gomel, M. K., and others. "Composite Cardiovascular Risk Outcomes of a Worksite Intervention Trial." *American Journal of Public Health,* 1997, *87,* 673–676.

Heaney, C. A., and Goetzel, R. Z. "A Review of Health-Related Outcomes of Multicomponent Worksite Health Promotion Programs." *American Journal of Health Promotion,* 1996, *11*(4), 290–307.

Heimendinger, J., and others. "The Working Well Trial: Baseline Dietary and Smoking Behaviors of Employees and Related Worksite Characteristics. The Working Well Research Group." *Preventive Medicine,* 1995, *24*(2), 180–193.

Linnan, L. A., and others. "Using Theory to Understand the Multiple Determinants of Low Participation in Worksite Health Promotion Programs." *Health Education and Behavior,* 2001, *28*(5), 591–607.

Patterson, R. E., and others. "Components of the Working Well Trial Intervention Associated with the Adoption of Healthful Diets." *American Journal of Preventive Medicine,* 1997, *13,* 271–276.

Sorensen, G., Emmons, K., Hunt, M. K., and Johnston, D. "Implications of the Results of Community Intervention Trials." *Annual Review of Public Health,* 1998, *19,* 379–416.

Sorensen, G., and others. "Work Site-Based Cancer Prevention: Primary Results from the Working Well Trial." *American Journal of Public Health,* 1996, *86*(7), 939–947.

Sorensen, G., and others. "Increasing Fruit and Vegetable Consumption Through Worksites and Families in the Treatwell 5-a-Day Study." *American Journal of Public Health,* 1999, *89*(1), 54–60.

U.S. Bureau of Labor Statistics. *Current Employment Statistics (CES).* Washington, D.C.: Government Printing Office, 2001.

Yen, L., and others. "Changes in Health Risks Among the Participants in the United Auto Workers-General Motors LifeSteps Health Promotion Program." *American Journal of Health Promotion,* 2001, *16*(1), 7–15.

APPENDIX A: WORKING WELL STUDY INVESTIGATORS AND COMMITTEE MEMBERS.

NATIONAL CANCER INSTITUTE (NCI)

Division of Cancer Prevention and Control. Program Director: Jerianne Heimendinger. Statisticians: Charles Brown, Don Corle. Fellows: Nancy Cotugna (1990), Susan Sullivan (1990–1991).

STUDY CENTERS

Brown University School of Medicine/Miriam Hospital. Principal Investigator: David B. Abrams. Co-Principal Investigator: Lois Biener. Co-Investigators: Karne M. Emmons, Laura Linnan. Statisticians: Joe Fava, Wayne Velicer. Project Director: Laura Linnan. Intervention Specialists: Edward Galuska, Mary Lynne Hixson, Sheila Jacobs, Suzanne Moriarty. Data Specialist: David Vampola, Kate Lapane (1989–1992). Research Associate: Janine Costa. Administrative Assistant: Mark Morgenstern.

Dana-Farber Cancer Institute/University of Massachusetts Medical School. Principal Investigator: Glorian Sorensen. Co-Principal Investigators: Jay Himmelstein, Judith Ockene. Co-Investigators: Katherine Hammond, James Hebert, Ruth Palumbo, Anne Stoddard. Project Director: Mary Kay Hunt. Evaluation Coordinator: Jean Hsieh. Intervention Coordinators: Lynda Graham-Meho, Elizabeth Harden, Jane Ellen Thompson. Nutrition Coordinator: Judith Phillips. Industrial Hygienist: Richard Youngstrom. Process Tracking Coordinator: Steve Potter. Administrative Assistant: Elizabeth Farr.

University of Florida at Gainesville. Principal Investigator: Jill Varnes. Co-Principal Investigator: Claudia Probart. Co-Investigator, Medical Consultant: David Schapira. Statistician: David Miller. Intervention Coordinators: Jeanine Lahey, Steve Livésay, Valerie Studnick (1990–1992). Interventionist/Tracking Coordinator: Susan Guckenberger. Office Manager, Data Manager: Kathy Galloway.

University of Texas M. D. Anderson Cancer Center. Principal Investigators: Ellen R. Gritz, W. Bryant Boutwell (1991–1993), Michael Ericksen (1989–1991). Co-Principal Investigator: Carlo DiClemente. Co-Investigators: Robert Chamberlain, Guy Parcel, Karen Basen-Engquist, John Foreyt, Larry Whitehead, Alan Herd, Jane Mayfield. Project Coordinator: Scott R. Cummings. Intervention Specialists: Scott R. Cummings, Ingrid Nielsen, James Eldridge, Bill Mann. Consultants: Karen Glanz, Robert Bertera.

STUDY COORDINATING CENTER

Fred Hutchinson Cancer Research Center. Principal Investigator: James Grizzle. Co-Investigators: Ziding Feng, Susan Kinne, Alan Kristal, Beti Thompson, Nicole Urban (1990–1992). Fellow: Ruth Patterson. Coordinating Center Managers: Sonya Olsen, Gwen Glaefke (1989–1992). Statistical Research Associates: Cynthia Lostoski, Steve Thomson, Dale McLerran. Database Manager: Allan Williams. Programmers: Stephanie Stafford, Peter Dueber, Lynette Brown (1990–1991). Cost Analysts: Shelly Hager, Addy Tseng, Carole Shaw (1990–1993). Support Staff: Catherine Cohen, Ellen Powell (1991–1992), Estella Bennett (1990–1992), Jenny Devaney (1990–1991).

APPENDIX B: PLANNED ACTIVITY FORM (PAF).

Activity Name:__ __

Worksite Name:_____ Worksite ID:__ __ __

Study Center ID:___

WWITS Assigned Activity Code __ __ __ __ __

CORE INTERVENTION *Circle one*

01 Direct Education

02 Information Materials

03 Self-Assessment with Feedback

04 Self-Help/Self-Management
If Code = 02, 03, 04, Circle *Mode of Delivery:*
  21 Lecture/Presentation
  22 Sample/Demo/Test/Measure
  23 Information Opportunity/Pickup
  24 Company-wide Distribution
  25 Home Mail

05 EAB Meetings **Circle** *Mode of Delivery:*
  26 Meeting
  27 Training

06 Co. Meeting/Presentation **Circle** *Mode of Delivery:*
  21 Lecture/Presentation
  26 Meeting

07 Environmental Policy **Circle** *Mode of Delivery:*
  26 Meeting
  27 Training
  28 Environmental Policy Notification/ Implementation
  29 Contact/Correspondence

08 Contest

09 EAB Organization

10 Event Coordination

11 Standard Program Contact Documentation

PART OF A LARGER EVENT? *Circle one*

1 WWW Kickoff __ __ __ __ __ *Enter Activity ID*
2 WW Health Fair __ __ __ __ __ *Enter Activity ID*
3 WW Campaign __ __ __ __ __ *Enter Activity ID*
4 Company-sponsored event _____
5 Other, specify _____
9 Not part of larger event

RISK FACTOR *Circle one*

1 Smoking
2 Nutrition
3 Exercise
4 Cancer Screening
5 Occupational Health
6 Weight Management
7 Multiple **List codes:** ___;___;___;___;___
8 Other, specify _____
9 Not application (e.g., EAB meetings, EAB organization, Event Coordination)

Form completed by: _____
ID code: __ __ __

Form entered by:
ID code: __ __ __

Activity Description (Include documentation for coding done above)

_____

_____

APPENDIX C: ACTIVITY CLOSEOUT FORM.

Activity: **50020**	Worksite: **902**	Study Center: 5

CANCER RISK LECTURES   **JET CITY SILICON**

PAF Date: 08/25/91   Interventionist: 77   LOTTA ENERGY

Form Completed by:_____   Form entered by:_____

ID Code:_____   ID Code:_____

Date form completed: ___/___/___   Date form entered: ___/___/___

THIS ACTIVITY IS: *[circle]*
- a. COMPLETE (All work and follow-up on activity is finished)
- b. Continuing (This is routine QUARTERLY CLOSEOUT)
- c. Canceled (Activity will not occur. Be sure to enter any time and materials expended)

Module A—Printed for Activities
    Act. Start Date: ___/___/___ End Date: ___/___/___ Follow-Up End Date: ___/___/___
OR

Module B—Printed for Events
    Event Start Date: ___/___/___ End Date: ___/___/___ Follow-Up End Date: ___/___/___

PARTICIPATION
    SEE MODULES ON PAGE 37

TIME AND EFFORT (Except Interventionist and EAB members)

Position Code	Description	Time (hh:mm)
_____	_____	___:___
_____	_____	___:___
_____	_____	___:___

1. Activity was conducted on *(circle)*
   - a. Employee time
   - b. Company time
   - c. Combination: APPROXIMATE PERCENT OF TIME SUBSIDIZED BY COMPANY__ __ __ %

2. Did the company donate or provide services or materials used for this activity (e.g., printing services, incentives, etc.)? *[circle one]* If yes, describe in Comments/Suggestions section.
   1. YES
   2. NO

3. IF PAF RISK FACTOR = MULTIPLE: Designate the ONE risk factor to be tracked for Process Objectives.
   1. Smoking
   2. Nutrition
   3. Exercise
   4. Cancer screen
   5. Occ. Health
   6. Weight Mgmt.
   7. Other (specify) _____

4. Indicate actual cost to employees (after subsidies or rebates) for participating in this activity.
   $ __ __ __.__ __.

   Comments and Suggestions:_____

CHAPTER SEVEN

Health Works for Women

Process Evaluation Results

Irene Tessaro, Marci Kramish Campbell, and Salli Benedict

Worksites provide an important community setting for reaching adults with health promotion interventions. Smoking cessation, dietary change, exercise, weight loss, and cardiovascular and cancer screenings are health behavior outcomes targeted in several large worksite health promotion and disease prevention trials (Erfurt, Foote, and Heirich, 1991; Jeffery and others, 1993; Abrams and others, 1994; Glasgow and others, 1995). Few worksite studies, however, have focused on women employed in blue-collar occupations in small- and medium-sized worksites, particularly in rural areas (Messing, 1997). In North Carolina, these worksites often lack comprehensive health promotion programs or resources such as cafeterias and fitness facilities (Leiss and Bert, 1995). Women working in blue-collar occupations in these companies tend to have elevated health risks because of the high prevalence of unhealthy behaviors and increased stress from jobs with high demand and low control (Messing, 1997). Women also face unique barriers to participation in traditional workplace health promotion programs, including lack of time, due to their need to balance multiple roles and responsibilities (Marcus and others, 1992).

This work was supported by grant U481CCU409660 from the Centers for Disease Control and Prevention, U.S. Public Health Service, awarded to the Center for Health Promotion and Disease Prevention, University of North Carolina, Chapel Hill. The authors wish to acknowledge the contributions of Health Works for Women coinvestigators Brenda DeVellis, Kristine Kelsey, and Leigh Belton, as well the contributions of additional investigators, including Alan Cross and David Farrell.

Health Works for Women (HWW) was a five-year worksite health promotion project that focused on rural, blue-collar women working in small- to medium-sized manufacturing industries. The project was funded from 1993 to 1998 through the CDC as the demonstration project of UNC's Center for Health Promotion and Disease Prevention. The process evaluation was important for formative assessment to design the intervention, monitor progress, and make midcourse corrections, and it was important for understanding the study outcomes. Process evaluation of one component of the HWW intervention—the Natural Helper program—was designed to answer the question How was a natural helper model of change adapted to a worksite setting? When we designed this project, there were no interventions that used a natural helper model in the workplace. Social support has been recognized as being important for facilitating behavior change in worksite health promotion programs (Fisher and others, 1994; Emmons, Linnan, Abrams, and Lovell, 1996; Zimmerman and Connor, 1989), but there has been little attempt to intervene at the social network level in the workplace (Gottleib and McLeroy, 1994). In addition, we knew of no studies that had combined two successful health promotion interventions—tailored health messages and natural helpers.

Description of Health Works for Women

Health Works for Women developed and evaluated an innovative intervention that addressed multiple health behaviors, including physical inactivity, unhealthy diet (high fat and low fruit and vegetable intake), and smoking, as well as breast and cervical cancer screening. An ecological framework (McLeroy, Bibeau, Steckler, and Glanz, 1988; Stokols, 1996) was used to target multiple levels of change—at (1) the *interpersonal* level, a social network intervention using the natural helping ability of women to support health promotion change at the worksite (Natural Helper program), and at (2) the *intrapersonal* level, using computer-generated, individually tailored health messages designed to inform women about health risks and to provide personalized feedback, strategies for change, and community resource information to initiate behavior change. Both components of the intervention were theory-based, using constructs from social cognitive theory (Bandura, 1986), social support theory (Israel, 1985), the health belief model (Strecher and Rosenstock, 1997), and the transtheoretical model (Prochaska, DiClemente, and Norcross, 1992).

Natural Helper Program

A natural helper model of change is a social network strategy designed to make behavioral and social change through naturally existing systems of social support

(Collins and Pancoast, 1976). The aims of a natural helper program are to identify those individuals to whom others turn for help and support and to strengthen their knowledge and skills in providing social support for behavioral and social change. The goal is to encourage natural helpers to enlarge their circle of influence through the natural networks that people have already established (Salber, 1979).

At the worksites, the natural helpers were identified by (1) women who were asked to name coworkers whom others often turned to for help and support, (2) managers who made recommendations to ensure that all networks of women and work areas in the workplace were included, and (3) women who identified themselves as someone with an interest in providing support and education to coworkers for health promotion change. We had expected to recruit between five and ten women volunteers at each worksite, but the program was able to identify and train 104 women (ranging from thirteen to thirty-six women per worksite) from among different social networks and shifts at the worksites. This represented 16.3 percent of all the women at the intervention worksites.

Natural helpers were asked to diffuse health information to women through their social networks, support other women in their efforts to make health promotion changes, and promote workplace activities and change. A series of six educational sessions for the natural helpers were offered over an eighteen-month period on-site and were scheduled immediately before or after the women's work shifts. All educational sessions were conducted by members of the project team and included a nurse, nutritionists, health educators, and graduate students in health education. The natural helpers received education on (1) the important role of support for making health behavior changes, (2) healthy eating, (3) fitness and exercise, (4) stress reduction, (5) women and cancer, and (6) weight management. Educational sessions involved group discussion and activities, as well as techniques to enhance skills in the targeted behavior areas.

Training materials used in the educational sessions included (1) information about targeted health behaviors and health education materials appropriate for the women, (2) resources for health promotion in the local community, such as low-cost mammography screening sites and places for exercise, (3) skill-building information about providing emotional support, listening, and helping with problem solving, and (4) skill building on how to work together as a group to organize worksite activities to promote healthy behaviors. The educational materials helped standardize the intervention, but the natural helpers decided exactly how to pass this information along, what educational and behavior change activities were most appropriate for their worksite, and what the best ways were to carry out these activities. Table 7.1 shows the number of natural helpers per worksite and the average number attending the six educational sessions by worksite. (See Tessaro and others, 2000, for more detailed information about the natural helpers intervention.)

TABLE 7.1. EDUCATIONAL TRAINING SESSION ATTENDANCE FOR NATURAL HELPERS.

	Natural Helpers		Average Attendance
	N	%	
Worksite 1	13	(6.3)	5.7
Worksite 2 (2 training groups)	21	(18.3)	12.0
Worksite 3 (3 training groups)	36	(17.4)	16.9
Worksite 4 (2 training groups)	34	(31.5)	18.9
Totals	104	(16.3)	

Tailored Health Messages

Individual computerized tailoring is a technique that combines health behavior change theory, communication theory, social marketing, and new technology to produce personally relevant health messages for each project participant. The tailoring framework for HWW incorporated demographic, psychosocial, behavioral, and community-specific resource information to address the factors that were considered most likely to predict change. The tailored feedback was presented in the format of a women's magazine, based on formative research showing that women's magazines were a primary source of health information for these women. Results from focus groups were used in combination with pertinent literature and the expertise of the project team to develop appropriate tailoring variables, the message content, language, and the literacy level for the tailored health messages.

Two individualized computer-tailored health messages were provided confidentially to all intervention group participants—the first one after participants filled out the baseline survey, and the second one after participants completed the six-month follow-up survey. Each magazine provided individualized feedback regarding all of the health behaviors targeted in the study—that is, fat, fruit, and vegetable consumption, aerobic, strengthening and flexibility exercise, cancer screening status, and (for smokers) readiness to quit smoking—showing current behaviors relative to recommended guidelines.

The information provided in the women's tailored health magazine integrated the individual and social network aspects of the intervention, and it used stories and graphics that depicted women making behavior changes in the context of social, worksite, and community support. A "buddy message" for women to give to those whom they identified as a support person to help them make health behavior changes was also included. After completing the six-month survey, de-layed intervention women received one individually tailored health magazine that was identical in content, format, and degree of tailoring to the magazines deliv-ered to the intervention group. They did not have the natural helpers program at their workplaces. (See Campbell and others, 2000, for more detailed information about the tailored health intervention.)

Psychosocial tailored feedback was focused only on the behavioral priority that each woman had selected. Based on the behavioral priority, psychosocial vari-ables used for tailoring included behavior-specific barriers, outcome expectations, stage of change, social support, informational needs, and community resources. In terms of behavioral priority for change, 16 percent of the women chose to work on healthy eating, 12 percent chose exercise, 51 percent chose both healthy eating and exercise, 9 percent chose smoking cessation (26 percent of current smokers), and 12 percent chose learning about cancer screening. This program may be the first to use a multibehavioral approach to tailoring based on partici-pant choice of behavioral priority (Campbell and others, 2000). The hypothesis was that tailoring health messages to focus on a woman's behavioral priority might result in greater success in achieving at least one behavior change, which in turn might be a "gateway" leading to increased motivation and confidence to tackle additional problem behaviors in the future (Emmons and others, 1994). The pos-sible drawback to tailoring health messages to behavioral priority is that women may not choose a behavior, such as smoking, that could have the highest objective impact on decreasing their health risks. Indeed, relatively few smokers in this study chose to work on quitting smoking, preferring to focus on healthy eating and ex-ercise (Campbell and others, 2000).

Methods. The project used a randomized two-group experimental design to test the effect of the two intervention components—the tailored health messages and the Natural Helper program—on changes in the multiple behaviors of phys-ical inactivity, unhealthy eating (high fat and low fruit and vegetable intake), and smoking, as well as breast and cervical cancer screening. Nine rural counties in eastern North Carolina, which had minority populations of at least 30 percent of the total county population, were selected for worksite recruitment. Workplaces were eligible for recruitment, based on the following criteria: (1) a small- to medium-sized company (125–350 workers) in a blue-collar textile or light manu-facturing industry, (2) a majority of women employees (at least 51 percent of the workforce), (3) no systematic health promotion program currently in place, and (4) no plans for immediate plant closure. From an original list of 132 worksites in the study counties, nineteen were deemed eligible for inclusion, based on these criteria. Seven worksites were not interested in participating and two expressed interest but could not commit to participation within the specified time period. Ten worksites—one pilot site and nine study sites—53 percent) agreed to participate in the study. Of the nine study sites, three were light manufacturing worksites and six were textile and apparel worksites. Four worksites were randomized to the intervention group and five were randomized to the delayed intervention condition. Intervention worksites were phased in over three years. The delayed intervention worksites were offered a menu of possible health education sessions for their employees on topics not directly related to the study objectives.

Measures. Women who agreed to participate in the study completed a ninety-two-question survey at three points during the intervention: baseline, six-month follow-up, and eighteen-month follow-up. Measures included demographic characteristics (age, ethnicity, education level), social support and social network characteristics, perceived health status, body mass index, targeted health behaviors of diet, physical activity, smoking, and cancer screening, stage of change for each targeted health behavior, and choice of behavioral priority for change. (See Campbell and others, 2000, for more details about the evaluation methods.)

Findings. Of the 859 baseline respondents, 660 women (77 percent) completed the six-month survey and 650 women (76 percent) completed the eighteen-month survey. In the overall sample, 53 percent of the women were forty years of age or younger, 58 percent were African American, and the majority were married and had a high school education or greater. Results showed that at the eighteen-month follow-up, the intervention group had increased fruit and vegetable consumption by 0.7 daily servings, compared with no change in the delayed group ($p < .05$). Significant differences in fat intake were observed at six months ($p < .05$) but not at eighteen months. The intervention group also demonstrated improvements in strengthening and flexibility exercise, compared with the delayed group. The rates of smoking cessation and cancer screening did not differ between study groups (Campbell and others, 2002).

Process Evaluation

A process evaluation can assess to what degree a program was implemented, including what activities were carried out, the degree to which the priority population was reached, and what the barriers were to adoption and implementation of the intervention. A process evaluation can also assume a formative role during the developmental phase of an intervention to better understand the context in which the intervention takes place and to identify determinants of, and facilitators for, the intended behavior change for the priority population (Patton, 1990). The process evaluation for HWW included both formative research to assist in the design of the intervention and an evaluation that assessed the implementation of the intervention for women in the worksites. Process evaluations are often qualitative in nature, using observation, personal interviews, and focus groups (Patton, 1990). For HWW, formative evaluation was done through focus groups and field notes, and personal interviews and process questions in the study survey helped explain how the Natural Helper program and the tailored health messages functioned to effect change.

Focus Groups

Methods. Focus groups were initially conducted in a pilot worksite to assist in the development of the study questionnaire, and they aided in designing the content, structure, and layout of the tailored health magazines and the natural helper training materials. Following administration of the baseline survey and prior to initiating the Natural Helper program at each intervention worksite, focus groups were conducted with women on all work shifts. The focus groups enabled the research team to better understand women's health concerns and the barriers to promoting healthy behaviors at each worksite, and they also enabled the researchers to learn about the support available through women's social networks, as well as being instrumental in developing the training sessions for the Natural Helper program.

An open-ended interview script was used for conducting the focus groups. Questions concentrated on (1) health issues of concern to women workers, including the major health issue women most wanted to do something about at their worksite, (2) the barriers to making health behavior changes and what actions could facilitate overcoming these barriers, including examples of change attempts by themselves and others, and (3) social support for health behavior change, including the people to whom women turn when they have health concerns, what others can do to help them make health behavior changes, and what they can do to help others make these changes. Descriptive exploratory methods were used in data analysis (Krueger, 1994), and data were coded deductively by using the initial organizing framework of the interview guide questions and were coded inductively by eliciting other patterns and themes.

Results. Thirteen focus groups were conducted at the four intervention worksites before and after each work shift. Seven of the focus groups were with women who worked the day shift, three were with women who worked the evening shift, and three were with women who worked the night shift. From six to twelve women participated in each group for a total of 121 women. Most women (85 percent) were line workers (machine operators, knitters, winders, trimmers, finishers, cutters, assemblers, setup persons, shippers, and processors); the others were supervisors and clerical or training staff. Three-fourths (75.8 percent) of the women at all the worksites had at least a high school diploma or GED, and the large majority had lived in the surrounding area most of their lives. The focus groups comprised European American women (43 percent), African American women (55 percent), and other—mostly Native American—women (2 percent). The socioeconomic characteristics of focus group participants were similar to those of the other women at the worksites.

The major health issues of concern for women in these workplaces centered on health-promoting behaviors such as exercise, healthy eating, weight loss, and smoking cessation. Stress, both physical and psychological, was also a major health issue for the women, particularly because of the multiple roles they played in their daily lives. It was clear that although the women saw the importance of changing unhealthy behaviors, they lacked the relevant information and skills to make changes that would fit in with the rest of their lives. Support was strong among these women, who had worked together for a long time, and they consistently mentioned that offering support was something others could do to help them make health changes as well as something they could do to help others make such changes. (See Tessaro and others, 1998, for more detailed information about the focus groups.)

Natural Helper Interviews

Methods. Personal open-ended interviews were conducted with natural helpers six months (time 1) and twelve months (time 2) after the initial educational training session, and a group interview was conducted at eighteen months, at which time the research team exited each worksite. Observation and field notes during the time in the worksites provided additional insights into program development and the experiences of the natural helpers. At the time 1 interview, fifty-two (75.4 percent) of the sixty-nine natural helpers were interviewed. Between the time 1 and time 2 interviews, an additional thirty-five women participated in the educational sessions. At the time 2 interview, seventy (67.3 percent) of the 104 natural helpers were interviewed. Eighty-two (76.9 percent) of the 104 natural helpers were personally interviewed at either six or twelve months, and forty completed both interviews. Interviews were conducted on a day that the women were allowed by worksite management to take off from the line in order to participate in the interviews. Women who were out sick, on vacation or other leave, working the weekend shift, no longer employed at the worksite, or otherwise constrained were not included in the interviewing.

Questions for the interviews focused on (1) how information about health promotion was spread (initiated, approached, in conversation, or through written materials); (2) to whom information was spread (family member[s], coworker[s], or friend[s]); (3) how many others the interviewees shared information with; (4) the barriers to sharing information with coworkers; and (5) group activities that involved targeted health issues. In the group interviews, the women were asked about their role as natural helpers, their coworkers' awareness of the Natural Helper program, changes in health promotion activities at the worksite since the program began, and how natural helpers would continue with the program after HWW.

Results. Information about health promotion was diffused by the natural helpers, mostly through general conversation with coworkers rather than through the proactive seeking out of coworkers. Natural helpers preferred to share health materials (manuals, recipes, handouts) with coworkers on a one-on-one basis, although contact persons who saw it as part of their larger role at the company also mentioned using bulletin boards and placing handouts by the time clock. Coworkers frequently asked natural helpers about what they had learned in the training sessions, and this was a major method of sharing information. As part of the training sessions, natural helpers were encouraged to develop group activities related to targeted health behaviors that would fit into their work situation. Initially, these activities were carried out on a limited basis, but they increased with time as women began to use the skills they had learned in the training sessions. For example, at one of the worksites, a lunchtime walking group was formed and the women mapped out a trail around the outside of the plant. At two of the worksites, natural helpers participated in a local walkathon.

Natural helpers reported that with time the focus of their diffusion of health promotion information shifted from their family members to their coworkers. Coworkers more frequently approached the natural helpers as they became known as people from whom others could seek health promotion information. This approach was consistent with the culture of the women, who, in focus groups, expressed their hesitancy about telling others to change their health behavior (Tessaro and others, 1998). Thus, over time, natural helping contacts became more responsive than proactive.

The major barrier to diffusion of health information by the natural helpers had to do with time constraints—caused by overtime work schedules, conflicting work shifts, and, in particular, evening and night shifts, as well as after-work family obligations. Such time constraints also limited natural helpers' ability to get together as a group for activities. As a result, written materials were often the preferred method of diffusing information about health promotion to women in their work areas, and coffee and lunch breaks were the best times for dissemination. Natural helpers had limited time to talk with the coworkers who were not in their immediate work areas. Since it was hard to leave their work areas, natural helpers mainly shared with people in their own circles and work areas.

One of the difficulties in evaluating natural helper interventions is in assessing how natural helpers "naturally" diffuse information to network members and offer support for behavior change. The research team felt that capturing what natural helpers were doing was best done through qualitative research methods. In the interviews, natural helpers were able to report how they shared health information with coworkers, but it was difficult for them to tell us exactly how many women this was with or what materials they shared with each person. They were doing this as part of their natural conversation with coworkers and not as part of a prearranged protocol. Because natural helpers were volunteers and were doing this on their own time, we did not ask them to keep logs of how many coworkers they had contacted about the targeted health behaviors, what information was distributed to coworkers, or what activities they initiated with coworkers. Instead, we asked coworkers about their exposure to the natural helper program on the follow-up survey.

Exposure to the Natural Helper Program

Exposure to the Natural Helper program can indicate how well the program was carried out and the extent to which women workers were reached with this component of the intervention.

Methods. As part of the eighteen-month follow-up survey, women workers from the intervention worksites who were *not* involved in the natural helper trainings were asked a series of questions about the Natural Helper program. They were asked if they had heard about the program (yes/no), if they had talked with or received written materials from a natural helper about the targeted health issues of exercise, healthy eating, weight management, stress management, women and cancer, smoking (yes/no to each of these), or if they had got together with coworkers about the targeted health issues (yes/no).

Results. Twenty-nine percent (N = 105) of the women who were *not* involved in the natural helper trainings had heard about the program at the workplace. The first (day) shifts were slightly more likely to report that they had heard of the program (45 percent), compared with the second (evening) and third (night) shifts (38 percent each) (see Table 7.2). Sixty-four percent of those who had heard of the program said that they had got together for group health-related activities

TABLE 7.2.   COWORKERS' EXPOSURE TO THE NATURAL HELPERS
PROGRAM (*N* = 105).

	Percentage Who		
	Received Written Materials from Natural Helpers About	Talked with Natural Helpers About	Got Together with Coworkers for
Exercise	78.3	80.2	64.8
Healthy eating	76.8	69.8	47.9
Weight management	50.7	46.5	43.7
Stress management	46.4	39.5	23.9
Smoking	34.8	26.7	16.9
Women and cancer	30.4	24.4	9.9

because of HWW. The women reported that, in order of frequency, they mostly received written materials, followed by discussions of health issues, and, less frequently, getting together for group activities. Exercise and healthy eating were the most frequently cited health behaviors around which women interacted with the natural helpers.

Exposure to Tailored Health Messages

The process evaluation of the tailored health messages was designed to assess measures of exposure and perceived impact. Questions were loosely based on the elaboration likelihood model, which suggests that factors such as attention, perceived personal relevance, and credibility of messages should increase information processing and ultimately lead to behavior change (Petty and Cacioppi, 1986). Previous studies of tailoring have used similar process measures (Skinner and others, 1999).

Methods. At the eighteen-month follow-up, women were asked a series of questions about the tailored health messages. They were asked if they remembered receiving the tailored health magazine (yes/no) and how much of the health information they had read, how much they had believed, how much they felt was written especially for them and caused them to think about making health changes, and how much the information helped them change their health habits (a lot, some, a little, or not at all).

Results. A total of 86.2 percent of the women in the intervention group recalled having received the tailored health information, versus 71.5 percent of the delayed

TABLE 7.3. PARTICIPANTS' EXPOSURE AND REACTIONS TO TAILORED HEALTH MESSAGES AT EIGHTEEN-MONTH FOLLOW-UP.

	Intervention	Delayed Intervention	
	N = 340	N = 270	
	%	%	P-value
Recalled receiving a personal health magazine	86.2	71.5	.009
Read the magazine*	76.0	66.0	.13
Believed the messages*	80.0	68.4	.12
Messages were written especially for the individual	47.4	34.8	.001
Messages caused the individual to think about behavior change*	47.4	37.7	.046
Messages caused actual behavior change*	35.8	31.2	.11

*Percentage represents the proportion who responded a lot versus some, a little, or not at all.

group (p < .05). Compared with the women in the delayed group, those in the intervention group reported significantly higher recall and personal relevance of the tailored health magazine and were more likely to say that the information caused them to think about changing their health behaviors (Table 7.3).

Lessons Learned About Process Evaluation

The process evaluation of HWW assisted the research team in understanding women's views about health behavior change, assisted in developing health education materials for the study, guided major changes in the original protocol, directed the implementation strategies of the natural helper and the tailored health message components, helped the research team understand study outcomes, and was used to develop a new five-year workplace-community intervention. The intervention as a whole (both the tailored health messages and the Natural Helper program) allowed a better understanding of how the use of an ecological framework to target individual behavioral and social change can affect multiple health behaviors in a natural setting (the worksite). Process evaluation of the Natural Helper program demonstrated the viability of using this model of change in a worksite setting.

LESSON 1. *Formative research can be used to develop culturally relevant program materials.*

Focus group findings were instrumental in developing the culturally tailored educational materials for the tailored health magazines and for the Natural Helper program. The focus group data were used in combination with pertinent literature and project team expertise to develop appropriate tailoring variables, message content, language, and literacy level for the tailored health messages. Original natural helper training and educational materials were developed by the project staff, and they relied heavily on information gathered from the focus groups. Included in the materials were health issues of concern to women at the worksites, barriers to change, what helped women change, and how women perceived the role of social support at the worksite.

LESSON 2. *Formative research can be used to develop intervention strategies and logistics.*

Formative research guided many of our logistical decisions as to how best to conduct the intervention in the work setting. For instance, we had planned to conduct the Natural Helper program outside the worksite in a community setting, but because time constraints were a major barrier, women preferred that meetings at the worksite take place before or after their shifts. We also learned that time off the production line for women to participate in the intervention would be a major barrier at worksites. Thus, both components of the intervention occurred outside of work hours: the tailored health magazines were sent to women's homes or were delivered at work, and the Natural Helper program was conducted either before or after work hours.

The strategies we used to recruit women for the Natural Helper program, the topics the program addressed, and the design of the training sessions themselves were all informed by focus group findings. More women than expected participated in the program, and we believe that our success may have been due to the fact that the health issues addressed and the strategies for addressing them came directly from the women. For example, the issue of stress, not originally targeted in the intervention, was incorporated into the educational sessions because of its importance to the women. Paying attention to what the women told us about the stress in their lives helped establish rapport and showed that we were listening to them.

Another reason for the high participation in the Natural Helper program may have been that our recruitment methods were inclusive. Reputational methods, similar to those used in recruiting natural helpers in other community programs, were used (Jackson and Parks, 1997), but we also used other methods to ensure that all of the social networks in the worksite were tapped and that the cultural norms of the women were respected. Our method of including all women who wanted to participate, and not just those named by others, was important so as not to disrupt the close friendships and working relationships among the women. This strong social support among women in the worksites was evident from the focus groups. And the importance of tapping all the networks of the women at the worksite was evident, given that the natural helpers reported in the personal interviews that information about health promotion was shared mostly with those in their own circles at the worksite.

LESSON 3. *Formative research can help tailor health promotion programs to individual worksites.*

Although there are similarities among all manufacturing workplaces, each workplace is unique. Using formative research methods allowed HWW to meet the needs of each workplace and to alter the intervention, based on needs expressed by the natural helpers and the workplace managers. Using formative research methods allows researchers to account for differences. For example, when natural helpers in several workplaces requested a "healthy eating for the holidays" session, we incorporated it. Because of the great interest in weight management (not a targeted behavior), we provided a training session and materials that reiterated the 5-a-day and low-fat behavior change strategies taught in the Healthy Eating session.

LESSON 4. *Process interviews with natural helpers can help evaluators learn how Natural Helper programs work.*

The natural helper interviews were able to show that the focus of diffusion of health promotion information in HWW started with family and friends, and, over time, it shifted to coworkers. Natural helpers reported that health promotion information was spread mainly in everyday conversation and not by the active seeking out of coworkers. These interviews also showed that as time went on, the natural helpers became known for their knowledge and coworkers more frequently approached them for this information. This approach was consistent with the culture of the women, who, in focus groups, expressed hesitancy to tell others to change their health behavior (Tessaro and others, 1998).

Two distinct patterns of the natural helping role were identified through the personal interviews with natural helpers. On the one hand, there were women who tended to get involved in the program because of a specific health concern or event of theirs or of others in their personal network; on the other hand, there were women who became involved within a broader conceptualization of health and prevention. Both types of natural helpers were able to take on the role of disseminating information about health promotion to coworkers, and this increased over time for both groups. The latter type of natural helper was characterized as being a *natural helper*—one who was sought out by others, was in contact with many others, and was more likely to be identified as a natural helper through reputational methods. But the interviews were able to show that both types of natural helper were able to take on the role of spreading health information to coworkers, and the longer they did this, the more others looked to them for information. We might not have seen this had formative evaluation not guided us to be inclusive in our recruitment methods.

LESSON 5. *Formative research methods alter researchers' priorities and require flexibility.*

Given the public health impact of smoking and the high rate of smoking in this population of women, smoking cessation was targeted as one of the main objectives of HWW. But study results showed that HWW did not have an impact on smoking rates. This lack of effect is not surprising, considering that our choice-based intervention approach resulted in little emphasis on smoking-related activities. Few women chose smoking as their behavioral priority for tailored health messages, and the natural helper trainings on smoking cessation were offered but were never implemented, because of lack of interest on the part of the natural helpers. Although smoking cessation was an issue of concern to women in the focus groups, when it came to choosing a health priority for the tailored health magazine, health eating and exercise were, together, the main interests of the women for behavior change. In addition, natural helpers expressed that they were not comfortable with or interested in trying to influence other women at their workplaces to quit smoking, which they viewed as a personal decision. Thus, neither component of the intervention was strongly influential toward changing smoking behavior. Intervention approaches targeted at the organizational or policy level may be needed in order to affect such behaviors as smoking.

LESSON 6. *Workplace interventions require adequate time for development, intervention, evaluation, and redevelopment phases.*

The original HWW research design proposed that we spend just six months in each workplace. Discussions with natural helpers and workplace managers clearly indicated that six months was too short a time to build rapport or organize and implement the Natural Helper program. Therefore, we made a midcourse correction to continue the intervention for eighteen months instead of the originally proposed six months. With the current emphasis on participatory action research and the understanding that building relationships with communities takes a great deal of time, we recommend that funding agencies recognize the importance of funding projects for five years or more. Budgets must reflect the need to spend time in communities, and they must provide adequate funding for staff members to spend time building relationships and implementing programs in communities.

LESSON 7. *Limited time is the most important perceived barrier to the practicing of healthy behaviors among the women in blue-collar worksites.*

The issue of limited time as a major barrier for women came up in the focus groups and was an important element in carrying out the Natural Helper program. Every component of the Natural Helper program was developed to emphasize strategies that do not take much time. "Quick and easy" strategies for increasing exercise, eating a healthy diet, and reducing stress were based on what women told us in focus groups. The time constraints faced by women working the evening and night shifts—mainly due to their family obligations—were especially problematic for their involvement in the natural helpers program. This was one reason why the Natural Helper program was more successful with women on the day shift. Because of the time issue, written materials were often the preferred method of diffusing information about health promotion to women in their work areas, and coffee and lunch breaks were the best times for dissemination. Natural helpers were encouraged as part of their role to initiate group activities appropriate for women at the worksite, but, given the time constraints and working schedules of the women, this was difficult. The tailored health messages were able to provide health information to women—even those women for whom there was limited (or no) time for involvement in health promotion activities at the worksite. This also shows the value of tapping multiple levels of change when designing interventions.

LESSON 8. *Process evaluation helped understand study outcomes.*

Formative research in the form of focus groups showed that the health behaviors women wanted most to change were in the areas of nutrition and physical activity. Baseline survey results confirmed that women most often chose these two behaviors as their priority health issues for change. On the follow-up survey, women reported that exercise and healthy eating were the most frequently cited health behaviors around which they interacted with the natural helpers. Thus, it probably is not surprising that nutrition and physical activity were the behaviors that showed the most positive outcomes in the study. The multiple process measures in the study gave a better understanding of these outcomes.

LESSON 9. *Process evaluation helped plan for program sustainability and institutionalization.*

In the natural helper interviews, women discussed how they were spreading health information and strategies to their families, churches, and communities. In addition, many natural helpers said that they would continue with their own attempts to practice healthy behaviors after HWW ended. They said that they had acquired skills for continuing to share information about health promotion and for supporting other women at work in their attempts at behavior changes. However, the formal Natural Helper program as a group effort is less likely to continue. To ensure program sustainability, a champion at each workplace would need to continue organizing the program and would need to enlist support from a local health department or other agency. The process evaluation of HWW was used to inform the development of another project, Health Works for Women/Health Works in the Community, which incorporates strategies for continuing this new program after funding ends.

Conclusion

The process and formative evaluation of HWW helped design an intervention appropriate for women in the worksite, showed what needed to be changed during the intervention, and, at the conclusion of the intervention, helped explain what was and was not successful. Both qualitative and quantitative methods were important for the evaluation. Using formative and process evaluation to understand the context in which the intervention took place and listening to the participants helped make HWW an intervention with positive behavior outcomes.

References

Abrams, D. B., and others. "Cancer Control at the Workplace: The Working Well Trial." *Preventive Medicine*, 1994, *23*, 15–27.

Bandura, A. *Social Foundations of Thought and Action: A Social Cognitive Theory.* Englewood Cliffs, N.J.: Prentice Hall, 1986.

Campbell, M. K., and others. "Tailoring and Targeting a Health Promotion Program to Address Multiple Health Behaviors Among Blue-Collar Women." *American Journal of Health Promotion*, 2000, *14*, 306–313.

Campbell, M. K., and others. "Effects of a Tailored Health Promotion Program for Female Blue-Collar Workers: Health Works for Women." *Preventive Medicine*, 2002, *34* (3), 313–323.

Collins, A. H., and Pancoast, D. L. *Natural Helping Networks: A Strategy for Prevention.* Washington, D.C.: National Association of Social Workers, 1976.

Emmons, K., Linnan, L., Abrams, D., and Lovell, H. J. "Women Who Work in Manufacturing Settings: Factors Influencing Their Participation in Worksite Health Promotion Programs." *Women's Health Issues*, 1996, *6*, 74–81.

Emmons, K., and others. "Mechanisms in Multiple Risk Factor Interventions: Smoking, Physical Activity, and Dietary Fat Intake Among Manufacturing Workers." *Preventive Medicine*, 1994, *23*, 481–489.

Erfurt, J. C., Foote, A., and Heirich, M. A. "Worksite Wellness Programs: Incremental Comparison of Screening and Referral Alone, Health Education, Follow-Up Counseling, and Plant Organization." *American Journal of Health Promotion*, 1991, *5*, 438–448.

Fisher, E. B., and others. "Social Support in Worksite Smoking Cessation: Qualitative Analysis of the EASE Project." *American Journal of Health Promotion*, 1994, *9*, 39–47, 75.

Glasgow, R. E., and others. "Take Heart: Results from the Initial Phase of a Work-Site Wellness Program." *American Journal of Public Health*, 1995, *85*, 209–216.

Gottlieb, N. H., and McLeroy, K. R. "Social Health." In M. P. O'Donnell and J. S. Harris (eds.), *Health Promotion in the Workplace*. (2nd ed.) Albany, N.Y.: Delmar, 1994.

Israel, B. "Social Networks and Social Support: Implications for Natural Helper and Community Level Interventions." *Health Education Quarterly*, 1985, *12*, 65–80.

Jackson, E. J., and Parks, C. P. "Recruitment and Training Issues from Selected Lay Health Advisor Programs Among African Americans: A Twenty-Year Perspective." *Health Education and Behavior*, 1997, *24*, 418–431.

Jeffery, R. W., and others. "The Healthy Worker Project: A Work-Site Intervention for Weight Control and Smoking Cessation." *American Journal of Public Health*, 1993, *83*, 395–401.

Krueger, R. A. *Focus Groups: A Practical Guide for Applied Research.* Thousand Oaks, Calif.: Sage, 1994.

Leiss, J. K., and Bert, M. S. *Private Sector Worksite Health Promotion Activities in North Carolina: Results from the 1994 Survey.* Special series report. Raleigh: North Carolina State Center for Health and Environmental Statistics, 1995.

Marcus, B., and others. "The Stages and Processes of Exercise Adoption and Maintenance in a Worksite Sample." *Health Psychology*, 1992, *11*, 386–395.

McLeroy, K. R., Bibeau, D., Steckler, A., and Glanz, K. "An Ecological Perspective on Health Promotion Programs." *Health Education Quarterly*, 1988, *15*, 351–377.

Messing, K. "Women's Occupational Health: A Critical Review and Discussion of Current Issues." *Women and Health*, 1997, *25*, 39–68.

Patton, M. Q. *Qualitative Evaluation and Research Methods.* (2nd ed.) Thousand Oaks, Calif.: Sage, 1990.

Petty, R., and Cacioppi, J. T. "The Elaboration Likelihood Model of Persuasion." *Advances in Experimental Social Psychology*, 1986, *19*, 123–205.

Prochaska, J., DiClemente, C., and Norcross, J. "In Search of How People Change: Applications to Addictive Behaviors." *American Psychologist*, 1992, *47*, 1102–1114.

Salber, E. "The Lay Health Advisor as a Community Health Resource." *Journal of Health Politics, Policy and Law*, 1979, *3*, 469–478.

Skinner, C., and others. "How Effective Are Tailored Print Communications?" *Annals of Behavioral Medicine*, 1999, *21*, 290–298.

Stokols, D. "Translating Social Ecological Theory into Guidelines for Community Health Promotion." *American Journal of Health Promotion*, 1996, *10*, 282–298.

Strecher, V. J., and Rosenstock, I. M. "The Health Belief Model." In K. Glanz, B. K. Rimer, and F. M. Lewis (eds.), *Health Behavior and Health Education: Theory, Research, and Practice.* San Francisco: Jossey-Bass, 1997.

Tessaro, I., and others. "Developing a Worksite Health Promotion Intervention: Health Works for Women." *American Journal of Health Behavior,* 1998, *22,* 434–442.

Tessaro, I., and others. "Adapting a Natural (Lay) Helper Model of Change for Worksite Health Promotion for Women." *Health Education Research,* 2000, *15,* 603–614.

Zimmerman, R. S., and Connor, C. "Health Promotion in Context: The Effects of Others on Health Behavior Change." *Health Education Quarterly,* 1989, *16,* 57–75.

APPENDIX A: PROCESS MEASURE FOR INTERVENTION
WORKSITES ONLY.

As part of *Health Works for Women,* several women at your workplace took part in a special "Natural Helpers" training to learn more about health issues and how to support coworkers with health changes.

If you are one of the women who took part in the Natural Helpers Training, skip to question #6 on the next page.

1. Have you heard about the Natural Helpers part of the *Health Works for Women* program?

   Yes
   No

2. Did you talk about any of the following with women who are Natural Helpers at your worksite? (Check all that are true for you)

   a. Exercise
   b. Healthy eating
   c. Weight management
   d. Stress management
   e. Women and cancer
   f. Smoking

3. Did you get any written material about any of the following from women who are Natural Helpers at your worksite? (Check all that are true for you)

   a. Exercise
   b. Healthy eating
   c. Weight management
   d. Stress management
   e. Women and cancer
   f. Smoking

4. Did you get together with women at your worksite to work on any of the following? (Check all that are true for you)

   a. Exercise
   b. Healthy eating
   c. Weight management
   d. Stress management
   e. Women and cancer
   f. Smoking

5. If you did get together with women at your worksite to work on any of the issues in question #4, do you think this was because of the *Health Works for Women* program in your worksite?

   Yes
   No

(Continued)

APPENDIX A: PROCESS MEASURE FOR INTERVENTION WORKSITES ONLY. (CONTINUED)

Process measure for all study worksites

6. Do you remember receiving a personal health newsletter with your name on it from the *Health Works for Women* program?

   Yes
   No (Skip to the end)

7. How much, if any, of the health information in the newsletter did you read?

   A lot
   Some
   A little
   None

8. How much did you believe the information in the newsletter?

   A lot
   Some
   A little
   None

9. How much of the information in the newsletter was written especially for you?

   A lot
   Some
   A little
   None

10. Did reading this information cause you to <u>think</u> about changing a health habit (such as changing your eating, exercising, or smoking habits)?

    A lot
    Some
    A little
    None

11. How helpful to you was this information in <u>actually changing</u> a health habit (such as changing your eating, exercising, or smoking habits)?

    A lot
    Some
    A little
    None

PART THREE

School-Related Process Evaluation Efforts

Process evaluation is well developed in the school setting. This may be because in schools the usual intervention program is a curriculum (or some equivalent thereof) that is delivered by teachers to students. In such cases, the contents and components of the intervention are clearly identified, as are the program implementers and the intended target audience. Furthermore, because of its structured nature, the school setting is conducive to process evaluation data collection—gathering, for example, observations about program implementation from questionnaires completed by administrators, teachers, and students.

Each of the three chapters included in this section illustrates a different approach to the process evaluation of school-based interventions. In Chapter Eight, Markham and colleagues illustrate the process evaluation of a curriculum, titled Safer Choices, which was designed to reduce sexual risk taking among students in five high schools in California and five high schools in Texas. This study measured four key components of process evaluation: (1) *completeness*—the amount of program activities that were implemented, (2) *fidelity*—the extent to which program activities adhered to the recommended content and methods, (3) *coverage*—the extent to which the target population participated in or received program activities, and (4) *reaction*—the target population's satisfaction with and reaction to program activities.

The curriculum was effective in reducing sexual risk taking, and the process evaluation indicated some of the reasons for implementation success, such as teacher training and teacher satisfaction with Safer Choices. Among the more interesting findings of the process evaluation was that female teachers were more likely to provide a thorough teaching of the lesson components and that knowing someone with HIV or AIDS was instrumental in this. Also related to this thoroughness was the teachers' perception of administrative support for the curriculum.

In Chapter Nine, Davis and colleagues discuss the implementation of a school-based program called Bringing It Home, which was designed to increase the consumption of fruit, juice, and vegetables (FJV) among fourth graders and their families. Lower-income African Americans consume less FJV than other Americans and are therefore at greater risk of becoming obese or contracting a chronic disease. The program described in this chapter was therefore directed at low-income African Americans, and it was implemented in a southeastern, urban, inner-city school system. Ninety-percent of these African American students, many of whom came from families that, compared with national norms, faced socio-economic disadvantage, participated in the free and reduced-price meal program. One of the innovative characteristics of the Bringing It Home program was that the fourth-grade children were used as change agents to bring home to their parents the nutrition messages taught in the classroom. Educational materials, including videotapes, were also used to convey the nutrition message to parents. The program was successful in increasing FJV consumption among experimental group participants, relative to the comparison group. A number of process evaluation components were assessed in this study, including

- How schools and families were recruited into the study
- How schools and participants were encouraged to stay in the study for its duration
- Aspects of the school and community environment that affected program implementation
- What resources were necessary for program implementation
- The extent to which comparison schools implemented nutrition education programs

Two aspects of the Bringing It Home process evaluation warrant special mention: (1) All of the intervention curriculum lessons were observed and rated by trained observers using pilot-tested structured observation forms. In terms of process evaluation methodology, observing intervention implementation by trained observers is the "gold standard." Frequently, such observations are not possible because of the expense associated with paying trained observers, and the cost of travel to the implementation sites. (2) The Bringing It Home project also used parent interviews and focus groups at the end of the study to gather information from parents about their perception of the facilitators and barriers to program success. This produced useful data for future program improvement.

In Chapter Ten, the final chapter in this section, Steckler and colleagues describe Pathways, a nutrition and physical activity trial conducted among schools on seven American Indian reservations in four geographic locations: Southern Arizona, Eastern Arizona, New Mexico, and South Dakota. The overall purpose of the Pathways program was to reduce dietary fat and increase fruit and vegetable consumption and physical activity among third-, fourth-, and fifth-grade students. There were four intervention components: (1) a physical activity curriculum, (2) a health education curriculum, (3) a food service worker training, and (4) family outreach. The intervention arm of the study included twenty-one schools, and there were twenty comparison schools. At the conclusion of the study, no difference was found in body mass index (BMI) between students in the intervention schools and those in the comparison schools. Although not statistically significant, there was a slightly higher rate of physical activity among intervention school students.

Twenty different instruments were used to collect process evaluation data in the Pathways study. Each instrument was designed to assess one or more components of process evaluation—such as *reach, dose,* or *fidelity.* One of the more innovative process evaluation methods used was the Food Service Kitchen Contact Form (Chapter Ten, Appendix A). This form listed thirteen behavior changes that the school food service workers were asked to implement, and the form was completed by a trained nutritionist two or three times per semester. As a result, the evaluators were able to calculate the percentage of food service changes for each year of the study. Another key process measure used in the Pathways study was the number of days that physical education was offered. The goal of the study was a minimum of thirty minutes of physical education at least three times per week. This goal was achieved, and in fact many of the intervention schools were able to offer physical education up to five days per week.

Each of the three studies included in this section of the book reports on the process evaluation of a school-based program. It is interesting that the projects varied in their conceptualization of the components of process evaluation. Each process evaluation was designed to meet the specific characteristics of the interventions they were designed to evaluate. For instance, in Chapter Nine, Davis and colleagues report that one of the key intervention elements was the use of educational materials, including videos, by parents. The researchers therefore assessed the extent to which the educational materials were received and were actually used by parents. Steckler and colleagues had to contend with schools that were in rural areas, were widely dispersed, and required extensive travel time to reach. Their process evaluation had to take this factor into consideration when designing their process evaluation measures. In fact, it will always be the case that the process evaluation methods used in any given study will vary, depending on the unique characteristics of the intervention being evaluated and the environment in which the project is carried out.

These three studies also illustrate the need for researchers to agree on and define the components of process evaluation early in the study planning process. Implementing a consistent approach to process evaluation may prove particularly useful in school settings, where a variety of comprehensive, excellent evaluation efforts have already been mounted, like those described in the following chapters.

CHAPTER EIGHT

Safer Choices, a School-Based HIV, STD, and Pregnancy Prevention Program for Adolescents

Process Evaluation Issues Related to Curriculum Implementation

Christine M. Markham, Karen Basen-Engquist, Karin K. Coyle, Robert C. Addy, and Guy S. Parcel

M any adolescents engage in behaviors that place them at increased risk of contracting sexually transmitted diseases (STD), including the human immunodeficiency virus (HIV). It is estimated that about two-thirds of all STDs in the United States occur among persons under twenty-five years of age, and that almost four million of the new STD cases each year occur among adolescents (U.S. Department of Health and Human Services, 2000). Approximately one-half of all new HIV infections in the United States occur among persons under the age of twenty-five (Centers for Disease Control and Prevention, 2001). In addition, each year, approximately one million teenage girls in the United States experience an unintended pregnancy—the highest teenage pregnancy rate among Western industrialized nations with available data (Card, 1999).

This research was conducted under Contract 200–91–0938 from the Centers for Disease Control and Prevention (CDC). The research team included individuals from the University of Texas's Center for Health Promotion and Prevention Research and its Health Science Center, in Houston, Education Training and Research Associates in California, and the CDC's Division of Adolescent and School Health.

Data from the 1999 Youth Risk Behavior Surveillance Survey (Kann and others, 2000), a biennial national survey of high school students, indicated that nearly two-thirds (65 percent) of high school seniors have had sexual intercourse, and 21 percent of these students reported four or more sexual partners. Among high school students who reported being currently sexually active, 58 percent reported using a condom during their last sexual intercourse, and only 16 percent reported that they or their partner used birth control pills before their last sexual intercourse (Kann and others, 2000).

School-based health education programs have been promoted as an efficient means of preventing risk behaviors that lead to unintended pregnancy, STD, and HIV infection (Kirby and others, 1994; Centers for Disease Control and Prevention, 1996). A growing number of school-based programs have had a significant impact on sexual risk behaviors (Kirby, 2001; Howard and McCabe, 1990; Kirby, Barth, Leland, and Fetro, 1991; Jemmott, Jemmott, and Fong, 1992; Walter and Vaughn, 1993; Main and others, 1994; St. Lawrence, Jefferson, Alleyne, and Brasfield, 1995). Safer Choices, a multicomponent HIV, STD, and pregnancy prevention program for high school students, is one of the few school-based health education programs to have effected a sustained long-term change in sexual behavior (Coyle and others, 1999, 2001; Basen-Engquist and others, 2001).

Safer Choices, based on social cognitive theory (Bandura, 1986), social influences models (McGuire and Papageoris, 1961; McGuire, 1972), and models of school change (Marsh and others, 1988), is designed to promote individual and schoolwide change related to sexual risk-taking behavior. It consists of five components (presented in Table 8.1): (1) school organization, (2) curriculum and staff development, (3) peer resources and school environment, (4) parent education, and (5) school-community linkages (Coyle and others, 1996, 1999). Evaluation study results indicate that approximately one year after the intervention, among students who had sex, Safer Choices students reported a reduction in the frequency of their unprotected sex and in the number of sexual partners with whom they had unprotected sex (Coyle and others, 2001). The program also positively influenced psychosocial variables related to sexual risk taking, including HIV/STD knowledge, condom use attitudes, norms and self-efficacy, the perceived risk of contracting HIV and other STD, and parent-child communication (Coyle and others, 2001; Basen-Engquist and others, 2001). In addition, students in Safer Choices schools reported that their school climate was significantly more supportive of HIV, STD, and pregnancy prevention, compared with that of comparison schools (Basen-Engquist and others, 2001).

The evaluation study included an intensive process evaluation to assess the implementation of program components, as well as individual and school

TABLE 8.1.   THE SAFER CHOICES PROGRAM.

Program Component	Description and Key Activities
School organization	This component featured a School Health Promotion Council involving approximately 8 to 14 teachers, students, parents, administrators, and community representatives. The council planned and conducted program activities.
Curriculum and staff development	The program curriculum featured a sequential, 20-session curriculum for ninth- and tenth-grade students (10 lessons at each grade level), which was implemented by teachers who received training and coaching from project staff. In-class peer leaders helped facilitate selected activities (e.g., small-group role playing).
Peer resources and school environment	This component involved the creation of a Safer Choices peer team or club at every school. Club members meet with an adult peer coordinator to plan and host six types of schoolwide activities designed to alter the normative culture of school (e.g., resource area, small media, group discussions, and drama productions). Project staff members also developed role model stories in which teens told their personal stories and modeled positive behaviors. The stories were printed in a monthly calendar for students.
Parent education	The parent education component featured parent newsletters, parent-child homework activities in the curriculum, parent education activities on campus, and parent involvement on the health promotion council.
School-community linkages	School-community linkage activities included homework assignments in the curriculum that required students to gather information about local resources and services, as well as resource guides that provided a list of local HIV, STD, and pregnancy-related services for adolescents.

characteristics associated with effective implementation. This chapter describes the theoretical framework and study design for the Safer Choices process evaluation. For illustrative purposes, we highlight process evaluation issues related to implementation of the Safer Choices curriculum, which represented the students' most intensive exposure to the program (Basen-Engquist and others, 2001). Examination of curriculum implementation and the factors that influenced it may provide an understanding of how the curriculum contributed to the overall success of the program. In this chapter, we discuss the strengths and limitations of several types of curriculum implementation measures, and we make recommendations for future school-based process evaluation studies.

Background

Safer Choices was evaluated in a randomized controlled trial conducted between 1992 and 1995 and involving ten high schools in Texas and ten high schools in California. Five schools in each state were randomly assigned to the Safer Choices program, and the remaining schools were assigned to a comparison condition. Comparison schools received a basic information-based HIV, STD, and pregnancy prevention curriculum that included five fifty-minute sessions covering information about the consequences of unprotected sex as well as information on contraception, STDs, and HIV (Basen-Engquist and others, 2001).

Overview of the Safer Choices Curriculum

As highlighted in Table 8.1, the Safer Choices program included a twenty-lesson curriculum for ninth- and tenth-grade students (ten lessons at each grade level), designed to affect attitudes, beliefs, social skills, functional knowledge, peer norms, and parent-child communication related to sexual risk-taking behavior. Curriculum activities included role-plays to practice refusal and communication skills, activities to address peer norms about sexual behavior, activities to increase risk perception related to pregnancy, STDs, and HIV infection, a condom demonstration to illustrate correct condom use, and student practice with condoms to enhance condom use skills. In-class peer leaders facilitated selected activities—such as small-group role-playing—and students completed several homework assignments to promote parent-child communication.

The Safer Choices curriculum was implemented during the 1993–94 and 1994–95 school years. For evaluation purposes, schools were asked to implement the curriculum in subject areas that were required instruction for the majority of the ninth- and tenth-grade students. In most schools, these subjects included science, English, physical education, health education, and social studies. Ninth- and tenth-grade teachers who taught these subjects were required to attend teacher training prior to curriculum implementation. During the first year of implementation (1993–94), all identified teachers were required to attend a four-day teacher training course. During the second year of implementation (1994–95), only new teachers were required to attend the full training, and returning teachers attended booster trainings to review teaching strategies and curriculum modifications. Teachers who did not attend the primary trainings received individual training from the project staff at their schools. In addition, teachers received ongoing coaching and support from the project staff during curriculum implementation to help them master the prescribed teaching strategies.

The teacher training design, based on social cognitive theory (Bandura, 1986), provided an overview of the Safer Choices program and an in-depth review of the twenty-lesson curriculum. The training included modeling and rehearsal of prescribed teaching strategies, such as facilitation of student role-plays and small group activities, effective use of peer leaders, and demonstration of proper condom use. On the final day of the training, teachers developed action plans for curriculum implementation and addressed potential barriers to implementation at their school. The teacher trainings were conducted separately for schools in California and Texas by a single training team to ensure consistency across sites. The team included expert trainers from ETR Associates who had experience in sexuality education, as well as members of the project staff.

Evaluation study results indicate that Safer Choices was effective at reducing sexual risk-taking behavior among high school students. Examination of process evaluation data may help us understand why individual components of the multicomponent program were effective. The following sections describe the overall framework for the Safer Choices process evaluation and investigate how aspects of curriculum implementation may have contributed to the program's overall effectiveness.

Process Evaluation

Process evaluation is an important but infrequently conducted component of evaluating the impact of health promotion interventions (Baranowski and Stables, 2000). Process evaluation data may be used to determine whether a program was implemented as intended, thus avoiding what has been termed a Type III error: evaluating a program that has not been adequately implemented (Basch and others, 1985; Resnicow and others, 1998). In school-based studies, process evaluation may also provide an understanding of how teachers use new health education curricula as well as provide insight into the individual- and school-level factors that influence implementation (Basch and others, 1985; Parcel and others, 1991; Rohrbach, Graham, and Hansen, 1993; Smith, McCormick, Steckler, and McLeroy, 1993). Process evaluation also provides useful feedback for program improvement, accountability to funding agencies, and data for conducting dose response and construct validity analyses (Basch and others, 1985; Resnicow and others, 1998).

Safer Choices Process Evaluation Study Design

The Safer Choices process evaluation was designed to assess program implementation, provide feedback to project staff members, and identify factors related to effective program delivery. Theoretical models used in designing, implementing, and analyzing the Safer Choices process evaluation included social cognitive theory (Bandura, 1986) and the concerns-based adoption model (Hall and Hord, 1987). Social cognitive theory holds that behavior is determined by the interaction of personal, environmental, and behavioral influences. Personal factors include cognitions such as attitudes, skills, outcome expectations, value expectancies, and perceived self-efficacy. Environmental factors include any aspect of the environment (social or physical) that supports or discourages a particular behavior, such as influential role models, social or normative support, or the availability of resources (Bandura, 1986).

The concerns-based adoption model proposes that behavior change involves a developmental process during which individuals experience varying concerns at different stages of implementation. For example, prior to implementing a new curriculum, teachers may be concerned primarily about the personal demands imposed on them. However, as they become more involved and comfortable with the curriculum, their concerns focus more on management issues, such as efficiency and scheduling. Ultimately, teachers' concerns will focus primarily on the impact the innovation has on others, such as the students (Hall and Hord, 1987).

These theories were applied in designing the process evaluation for individual program components. For example, constructs from social cognitive theory were used to design the teacher training and to develop questionnaires used to evaluate the training's impact on teachers. In addition to these theoretical models, four implementation factors were used to guide the development of the process evaluation:

1. *Completeness*—the amount of program activities that were implemented (Basen-Engquist and others, 1994)

2. *Fidelity*—the extent to which program activities adhered to recommended content and methods (Basen-Engquist and others, 1994)
3. *Coverage*—the extent to which the target population participated in or received program activities (Rossi and Freeman, 1993)
4. *Reaction*—the target population's satisfaction with and reaction to program activities

Multiple instruments were used to collect process data. Respondents included students, teachers, school administrators, parents, and community organization representatives. Instruments included contact and activity logs, questionnaires, classroom observations, meeting minutes and attendance sheets, in-person interviews, and focus groups. Table 8.2 provides a summary of process evaluation instruments and their purpose, arranged by respondent.

Process evaluation data were used for several purposes: (1) for program revision and dissemination, (2) to provide implementation feedback to school districts and the funding agency, and (3) to enhance the validity of the summative evaluation. For example, feedback from teachers and students following the first year of intervention was used to refine curriculum activities prior to the 1994–95 implementation phase. Results from student curriculum questionnaires were presented to school district personnel and the funding agency prior to the availability of student outcome data as an indication of program satisfaction, and teacher, student, and administrator comments were used to promote program dissemination. The remainder of the chapter illustrates how process evaluation data were used to explore the implementation and effectiveness of curriculum implementation and to assess how the curriculum may have contributed to student outcomes.

Process Evaluation of Curriculum Implementation

Process evaluation objectives for the Safer Choices curriculum implementation were to assess the completeness, fidelity, and coverage of implementation and to assess teacher and student reactions to the curriculum. In addition, exploratory analyses were conducted to assess the effectiveness of the Safer Choices teacher training in increasing cognitive variables related to implementation—such as self-efficacy and outcome expectations, the effect of teacher variables on curriculum implementation, and the extent to which self-reported measures of completeness (teacher curriculum logs) concurred with observational measures. These objectives stemmed from prior research in school-based health promotion.

Several studies have shown that the completeness and fidelity of teacher implementation are associated with student outcomes (Basch and others, 1985; Bush and others, 1989; Tortu and Botvin, 1989; Botvin and others, 1990; Parcel

TABLE 8.2.   PROCESS EVALUATION INSTRUMENTS BY RESPONDENT AND PURPOSE.

Respondent	Process Evaluation Instrument	Purpose of Instrument
Safer Choices Staff		
Project staff	Contact log	Completeness, fidelity, coverage, reaction
Curriculum coaches	Teacher coaching log	Completeness, fidelity, coverage
Classroom observers	Classroom observation form	Completeness, fidelity, coverage
School Personnel		
Site coordinator	Activity log	Completeness, fidelity, coverage
	Interview	Completeness, fidelity, reaction
Peer coordinator	Activity log	Completeness, fidelity, coverage
	Interview	Completeness, fidelity, reaction
Peer resource group	Member questionnaire	Completeness, fidelity, reaction
	Membership forms	Completeness, fidelity, coverage
	Meeting attendance lists	Completeness, fidelity, coverage
	Meeting minutes	Completeness, fidelity, coverage, reaction
School Health Promotion Council members	Member questionnaire	Completeness, fidelity, reaction
	Membership forms	Completeness, fidelity, coverage
	Meeting attendance lists	Completeness, fidelity, coverage
	Meeting minutes	Completeness, fidelity, coverage, reaction
	Exit interview	Reaction
School administrator	Interview	Completeness, fidelity, reaction
Parent representative	Interview	Completeness, fidelity, reaction
Curriculum teachers	*Teacher questionnaire:*	
	Preteacher training	Completeness, fidelity
	Postteacher training	Completeness, fidelity, reaction
	Postimplementation	Completeness, fidelity, reaction
	Curriculum logs	Completeness, fidelity, coverage
	Focus groups	Reaction
Curriculum peer leaders (students)	Pre- and posttraining questionnaire	Completeness, fidelity, coverage, reaction
	Focus groups	Reaction
Students	Homework verification forms	Completeness, fidelity, coverage
	Student curriculum questionnaire	Completeness, reaction
	Focus groups	Reaction
	Student outcome questionnaire	Outcomes, coverage

and others, 1991; Ross and others, 1991; Rohrbach, Graham, and Hansen, 1993). Studies have also shown that teacher implementation may be influenced by internal factors, such as self-efficacy, preparedness, and teaching methods compatibility (Ross and others, 1991; Rohrbach, Graham, and Hansen, 1993), as well as external factors, such as administrative support and turbulence in the school environment (Rohrbach, Graham, and Hansen, 1993; Smith, McCormick, Steckler, and McLeroy, 1993). Teachers who receive preimplementation teacher training, particularly in-person training based on cognitive-behavioral theory, are more likely to implement curricula as intended (Tortu and Botvin, 1989; Perry, Murray, and Griffin, 1990; Parcel and others, 1991; Basen-Engquist and others, 1994; Smith, McCormick, Steckler, and McLeroy, 1993). Finally, previous studies have emphasized the need for closer examination of methodological issues related to curriculum evaluation, especially the degree of correspondence between teacher-reported measures of implementation, such as curriculum logs and interviews, and observational data (Resnicow and others, 1998).

For the process evaluation, completeness was operationalized as the percentage of curriculum activities taught (Basen-Engquist and others, 1994). Fidelity was operationalized as the amount (the percentage for teacher curriculum logs and the mean for classroom observations) of the prescribed teaching strategies that were used. Coverage was operationalized as the percentage of students who participated in curriculum activities. Reaction was operationalized as the percentage of teachers or students who endorsed curriculum satisfaction items on teacher and student questionnaires.

Several instruments were used to assess curriculum implementation. This chapter presents data from teacher questionnaires, curriculum logs, classroom observations, and program exposure items on student questionnaires.

Teacher Questionnaire. The teacher questionnaire included questions on cognitive variables hypothesized to be affected by training and to have an impact on curriculum implementation. The variables, identified from social cognitive theory, included self-efficacy, outcome expectations, student reaction, administrative support, and the perceived importance of teaching strategies (value expectancy). Questions for each construct were stated in reference to each of six activities involved in teaching the curriculum: (1) teaching about sexuality, (2) demonstrating condom use, (3) implementing small group activities, (4) doing role-plays, (5) implementing parent/guardian-student homework activities, and (6) using peer leaders. The response format, excluding perceived importance, was on a 4-point Likert scale ranging from *strongly disagree* to *strongly agree*. Perceived importance items were measured on a 5-point scale, ranging from *not at all important* to *extremely important*. (See the example in Appendix A.)

For illustrative purposes, teacher questionnaire data presented here are from the first year of implementation only (1993–94). The questionnaire was administered before and after teacher training in Fall 1993 and was again administered at postimplementation, following the first semester of curriculum implementation, and the five cognitive scales were administered at each time point. Internal reliability for each scale fell within acceptable ranges at all administrations (Cronbach's alpha for self-efficacy ranged from 0.66 to 0.81; for outcome expectations, from 0.76 to 0.82; for student reaction, from 0.60 to 0.66; for administrative support, from 0.74 to 0.77; and for perceived importance, from 0.66 to 0.80). In addition to these core items, the pretraining questionnaire included ten demographic items, including gender, years of teaching experience, main subject taught, and previous experience in HIV, AIDS, or sexuality education. The postimplementation questionnaire included fifteen items to assess teacher satisfaction with the curriculum. These items were scored on a 5-point response scale ranging from *strongly disagree* to *strongly agree*.

All questionnaires were confidential, and a code number was used to identify each teacher and link data from the pretraining, posttraining and postimplementation administrations. Of the 115 teachers who implemented the curriculum in 1993–94, 111 (97 percent) completed pretraining questionnaires, 107 (93 percent) completed posttraining questionnaires, and sixty-seven (58 percent) completed postimplementation questionnaires.

Curriculum Log. A curriculum log was used to assess the completeness and fidelity with which a teacher implemented the curriculum. For each lesson, teachers were asked to check whether or not they did an activity, whether or not they used teaching strategies critical to the success of the lessons as directed in the curriculum (for example, small group activities, the involvement of peer leaders, role-plays, and large group discussions), and whether or not they made modifications to the lesson. Sample curriculum log pages are included in Appendix B.

The importance of completeness and fidelity in curriculum implementation was emphasized during teacher training. The importance of completing the log was also emphasized and was reiterated throughout curriculum implementation. Teachers completed curriculum logs for both years of the intervention, returning them to the school's site coordinator in a prelabeled envelope. Project staff members also visited schools and collected logs from teachers who had not returned them to the site coordinator. Of the 115 teachers who implemented the curriculum in 1993–94, eighty-two (72 percent) returned curriculum logs, whereas, in 1994–95, eighty-two out of 112 teachers (73 percent) returned curriculum logs.

Teacher Observation Form. Classroom observations were used as an independent method of assessing the completeness and fidelity of curriculum instruction, and outside observers were trained to monitor two to three key lessons conducted by each teacher. These lessons were chosen because they included at least three of the following teaching strategies: role-plays, small group activities, the use of peer leaders, and large group discussions. Lessons 2, 3, and 7, all focusing on refusal skills, were observed in 1993–94. Lessons 5 and 6, focusing on refusal skills, and Lesson 7, focusing on correct and consistent condom use, were observed in 1994–95.

The observation instrument was developed using previous classroom observation instruments as a guide (see, for example, Kerr, Kent, and Lam, 1985). It included a checklist of activities conducted during the lesson to measure the completeness of implementation. Each lesson was divided into four or more subactivities or *phases* to measure fidelity of implementation, each phase was broken down into the individual steps required to teach a behavioral strategy effectively, and each step was rated on a scale of 0 to 2, with 0 corresponding with "did not complete the activity/criteria at all," 1 corresponding with "partially completed the activity/criteria," and 2 corresponding with "fully completed the activity/criteria." Fidelity was calculated using the mean phase score for each lesson observed. Sample pages from a teacher observation form are included in Appendix C.

Observers completed approximately ten hours of training prior to data collection. The training process was developed to ensure the reliability of observations. Observers practiced coding curriculum implementation by using videotaped lessons. During the training, the coding was discussed and discrepancies were resolved to help ensure reliability. Interrater reliability was calculated and observers who had interrater reliability estimates below 0.75 were given additional practice and asked to rate a second tape for reliability. Any observers who did not reach interrater reliability estimates of 0.75 following the extra practice were not used for data collection.

All observations were scheduled in advance with teachers' permission. A consent and scheduling form was used to obtain teachers' preferred dates for observation as well as their consent for conducting the observations. Of the 115 teachers who implemented the curriculum in 1993–94, seventy-seven (68 percent) were observed conducting one or more lessons. In 1994–95, the number of observations was reduced to decrease the burden on teachers and project staff members. Observations were required for teachers who were new to the curriculum and also for tenth-grade teachers because activities in the tenth-grade curriculum were different from those of the previous year. In 1994–95, forty-five out of eighty-eight teachers (51 percent) were observed conducting one or more lessons.

Student Questionnaire. The student questionnaire used to measure outcome variables also included a section to assess students' exposure to selected curriculum activities, including skits on *how to say no* and talking to one's partner about condom use, class members modeling how to say no, condom demonstrations, parent-child homework, and presentations by HIV-positive persons. Students in intervention and comparison schools completed program exposure items late in Spring 1994 and 1995. A total of 3,560 students (92 percent of the cohort) completed student exposure items in 1994; 3,120 students (81 percent) completed student exposure items in 1995.

These four instruments—teacher questionnaires, curriculum logs, classroom observations, and student questionnaires—represent the primary methods used to assess curriculum implementation. The following section describes the analytical methods used to examine these process data and presents results for each of the process evaluation objectives related to curriculum implementation.

Analyses and Results

The primary objectives of the curriculum process evaluation were to assess the completeness and fidelity of implementation, coverage, and participant reaction, and to examine exploratory research questions related to implementation. One hundred and fifteen teachers implemented the curriculum in 1993–94, and 112 implemented it in 1994–95. Almost 60 percent of the teachers who implemented the curriculum in the first year also implemented it in the second year. The majority of teachers who did not implement the curriculum in the second year were not able to because they changed subject areas or because they changed schools.

Demographic information for teachers who attended teacher training in 1993 is presented in Table 8.3. Teachers reported instructing a wide range of subjects, which resulted primarily from curriculum placement to maximize ninth- and tenth-grade coverage. These subjects were collapsed into five categories: (1) language arts—such as English, German, modern languages, reading, and theater arts, (2) physical science—such as biology, chemistry, physics, and environmental science, (3) health—such as general health and physical education, (4) social sciences—such as government science, economics, history, home economics, social studies, U.S. history, and world history, and (5) other subjects—such as special education and typing.

Of the teachers who reported demographic information, 54 percent were female, 65 percent were Caucasian, 41 percent primarily taught physical science disciplines, 24 percent taught language arts, and 12 percent taught health or physical education. Sixty percent took one or more health courses in college, 13 percent either majored or minored in health education, and 65 percent knew or had known

TABLE 8.3. DEMOGRAPHICS OF TEACHERS ATTENDING TEACHER TRAINING IN FALL 1993.

	Combined Teachers in Texas and California	
	N	%
Gender		
Male	57	46.0
Female	67	54.0
Race/Ethnicity		
White (non-Hispanic)	80	64.5
African American	23	18.6
Hispanic	9	7.3
Asian	4	3.2
Other	8	6.5
Subject Area Taught		
Language arts	29	24.2
Physical science	49	40.8
Health	14	11.7
Social sciences	21	17.5
Other	7	5.8
Highest Completed Degree		
Bachelor's	60	49.6
Master's	59	48.8
Doctorate	2	1.7
College Health Education Background		
Majored in health education	10	8.2
Minored in health education	6	4.9
Had ≥ 1 health course	73	59.8
None	33	27.1
Know/Knew Person with AIDS/HIV		
Yes	81	64.8
No	44	35.2
Prior AIDS/HIV/Sexuality Teaching Experience		
Yes	53	42.4
No	72	57.6
Perceived Fit of AIDS/HIV/Sexuality with Other Topics Taught		
Excellent fit	57	46.0
Fair fit	37	30.0
Poor fit	17	13.7
No fit	13	10.5

someone living with HIV or AIDS. Fifty-eight percent had no previous experience teaching HIV or sexuality education, and 46 percent felt that HIV/AIDS or sexuality education was an excellent fit with other topics that they taught. Years of teaching experience ranged from 0 to 43, with a mean value of 14.4 years ($SD = 10.52$).

Completeness and Fidelity of Implementation

The completeness and fidelity of curriculum implementation were assessed by using two independent methods: teacher-reported data from the teacher curriculum logs and observational data from the classroom observations. The curriculum logs provided a measure of implementation across all curriculum lessons. The observations provided an assessment of implementation for selected curriculum lessons.

Curriculum Logs. Using data from the curriculum logs, completeness was measured by the percentage of curriculum activities that teachers reported conducting. Fidelity was measured by the percentage of prescribed teaching strategies (role-plays, small group work, large group discussion, and the use of peer leaders) reported by teachers during the curriculum. Not all teachers completed information for every lesson; therefore, teachers who reported information for at least two-thirds of the curriculum (seven out of ten lessons) were included in the analyses. In 1993–94, completeness data were analyzed for eighty out of eighty-two teachers (70 percent of all curriculum teachers) who returned logs, and fidelity data were analyzed for seventy-one out of eighty-two (62 percent of all curriculum teachers). In 1994–95, completeness data were analyzed for seventy-one out of eighty-two teachers (63 percent of all curriculum teachers) who returned logs, and fidelity data were analyzed for fifty-seven out of eighty-two (51 percent of all curriculum teachers). Results are presented in Table 8.4.

With regard to completeness, in 1993–94, Texas teachers reported completing 90 percent of the prescribed activities, and California teachers reported completing 84 percent. In 1994–95, the percentage rose to 93 percent in Texas and 95 percent in California. With regard to fidelity, in 1993–94, Texas teachers reported implementing 88 percent of the required teaching strategies, whereas California teachers reported implementing 80 percent. In 1994–95, the percentages changed to 81 percent and 83 percent in Texas and California, respectively. These data suggest that the completeness of curriculum implementation was relatively high across sites and throughout the intervention.

Classroom Observations. Using data from the classroom observations, completeness was measured by calculating the percentage of required activities conducted for each lesson observed. Fidelity was measured by calculating the mean phase score for each lesson observed. Results are presented in Table 8.5.

TABLE 8.4. COMPLETENESS AND FIDELITY OF CURRICULUM IMPLEMENTATION, MEASURED BY TEACHER CURRICULUM LOGS.

	Texas			*California*		
Completeness	N	M (SD) %	Range %	N	M (SD) %	Range %
1993–1994	46	90 (11.2)	38–100	34	84 (11.4)	57–97
1994–1995	34	93 (7.4)	77–100	37	95 (6.7)	71–100
Fidelity						
1993–1994	37	88 (15.4)	38–100	34	80 (13.0)	44–100
1994–1995	27	81 (16.1)	49–100	30	83 (13.2)	47–100

TABLE 8.5. COMPLETENESS AND FIDELITY OF CURRICULUM IMPLEMENTATION, MEASURED BY CLASSROOM OBSERVATIONS.

	Texas			*California*		
Completeness **1993–1994**	N	M (SD) %	Range %	N	M (SD) %	Range %
Lesson 2	14	90 (0.1)	60–100	42	99 (0.1)	80–100
Lesson 3	13	74 (0.3)	33–100	21	82 (0.2)	33–100
Lesson 7	10	70 (0.3)	00–100	4	94 (0.1)	75–100
1994–1995						
Lesson 5	7	79 (0.2)	50–100	16	91 (0.2)	50–100
Lesson 6	9	81 (0.2)	50–100	16	93 (0.1)	67–100
Lesson 7	12	82 (0.1)	60–100	2	80 (0.3)	60–100
Fidelity **1993–1994**	N	M (SD)	Range	N	M (SD)	Range
Lesson 2	17	1.1 (0.4)	0.2–1.8	41	1.3 (0.3)	0.8–1.8
Lesson 3	17	1.0 (0.5)	0.2–1.7	26	1.1 (0.4)	0.3–1.7
Lesson 7	11	0.7 (0.4)	0.1–1.3	3	1.2 (0.3)	0.9–1.5
1994–1995						
Lesson 5	9	1.4 (0.4)	0.8–1.8	13	1.4 (0.3)	0.6–1.9
Lesson 6	9	1.2 (0.4)	0.8–1.8	14	1.3 (0.3)	0.6–1.8
Lesson 7	12	1.5 (0.4)	0.9–2.0	2	1.4 (0.1)	1.4–1.5

Completeness data indicate that teachers taught between 70 and 99 percent of required activities in 1993–94, and between 79 and 91 percent in 1994–95. Fidelity data, measured on a scale from 0 to 2, indicate that fidelity of implementation for the three observed lessons ranged across sites from mean phase scores of 0.7 to 1.3 in 1993–94 and 1.2 to 1.5 in 1994–95. These data suggest that the completeness and fidelity of implementation was moderate in 1993–94 and relatively high in 1994–95. Fidelity of implementation—that is, the degree to which teachers implemented activities as prescribed and without modification—appears to have increased at both sites in 1994–95, suggesting that teachers were more comfortable with the curriculum. However, because of low sample sizes, this effect could not be tested for significance.

Table 8.5 indicates that the number of observations completed for Lesson 7 in both years was low. This resulted primarily from the observation protocol, which stated that teachers should be observed conducting two of the three key lessons. Observations tended to be completed on the earlier lessons (Lessons 2 and 3 in 1993–94 and Lessons 5 and 6 in 1994–95) to identify teachers in need of additional coaching.

Coverage

Coverage data were used to provide an estimate of the percentage of students in Safer Choices program schools who participated in selected curriculum activities, such as role-plays, condom demonstrations, a presentation by an HIV-positive person, and parent-child homework activities. Coverage data therefore provide a useful means of evaluating student exposure to an intervention. The data also provide an estimate of the percentage of students in comparison schools who were exposed to similar types of activities. Coverage was assessed by using program exposure items included in the Safer Choices student questionnaire. Results are presented in Table 8.6 and indicate relatively high participation among students in the Safer Choices schools. They also indicate that a smaller proportion of students in comparison schools participated in similar activities at their schools. For example, in 1993–94, 79 percent of Safer Choices students in Texas and 89 percent of those in California reported participating in skits on how to say no, compared with 17 percent and 10 percent of comparison school students in Texas and California, respectively. Similarly, 75 percent of Safer Choices students in Texas and 92 percent of those in California reported seeing a condom demonstration, compared with 25 percent and 21 percent of comparison school students in Texas and California, respectively. Results are comparable for 1994–95.

Teacher Satisfaction

Factors related to teacher satisfaction following curriculum implementation were identified by using data from the 1993–94 postimplementation teacher questionnaires ($n = 67$; 58 percent of teachers). Subscales were formed by using an exploratory factor analysis with oblique rotation on fifteen items from the

TABLE 8.6. PERCENTAGE OF STUDENTS WHO PARTICIPATED IN SELECTED ACTIVITIES, MEASURED BY STUDENT QUESTIONNAIRES.

| | Comparison Schools | | | | Safer Choices Schools | | | |
| | Texas | | California | | Texas | | California | |
	N	% Yes	N	% Yes	N	% Yes	N	% Yes
1993–1994 Variable								
Do skits on "How to say No"	637	17	1,079	10	753	79	1,086	89
Condom demonstration	638	25	1,075	21	754	75	1,072	92
Talk with students your age about sex	639	37	1,080	34	755	70	1,085	66
Do skits on talking with partner	636	18	1,083	8	751	72	1,086	83
Classmates teach "How to say No"	636	20	1,076	12	754	75	1,078	80
Homework on talking with parent	635	16	1,075	14	754	64	1,073	77
Homework on buying condoms	636	6	1,080	5	755	35	1,072	52
See video about teens with HIV	637	45	1,075	78	754	65	1,070	91
1994–1995 Variable								
Do skits on "How to say No"	531	15	1,003	9	615	66	966	78
Condom demonstration	531	26	1,001	14	614	67	961	82
Do skits on talking with partner	533	12	1,003	8	617	64	963	74
Classmates teach "How to say No"	533	17	1,002	9	615	65	959	75
Homework on talking with parent	533	11	995	11	609	52	963	71
See video about condom use	533	36	999	26	612	54	953	68
HIV+ speaker	532	21	998	16	614	69	957	77
Learn about STD & pregnancy testing	532	46	997	27	611	67	951	78

questionnaire (Appendix A: items 31–45). The initial factor analysis retained three factors that accounted for slightly over 50 percent of the total variance. One item (item 42: "The content on how to prevent HIV, STD, and pregnancy seemed relevant to most of my students") had loadings of 0.33 to 0.36 across all three factors. Consequently, this item was omitted and the remaining items were refactored. Results are presented in Table 8.7.

The first factor, labeled *satisfaction with curriculum content*, consisted of seven items focusing on the curriculum's age appropriateness, cultural sensitivity, student reaction, role-play realism, and student involvement (items 33, 37–39, and 43–45). This factor had a Cronbach's alpha of 0.81. The second factor, labeled *satisfaction with materials and preparation*, consisted of three items focusing on organization and format of the curriculum, as well as adequacy of teacher preparation (items 31, 32, 40), and had a Cronbach's alpha of 0.67. The third factor, labeled *problems with student involvement*, consisted of two items focusing on the difficulties of getting

TABLE 8.7.   LOADINGS FROM EXPLORATORY FACTOR ANALYSIS (WITH OBLIQUE ROTATION) USING TEACHER SATISFACTION ITEMS FROM POSTIMPLEMENTATION TEACHER QUESTIONNAIRES (*N* = 67).

Factor 1: Satisfaction with curriculum content (Cronbach's alpha = 0.81)	
Q33: Role-plays were realistic	0.823
Q37: Students participated in large group discussion	0.516
Q38: Students responsive to peer leaders	0.649
Q39: Student activities appropriate for grade level	0.722
Q43: Curriculum content culturally sensitive	0.610
Q44: No problems implementing curriculum	0.537
Q45: Students responded positively to curriculum	0.572
Factor 2: Satisfaction with curriculum materials and preparation (Cronbach's alpha = 0.67)	
Q31: Curriculum clearly written	0.789
Q32: Curriculum format easy to follow	0.756
Q40: Preparation adequate for teaching curriculum	0.629
Factor 3: Problems with student involvement (Cronbach's alpha = 0.66)	
Q34: Difficulty involving students in role-plays	0.615
Q35: Difficulty involving students in small group work	0.689
Single-Item Factors	
Q36: Discomfort in presenting curriculum content	
Q41: Curriculum should contain more on abstinence	

students involved in activities (items 34 and 35). The Cronbach's alpha for this factor was 0.66. Item 36 ("I was uncomfortable presenting the content of the curriculum") and item 41 ("This curriculum should include more content about abstinence") were initially considered as contributing to factor 3; however, low factor loadings relative to items 34 and 35 raised questions about their retention. Reliability of the subscale with and without the items was examined. The reliability dropped to unacceptable levels when items 36 and/or 41 were retained on factor 3 (Cronbach's alpha dropped from 0.66 to 0.52 with item 35, to 0.41 with item 41, and to 0.46 with both items). In addition, the content of these two items appeared to represent qualitatively different constructs, compared with items 34 and 35. Consequently, items 36 and 41 were retained as single-item factors.

Table 8.8 presents mean values for teacher satisfaction scales and retained individual items by site. The items were scored on a 5-point scale, with 1 corresponding to *strongly disagree* and 5 corresponding to *strongly agree*. Overall, teachers were generally satisfied with curriculum content [$M = 4.0$ ($SD = 0.60$) in Texas, $M = 3.5$ ($SD = 0.69$) in California], and with curriculum materials and preparation [$M = 4.1$ ($SD = 0.70$) in Texas, $M = 4.0$ ($SD = 0.54$) in California]. They also reported little discomfort presenting the curriculum content [$M = 1.8$ ($SD = 1.02$) in Texas, $M = 1.9$ ($SD = 1.14$) in California] and did not appear to have difficulty getting students involved [$M = 2.2$ ($SD = 0.97$) in Texas, $M = 1.9$ ($SD = 0.85$) in California]. Teachers were generally noncommittal or only in slight agreement about the need to include more information about abstinence [$M = 3.4$ ($SD = 1.29$) in Texas, $M = 3.0$ ($SD = 1.17$) in California].

TABLE 8.8.   TEACHER SATISFACTION AFTER CURRICULUM
IMPLEMENTATION, MEASURED BY FOLLOW-UP TEACHER
QUESTIONNAIRES, 1994.

Variable	Texas			California		
	N	M (SD)	Range	N	M (SD)	Range
Satisfaction with curriculum content	46	4.0 (0.60)	3.0–5.0	30	3.5 (0.69)	1.8–4.9
Satisfaction with materials and preparation	46	4.1 (0.70)	2.3–5.0	30	4.0 (0.54)	3.0–5.0
Problems with student involvement	46	2.2 (0.97)	1.0–5.0	30	2.6 (0.85)	1.0–4.0
Discomfort in presenting content	46	1.8 (1.02)	1.0–5.0	30	1.9 (1.14)	1.0–5.0
Need for more content on abstinence	46	3.4 (1.29)	1.0–5.0	30	3.0 (1.17)	1.0–5.0

These data indicate that, in general, teachers were satisfied with curriculum content and preparation and had a positive experience during curriculum implementation.

Impact of Teacher Training on Teacher Attitudes

One of the exploratory research questions focused on the impact of training on teacher attitudes related to curriculum implementation. The preimplementation training was designed to have an impact on the cognitive variables identified by social cognitive theory as being critical to effective implementation. Data from teacher questionnaires (pretraining, posttraining, and postimplementation) were examined to assess the impact of teacher training on selected cognitive variables immediately following training (posttraining) and after curriculum implementation (postimplementation).

Mean scores for each variable were calculated for each set of questionnaires. Scores were calculated for all subjects who responded to at least four out of six items for each scale. Dependent t-tests were conducted to assess the impact of teacher training on cognitive variables immediately following training and after curriculum implementation. Difference scores between posttraining and pretraining, postimplementation, and posttraining were calculated and tested.

Table 8.9 presents mean values for teacher cognitive variables reported after pre- and posttraining and postcurriculum implementation in 1993–94, together with difference score calculations. The comparison of pre- and posttraining data indicates that teacher training had a positive impact on teachers' self-efficacy ($t_{104} = 3.61$; $p < 0.001$), outcome expectations ($t_{100} = 4.05$; $p < 0.001$), perception of student reactions ($t_{97} = 3.47$; $p < 0.001$), and importance of teaching strategies ($t_{100} = 3.33$; $p < 0.01$).

The comparison of posttraining and postimplementation data indicates that curriculum implementation itself did not have a significant impact on these cognitive variables during the implementation period. No significant difference between posttraining and postimplementation scores were observed for self-efficacy, outcome expectations, perceived student reaction, or the importance of teaching strategies. However, teachers' perception of administrative support did increase following implementation ($t_{59} = 4.06$; $p < 0.001$).

Impact of Teacher Variables on Curriculum Implementation

The extent to which individual teacher variables influenced curriculum implementation was assessed by using 1993–94 data from posttraining teacher questionnaires and classroom observations. Bivariate analyses were conducted to assess

TABLE 8.9. TEACHER ATTITUDES MEASURED BY TEACHER QUESTIONNAIRES (PRE- AND POSTTRAINING AND POSTIMPLEMENTATION) AND DIFFERENCE SCORES BETWEEN POSTTRAINING/PRETRAINING QUESTIONNAIRES AND POSTIMPLEMENTATION/POSTTRAINING QUESTIONNAIRES.

Teacher Attitude	Pretraining			Posttraining			Postimplementation		
	N	M (SD)	Range	N	M (SD)	Range	N	M (SD)	Range
Self-efficacy	125	3.2 (0.49)	1.8–4.0	107	3.3 (0.44)	1.2–4.0	76	3.4 (0.40)	2.3–4.0
Outcomes expectations	122	3.2 (0.45)	2.0–4.0	106	3.4 (0.44)	1.5–4.0	75	3.3 (0.45)	2.3–4.0
Student reaction	122	3.0 (0.41)	1.8–4.0	103	3.1 (0.35)	2.3–3.8	76	3.1 (0.42)	1.8–4.0
Administrative support	121	3.2 (0.43)	1.8–4.0	104	3.3 (0.38)	1.8–4.0	74	3.5 (0.39)	2.7–4.0
Importance of teaching strategies	122	3.7 (0.71)	1.8–5.0	106	3.9 (0.63)	1.7–5.0	76	3.9 (0.57)	2.3–5.0

Teacher Attitude	Posttraining/Pretraining Difference				Postimplementation/Posttraining Difference			
	N	M (SD)	Range	t	N	M (SD)	Range	t
Self-efficacy	105	0.2 (0.49)	−2.8–1.3	3.61***	64	0.1 (0.45)	−1.1–2.2	1.07
Outcomes expectations	101	0.2 (0.47)	−2.5–1.3	4.05***	62	−0.1 (0.48)	−1.3–1.3	−1.19
Student reaction	98	0.2 (0.42)	−1.5–1.2	3.47***	61	−0.0 (0.45)	−1.3–0.8	−0.28
Administrative support	99	0.1 (0.41)	−1.5–1.2	1.78	60	0.2 (0.42)	−1.0–1.8	4.06***
Importance of teaching strategies	101	0.2 (0.72)	−3.3–1.8	3.33**	63	−0.0 (0.64)	−1.3–2.7	−0.13

*$p < .05$

**$p < .01$

***$p < .001$

the association between teachers' cognitive and demographic variables regarding the completeness and fidelity of the implementation, as measured for Lesson 2. This lesson was selected because it had the single largest number of observations ($n = 50$). The cognitive variables examined were self-efficacy, outcome expectations, the perceived administrative support, the perceived student reaction, and the perceived importance of teaching strategies. The demographic variables examined were gender, race/ethnicity, the highest degree completed, college health education background, years of teaching experience, having known or not having known a person with HIV or AIDS, prior experience in HIV or sexuality education, and the perceived fit of HIV or sexuality education with other topics taught. Pearson correlation coefficients were first calculated and variables that were significant at the $p < 0.05$ level were retained for multivariate regression models.

Table 8.10 presents correlations significant at $p < 0.05$. Among demographic variables, only gender was associated with curriculum completeness ($r = 0.29$). Female teachers, compared with male teachers, were observed conducting a greater number of prescribed activities. Among teacher cognitive variables, only administrative support was positively associated with curriculum completeness ($r = 0.37$). Teachers who perceived greater support from their school administration regarding curriculum implementation conducted a greater number of required activities. Gender ($r = 0.40$) and knowing or having known someone with HIV or AIDS ($r = 0.33$) were positively associated with observed fidelity of implementation. Length of teaching experience was negatively associated with fidelity ($r = -0.47$). None of the cognitive variables was associated with fidelity at $p < 0.05$.

TABLE 8.10. PEARSON CORRELATION COEFFICIENTS FOR SELECTED TEACHER VARIABLES RELATED TO COMPLETENESS AND FIDELITY OF CURRICULUM IMPLEMENTATION FOR LESSON 2, 1993–94.

	N	r
Completeness		
Gender	50	0.29*
Administrative support	43	0.37*
Fidelity		
Gender	49	0.40**
Years of teaching experience	49	−0.47***
Know someone with HIV or AIDS	49	0.33*

*$p < .05$

**$p < .01$

***$p < .001$

When gender and administrative support were entered into a regression model to examine their impact on curriculum completeness, gender no longer remained significant at $p < 0.05$. Administrative support alone explained 13.9 percent of the observed variance for curriculum completeness in Lesson 2. A significant interaction between gender and administrative support was not observed. Gender, years of teaching experience, and knowing or having known someone with HIV or AIDS were entered into a multivariate regression model to determine what percentage of curriculum fidelity could be explained by key demographic variables. These three variables remained significant in the multivariate model (years of teaching experience and knowing someone with HIV or AIDs at $p < 0.02$, gender at $p < 0.007$), and together explained 39 percent of the observed variance in the Lesson 2 curriculum fidelity [$F_{(3, 45)} = 9.69, p < 0.0001$]. Teachers who were female, knew someone with HIV or AIDS, and had fewer years of teaching experience were more likely to implement the curriculum as prescribed.

Comparison of Teacher Curriculum Logs and Classroom Observations

The final exploratory research question addressed in the process evaluation was to examine the extent to which teacher reports of implementation agreed with observation data as a measure of curriculum implementation completeness. McNemar's test for correlated proportions (exact test) was used to assess the reliability of self-reported teacher curriculum logs, compared with classroom observations as a measure of the completeness of implementation. Data from 1994–95 teacher curriculum logs and classroom observations were used for these calculations because inconsistent data entry procedures precluded us from linking 1993–94 curriculum logs and observations at the individual teacher level.

Table 8.11 presents a comparison of implementation data from self-reported teacher curriculum logs and independent classroom observations for three lessons observed in 1994–95 (Lessons 5, 6, and 7). To be included in the analysis, teachers had to have returned a curriculum log and to have completed at least one classroom observation. This reduced the sample to thirty-four teachers (30 percent of teachers who taught in 1994–95). Curriculum logs and classroom observations were in agreement that 86 percent of the required activities were conducted and that 3 percent of the required activities were not conducted (homework review, preparation for the next class, and showing a video about condoms). Compared with classroom observations, curriculum logs provided discrepant reports of implementation for 12.4 percent of the activities. Of these discrepant reports, curriculum logs overreported 8.6 percent of the completed activities, compared with classroom observations, and they underreported 3.8 percent of the completed activities. The activities most likely to be overreported by teachers included the use

TABLE 8.11. COMPLETENESS OF CURRICULUM IMPLEMENTATION: COMPARISON OF TEACHER SELF-REPORT FROM CURRICULUM LOGS AND CLASSROOM OBSERVATIONS, 1994–95 (N = 34 PAIRS).

	Teacher and Observer Agree Activity Taught	Teacher and Observer Agree Activity Not Taught	Teacher Reports Activity—Activity Not Observed	Teacher Does Not Report Activity—Activity Observed
Lesson 5: Homework review	12	2	2	0
Lesson 5: Review of refusal skills	17	0	0	0
Lesson 5: Peer leader demonstration	13	0	3	0
Lesson 5: Student role-plays	16	0	0	1
Lesson 6: Reviewing refusal skills	18	0	1	0
Lesson 6: Peer leader demonstration	16	0	2	1
Lesson 6: Student role-plays	17	0	0	1
Lesson 6: Unscripted role-plays	13	0	1	2
Lesson 6: Preparation for next class	11	1	3	1
Lesson 7: Review of contraceptive methods	8	0	0	0
Lesson 7: Video on condoms	3	2	2	1
Lesson 7: Condom demonstration	7	0	1	0
Lesson 7: Student practice condom use	7	0	1	0
Totals	158 (85.9%)	5 (2.9%)	16* (8.6%)	7* (3.8%)

*χ^2_1 = 2.78, not significant at $p \leq 0.05$

of peer leaders, preparation for the next class, homework review, and showing a video about condoms. The activities most likely to be underreported included role-plays, peer leader demonstrations, and showing a video about condoms. However, McNemar's exact test indicated that the difference between the over- and under-reporting of activities was not significant at $p < 0.05$. This suggests that teacher self-reported curriculum logs neither significantly over- nor underreported activities and that the logs provided a reliable method for evaluating the completeness of curriculum implementation, compared with independent classroom observations. This test was not conducted on fidelity measures because of incongruent response formats between curriculum logs and observation reports.

Discussion

The Safer Choices evaluation study included an intensive process evaluation designed to assess program implementation and examine how individual intervention contributed to the program's success. In this chapter, we have focused on process evaluation issues related to curriculum implementation, as this represented students' most intensive exposure to the program (Basen-Engquist and others, 2001).

Process evaluation data suggest that the Safer Choices curriculum was implemented with a relatively high degree of completeness, fidelity, and coverage. In addition, teacher reactions to curriculum materials, content, and training were generally positive. Several factors may have contributed to these results. First, all schools were required to appoint a site coordinator and school health promotion council, which included teachers and school administrators, to plan and oversee program implementation at their school. Individual teachers were also required to complete implementation plans during teacher training. Previous studies have shown that involving teachers in curriculum planning and appointing a school site coordinator have a positive impact on the implementation of school-based curricula (Parcel and others, 1991; Smith, McCormick, Steckler, and McLeroy, 1993).

Second, consistent with previous research (Perry, Murray, and Griffin, 1990; Rohrbach, Graham, and Hansen, 1993; Smith, McCormick, Steckler, and McLeroy, 1993), positive administrative support influenced implementation. Among curriculum teachers, perceived administrative support increased significantly following the first semester of implementation and was one of the few variables to predict curriculum completeness. Student perceptions regarding the supportiveness of the school climate for HIV, STD, and pregnancy prevention also increased (Basen-Engquist and others, 2001). Administrative support may be especially important for the implementation of sexuality education curricula because of the sensitive nature of their content.

Third, prior to implementation, Safer Choices teachers received four days of intensive training, which included modeling and the practice of key teaching strategies. Results show that teacher training had a significant impact on the enhancement of cognitive variables, such as self-efficacy and outcome expectations. Previous studies have shown that preimplementation training—in particular training based on social cognitive theory—has a positive impact on curriculum implementation (Tortu and Botvin, 1989; Perry, Murray, and Griffin, 1990; Parcel and others, 1991; Ross and others, 1991; Smith, McCormick, Steckler, and McLeroy, 1993; Basen-Engquist and others, 1994).

Certain demographic variables (being female, knowing or having known someone with HIV/AIDS, having fewer years of teaching experience) were more likely to predict fidelity of implementation than teacher cognitive variables, with the exception of perceived administrative support. Having fewer years of teaching experience may represent a generational factor, in that less experienced teachers are generally younger and may be more comfortable implementing sexuality education curricula. In addition, teachers who have been more recently trained may be more comfortable with the types of teaching strategies used in the curriculum (such as role-plays and peer leaders), which are a departure from more traditional didactic methods. In contrast with other studies, a background in health education was not a prerequisite for complete implementation (Smith, McCormick, Steckler, and McLeroy, 1993; Ross and others, 1991). This indicates that teachers in other disciplines can successfully implement HIV prevention curricula with adequate training and support.

Lessons Learned About Process Evaluation

Experience in developing and implementing the Safer Choices process evaluation provided some insights into the strengths and limitations of selected curriculum implementation measures.

LESSON 1. *The use of teacher logs is reliable but can be improved.*

Although teacher curriculum logs appear to provide a reliable, cost-effective method of documenting curriculum implementation, several steps can be taken to improve reporting compliance. Teachers were informed at teacher training of the purpose and importance of completing logs and were periodically reminded during implementation. And collecting logs at intervals throughout implementation, rather than at the end of the curriculum, may have increased their reliability. Resnicow and others (1998) also recommend offering incentives for the completion of logs and assuring teachers that there will be no adverse consequences if they report low implementation rates.

LESSON 2. *The selective use of classroom observations is recommended.*

Classroom observations provide a valuable, independent assessment of the completeness and fidelity of implementation. However, some curriculum teachers may perceive them as intrusive and judgmental, and they may alter their implementation in response to the observation. Informing teachers of the purpose and nature of observations during teacher training, scheduling observations at the teacher's convenience, and providing positive feedback following observation helped alleviate such perceptions. Observations are also resource-intensive, as they require additional personnel and training. Selecting lessons for observation that include critical teaching strategies provides a cost-effective method of assessing the completeness and fidelity of curriculum implementation.

LESSON 3. *Student exposure is difficult to assess.*

The inclusion of program exposure items on student outcome questionnaires—the approach used in Safer Choices—provides an efficient method of measuring curriculum participation. However, it is often impossible to assess whether students took part in specific activities in the context of the curriculum under study or in the context of another program. Having teachers complete student attendance lists for each lesson, possibly incorporated into the curriculum log, could provide a more accurate method of documenting student exposure to individual activities. However, with large samples, the data entry and management may be tedious.

LESSON 4. *Process evaluation is resource-intensive.*

The Safer Choices process evaluation was extremely intensive, collecting data from multiple sources via multiple instruments. In retrospect, some instruments were completed sporadically and provided less information than others—such as homework verification forms. Administering multiple instruments and ensuring that all were completed at comparable levels across schools also required substantial effort from the research staff. In developing process evaluation protocols, investigators are advised to prioritize the research questions they wish to address in order to minimize the burden on subjects and staff members.

LESSON 5. *Multiple links between process evaluation datasets are recommended.*

Finally, in collecting and entering data from various process evaluation instruments and sources, steps should be taken to ensure that information from disparate datasets are linked. For example, in the current analysis, it was not possible to link teacher questionnaire data directly to student outcome data, making it impossible to assess the impact of the curriculum component alone on individual student behavior change. We attempted to do this by asking students to write on the student questionnaire the name of the teacher they had for HIV education, but in retrospect, this approach yielded too much missing or incorrect information.

Areas for Further Research

Although this chapter provides an assessment of how well the Safer Choices curriculum was implemented, further research is needed to assess how this component interacted with other Safer Choices components to produce positive student outcomes. For example, were students who participated in curriculum activities more likely to participate in schoolwide events hosted by the peer resource groups? Were parents whose children received the curriculum more likely to participate in parent education activities? Such an investigation would provide a greater understanding of the dynamics generated by a multicomponent program. Further research is also needed to understand how demographic and environmental factors mediate the influence of teacher variables—such as self-efficacy and outcome expectations—on curriculum implementation. More research is also needed to assess the reliability of common curriculum evaluation instruments—in particular, teacher logs and student exposure measures.

Conclusion

Process evaluation data presented in this chapter indicate that the Safer Choices curriculum was implemented with a high degree of completeness, fidelity, and coverage. In addition, teachers reported high satisfaction with curriculum content and training, and they reported positive administrative support for curriculum implementation. These factors may help explain how the curriculum contributed to overall program success. This chapter also provides a model for designing, implementing, and analyzing a process evaluation to assess the implementation of a school-based health education curriculum, and it provides some lessons learned regarding process evaluation methodology. The instruments and process evaluation model presented here may be adapted to other school-based health education areas.

References

Bandura, A. *Social Foundations of Thought and Action: A Social Cognitive Theory.* Englewood Cliffs, N.J.: Prentice-Hall, 1986.

Baranowski, T., and Stables, G. "Process Evaluation of the 5-a-Day Projects." *Health Education and Behavior,* 2000, *27*(2), 157–166.

Basch, C. E., and others. "Avoiding Type III Errors in Health Education Program Evaluations: A Case Study." *Health Education Quarterly,* 1985, *12*(4), 315–331.

Basen-Engquist, K., and others. "The Effect of Two Types of Teacher Training on Implementation of Smart Choices: A Tobacco Prevention Curriculum." *Journal of School Health,* 1994, *64*(8), 334–339.

Basen-Engquist, K., and others. "Schoolwide Effects of a Multicomponent HIV, STD, and Pregnancy Prevention Program for High School Students." *Health Education and Behavior,* 2001, *28*(2), 166–185.

Botvin, G. J., and others. "Preventing Adolescent Drug Abuse Through a Multimodal Cognitive-Behavioral Approach: Results of a Three-Year Study." *Journal of Consulting and Clinical Psychology,* 1990, *58*(4), 437–446.

Bush, P. J., and others. "Cardiovascular Risk Factor Prevention in Black School Children: The 'Know Your Body' Evaluation Project." *Health Education Quarterly,* 1989, *16*(2), 215–227.

Card, J. J. "Teen Pregnancy Prevention: Do Any Programs Work?" *Annual Reviews in Public Health,* 1999, *20*, 257–285.

Centers for Disease Control and Prevention. "School-Based HIV-Prevention Education—United States, 1994." *Morbidity and Mortality Weekly Report,* 1996, *45*(35), 760–764.

Centers for Disease Control and Prevention. *HIV Prevention Strategic Plan through 2005.* Atlanta, Ga.: Centers for Disease Control and Prevention, Jan. 2001.

Coyle, K., and others. "Safer Choices: A Multicomponent School-Based HIV/STD and Pregnancy Prevention Program for Adolescents." *Journal of School Health,* 1996, *66*(3), 89–94.

Coyle, K., and others. "Safer Choices: Reducing Teen Pregnancy, HIV and STDs." *Public Health Reports,* 2001, *116* (supp. 1), 82–93.

Coyle, K. K., and others. "Short-Term Impact of Safer Choices: A Multicomponent, School-Based HIV, Other STD, and Pregnancy Prevention Program." *Journal of School Health,* 1999, *69*, 181–188.

Hall, G. E., and Hord, S. M. *Change in Schools: Facilitating the Process.* New York: State University of New York Press, 1987.

Howard, M., and McCabe, J. "Helping Teenagers Postpone Sexual Involvement." *Family Planning Perspectives,* 1990, *22*(1), 21–26.

Jemmott, J. B. III, Jemmott, L. S., and Fong, G. T. "Reductions in HIV Risk-Associated Sexual Behaviors Among Black Male Adolescents: Effects of an AIDS Prevention Intervention." *American Journal of Public Health,* 1992, *82*(3), 372–377.

Kann L., and others. "Youth Risk Behavior Surveillance—United States, 1999." *Morbidity and Mortality Weekly Report,* 2000, *49*(SS05), 1–96.

Kerr, D. M., Kent, L., and Lam, T.C.M. "Measuring Program Implementation with a Classroom Observation Instrument." *Evaluation Review.* 1985, *9*(4), 461–482.

Kirby, D. *Emerging Answers: Research Findings on Programs to Reduce Teen Pregnancy.* Washington, D.C.: National Campaign to Prevent Teen Pregnancy, 2001.

Kirby, D., Barth, R., Leland, N., and Fetro, J. "Reducing the Risk: A New Curriculum to Prevent Sexual Risk Taking." *Family Planning Perspectives,* 1991, *23*(6), 253–263.

Kirby, D., and others. "School-Based Programs to Reduce Sexual Risk Behaviors: A Review of Effectiveness." *Public Health Report,* 1994, *109*(2), 339–360.

Main, D. S., and others. "Preventing HIV Infection Among Adolescents: Evaluation of a School-Based Education Program." *Preventive Medicine,* 1994, *23,* 409–417.

Marsh, D., and others. *Building Effective Middle Schools: A Study of Middle School Implementation in California Schools.* Los Angeles: University of Southern California, 1988.

McGuire, W. "Social Psychology." In P. C. Dodwell (ed.), *New Horizons in Psychology.* Harmondsworth, England: Penguin Books, 1972.

McGuire, W., and Papageoris, D. "The Relative Efficacy of Various Types of Prior Belief-Defense in Producing Immunity to Persuasion." *Journal of Abnormal Social Psychology,* 1961, *62,* 237–337.

Parcel, G. S., and others. "Enhancing Implementation of the Teenage Health Teaching Modules." *Journal of School Health,* 1991, *61*(1), 35–42.

Perry, C. L., Murray, D. M., and Griffin, G. "Evaluating the Statewide Dissemination of Smoking Prevention Curricula: Factors in Teacher Compliance." *Journal of School Health,* 1990, *60*(10), 501–504.

Resnicow, K., and others. "How Best to Measure Implementation of School Health Curricula: A Comparison of Three Measures." *Health Education Research,* 1998, *13*(2), 239–250.

Rohrbach, L. A., Graham, J. W., and Hansen, W. B. "Diffusion of a School-Based Substance Abuse Program: Predictors of Program Implementation." *Preventive Medicine,* 1993, *22,* 237–260.

Ross, J. G., and others. "Design of the Teenage Health Teaching Modules Evaluation." *Journal of School Health,* 1991, *61*(1), 21–25.

Rossi, P. H., and Freeman, H. E. *Evaluation: A Systematic Approach.* (5th ed.) Thousand Oaks, Calif.: Sage, 1993.

St. Lawrence, J. S., Jefferson, K. W., Alleyne, E., and Brasfield, T. L. "Comparison of Education Versus Behavioral Skills Training Interventions in Lowering Sexual HIV Risk Behavior of Substance-Dependent Adolescents." *Journal of Consulting and Clinical Psychology,* 1995, *63*(2), 221–237.

Smith, D. W., McCormick, L. K., Steckler, A. B., and McLeroy, K. R. "Teachers' Use of Health Curricula: Implementation of Growing Healthy, Project SMART, and the Teenage Health Teaching Modules." *Journal of School Health,* 1993, *63*(8), 349–354.

Tortu, S., and Botvin, G. J. "School-Based Smoking Prevention: The Teacher Training Process." *Preventive Medicine,* 1989, *18,* 280–289.

U.S. Department of Health and Human Services. *Healthy People 2010: Understanding and Improving Health.* Washington D.C.: Government Printing Office, 2000.

Walter, H. J., and Vaughn, R. D. "AIDS Risk Reduction Among a Multi-Ethnic Sample of Urban High School Students." *Journal of the American Medical Association,* 1993, *270*(6), 725–730.

APPENDIX A: TEACHER SURVEY: FOLLOW-UP.

Items 1 through 30 are statements about ways of teaching about HIV, STD, and pregnancy prevention. Please indicate whether you agree or disagree with each statement by circling the appropriate number.

	Strongly Disagree	Disagree	Agree	Strongly Agree
1. Assigning homework activities on HIV, other STD, and pregnancy prevention that students do with their parents would be encouraged by the administrators in my school.	1	2	3	4
2. I am confident that I can get students to do an assignment that involves them talking with their parents about HIV, other STD, and pregnancy prevention.	1	2	3	4
3. I am confident that I can effectively use small groups for curriculum activities.	1	2	3	4
4. Using student peer leaders to teach about HIV, STD, and pregnancy will make it more likely that the lessons will be effective in getting students to avoid unprotected sex.	1	2	3	4
5. My students like to have condoms demonstrated in the classroom.	1	2	3	4
6. I am sure that I can effectively demonstrate how to use a condom in my classroom.	1	2	3	4
7. I am confident that I can talk comfortably about sexuality in the classroom.	1	2	3	4
8. Using small group activities in teaching about HIV, STD, and pregnancy will provide students with the skills they need to avoid unprotected sex in the future.	1	2	3	4
9. The administrators in my school support the idea of using student peer leaders to teach some classroom activities about HIV, STD, and pregnancy prevention.	1	2	3	4

(Continued)

APPENDIX A: TEACHER SURVEY: FOLLOW-UP. (CONTINUED)

	Strongly Disagree	Disagree	Agree	Strongly Agree
10. The administrators in my school support the idea of using role-play activities in the classroom.	1	2	3	4
11. Students react favorably to talking about sexuality in the classroom.	1	2	3	4
12. Having students role-play situations like how to negotiate with a partner about whether to have sex or use a condom will help them avoid unprotected sex in real life.	1	2	3	4
13. Assigning activities in which students talk with their parents about HIV, STD, and pregnancy will help students make better decisions about their sexual behavior.	1	2	3	4
14. Doing small group activities in the classroom is a teaching method that is acceptable to my school's administrators.	1	2	3	4
15. Students enjoy doing role-play activities.	1	2	3	4
16. Seeing a condom demonstration will help students use one effectively when they need to.	1	2	3	4
17. If I demonstrated how to use a condom in the classroom, the school administrators would not approve.	1	2	3	4
18. The administrators in my school support teachers who teach about sexuality in the classroom.	1	2	3	4
19. I am confident I can successfully facilitate role-playing exercises in the classroom.	1	2	3	4
20. Receiving instruction about sexuality helps students learn to protect themselves from sexually transmitted diseases, including HIV.	1	2	3	4

APPENDIX A: (CONTINUED)

	Strongly Disagree	Disagree	Agree	Strongly Agree
21. Students enjoy doing classroom activities in small groups.	1	2	3	4
22. Students like to do homework activities involving their parents.	1	2	3	4
23. I am confident that I can use student peer leaders effectively to teach some STD and HIV education activities.	1	2	3	4
24. Students respond well when other students are used as peer leaders to guide teaching activities.	1	2	3	4

How important is each of the following in teaching about HIV, STD, and pregnancy?

	Not at All Important	Slightly Important	Important	Very Important	Extremely Important
25. Using student peer leaders to teach some of the classroom activities	1	2	3	4	5
26. Doing small group activities about HIV, other STD, and pregnancy	1	2	3	4	5
27. Demonstrating how to use a condom	1	2	3	4	5
28. Doing role-play activities about how to avoid unprotected sex	1	2	3	4	5
29. Having students do homework assignments about HIV, STD, and pregnancy with their parents	1	2	3	4	5
30. Teaching about sexuality	1	2	3	4	5

(Continued)

APPENDIX A: TEACHER SURVEY: FOLLOW-UP. (CONTINUED)

The next questions ask for your reactions to the HIV/STD and Pregnancy Prevention Education unit you just completed.

	Strongly Disagree	Disagree	Not Sure	Agree	Strongly Agree
31. The HIV/STD and pregnancy prevention curriculum was written clearly.	1	2	3	4	5
32. The organization and format of the lessons were easy to follow.	1	2	3	4	5
33. The role-play situations were realistic.	1	2	3	4	5
34. I had difficulty getting students involved in the role-plays.	1	2	3	4	5
35. I had difficulty getting students involved in the small group activities.	1	2	3	4	5
36. I was uncomfortable presenting the content of the curriculum.	1	2	3	4	5
37. Most of my students participated in the large group discussions.	1	2	3	4	5
38. Most of my students were responsive to the peer leaders.	1	2	3	4	5
39. The student activities were appropriate for the grade level.	1	2	3	4	5
40. I felt adequately prepared to teach this curriculum.	1	2	3	4	5
41. This curriculum should include more content about abstinence.	1	2	3	4	5
42. The content on how to prevent HIV, STD, and pregnancy seemed relevant to most of my students.	1	2	3	4	5
43. The curriculum content was culturally sensitive and appropriate for my students.	1	2	3	4	5
44. There were no problems with implementing this curriculum.	1	2	3	4	5
45. My students responded positively to the curriculum.	1	2	3	4	5

APPENDIX B: TEACHER CURRICULUM LOG: NINTH GRADE.

Curriculum Log Consent

You are invited to complete a questionnaire regarding the implementation of the classroom curriculum for the Safer Choices project. The questionnaire (log) asks you to keep track of the lessons and activities you teach as you are implementing the curriculum.

You will be asked to complete this log each semester you teach the curriculum (up to four times over the next two years). You will receive the log along with the curriculum materials. The log will take no more than forty minutes to complete each time.

Completing the log is voluntary and is an indication of your consent to participate in this activity. You will be asked to put your name and the name of your school directly on the log so that the information from each log you complete can be linked. The information you provide is *confidential*. The University of Texas Health Science Center and the Centers for Disease Control and Prevention (CDC) guarantee that it will be held in strict confidence, will be used only for purposes stated in the study, and will not be disclosed or released to anyone other than authorized staff members of the CDC without the consent of the individuals in accordance with Section 308(d) of the Public Health Service Act (42 U.S.C. 242m).

Your help in completing the log is important. The information you provide will be used to determine the extent to which the curriculum was implemented in the classroom and to identify ways to improve the curriculum.

If you have questions about participating in this survey or would like additional information, please contact Karen Basen Engquist at (713) 792-8540.

Public reporting burden for this collection of information is estimated to average forty minutes per response, including the time for reviewing instructions, searching existing data sources, gathering and maintaining the data needed, and completing and reviewing the collection of information. Send comments regarding this burden estimate or any other aspect of this collection of information, including suggestions for reducing the burden, to PHS Reports Clearance Officer: ATTN: PRA; Hubert H. Humphrey Bldg. Rm. 721-B; 200 Independence Ave., SW, Washington, D.C. 20201, and to the Office of Management and Budget: Paperwork Reduction Project (0920-0327), Washington, D.C. 20506.

Teacher Curriculum Log
Ninth Grade

Name:	
School:	
Dept.:	

Number of students in each class period: (please indicate any planning period with a P)									
Period	0	1	2	3	4	5	6	7	8
grade 9									
grade 10									
grade 11									
grade 12									
TOTAL									
# excused by parent									

(Note: excused students are those not allowed to participate in program)

Preparation: Setting the Stage	CLASS PERIOD (write in period #)					
Date began preparation						
Date ended preparation						

Which parts of the preparation did you do?

(please check Y or N)

Part I: Notifying parents/guardians	Y		N
Part II: Selecting Peer Leaders	Y		N
Part III: Establishing Ground Rules	Y		N
Part IV: Setting up Question Box	Y		N
Part V: Explaining Project Paradigm	Y		N

Did you make any changes in the Preparation? If yes, what changes?	Y		N

CLASS #1—<u>Not</u> Everybody's Having Sex	
Dates you did lesson	
Periods in which you did lesson	

Which parts of Class #1 did you teach?   (please check Y or N)

	Y		N
Part I: Why Young Women/Men Choose Not to Have Sex	Y		N
Part II: Influences on Decisions	Y		N
Part III: Expressing Love and Affection	Y		N
Part IV: Homework Assignment: Then and Now	Y		N

Strategies used: (please check Y or N)

	Y		N
—Small group activities	Y		N
—Use of peer leaders	Y		N
—Role-playing	Y		N
—Large group discussion	Y		N

(Not all strategies are included in every lesson.)

Did you make any changes in Class #1?	Y		N

If yes, what changes?

APPENDIX C: SAFER CHOICES OBSERVATION FORM:
CLASS 3 REFUSAL SKILLS.

School: _____

Teacher: _____

Class Period: _____   Length of Period (in minutes): _____

Date: _____   Name of Observer: _____

Lesson Activities: Indicate which of the activities were completed by the teacher during the class period you observed by putting a Y for YES or an N for NO. Also, note any deviations from the lesson that occurred.

_____   Review characteristics of a clear NO statement
_____   More ways to say NO (alternative and delay)
_____   Responding to one-liners
_____   Role-playing in small groups
_____   Two Peer Leaders modeled the use of alternative actions and delaying tactics using the role-play Trying to Slow Down—Part 2
_____   One Peer Leader modeled different refusal skills in response to one-line pressure statements
_____   Deviated from lesson plan in following ways:
             _____
             _____

SCORING: Use the following scoring system to indicate the extent to which teachers implemented each phase and step of guiding group discussions:

0 = Did not complete the activity/criteria at all: Use for teachers who do not complete the criteria for teaching how to use effective NO statements. For example, if a teacher does not review the characteristics of alternative actions, that teacher would receive a score of "0" for "reviewed characteristics of alternative action."

1 = Partially completed activity/criteria: Use for teachers who partially complete the criteria. For example, if a teacher writes the name of the skill suggesting an alternative action on the chalkboard but students cannot read it because it is too small or illegible, that teacher would receive a score of "1" for "wrote name of skill on chalkboard or used other visual."

2 = Fully completed activity/criteria: Use for teachers who fully complete the criteria.
NA = Not applicable: Use for criteria that don't occur because they are dependent upon certain student behaviors. For example. if students do not have any questions regarding alternative actions or delay statements, mark NA for "addressed questions in a manner consistent with the explanation of using clear NO messages." Items that may need to be scored as Not Applicable include parentheses ( ).

Skip step completely: Some teachers may skip an entire step. If this occurs, mark "skipped step completely," and assign the score of "0" to each substep.

Draft: 10-26-93

APPENDIX C: (CONTINUED)

RATINGS OF OBSERVATION

NOTE: The beginning of Class #3 provides students with practice in using clear NO statements. This refusal skill was introduced in the previous class.

PART I: REVIEW AND PRACTICE OF CLEAR NO STATEMENTS

Note time when review and practice of clear NO statements is started: _____

☐ Phase A. Conduct small group practice (Part I, Section C)

Step 1. Prepare for role-play practice in pairs

_____ Described the task for students <u>before</u> handing out role-play sheet (e.g., write responses to pressure lines individually, then work in pairs taking turns reading role-play lines)

_____ Divided students into pairs, using efficient method of getting students into pairs

_____ Had students construct their responses to pressure lines

_____ Identified roles (person reading pressure lines, person reading refusals) and instructed students to decide who will play which role first

_____ **Skipped step completely**

Step 2. Enact in small groups

_____ Walked from pair to pair to check on students' use of skills

(_____) Coached students as needed if students were practicing skill incorrectly

_____ Watched the time and reminded students to switch roles after each reading of the role-play

_____ **Skipped step completely**

Step 3. Small group discussion

(_____) Prompted students as needed to initiate discussion when role-playing complete

(_____) Reminded students as needed to discuss how it felt to play each role

(_____) Reminded students as needed to give each other feedback on the characteristics of the skills that were or weren't in place during the demonstration

_____ **Skipped step completely**

Draft: 10-26-93

APPENDIX C: SAFER CHOICES OBSERVATION FORM: CLASS 3 REFUSAL SKILLS. (CONTINUED)

☐ Phase B. Guide large group discussion (Part I, Section D)

Step 1. Debrief skill practice experience

_____ Called students back together to guide large group discussion
_____ Asked students to identify feelings about skill practice (e.g., what was easy, what was hard)
_____ Asked students how the situation is or is not like real life
_____ Elicited responses to same question from several students—as time permitted
_____ Used a combination of comprehension and open-ended questions
_____ Avoided making judgmental responses regarding students' comments
_____ **Skipped step completely**

Note time when review and practice of clear NO statements ends: _____

PARTS II–IV: ALTERNATIVE AND DELAY TACTICS

Note time when instruction of alternative and delay tactics is started: _____

☐ Phase A. Explain the skill—Suggesting an Alternative Action

Step 1. Name the skill (Part II, Section A)

_____ Used label consistent with the label in curriculum (Suggesting an Alternative Action)
_____ Wrote the name of skill on chalkboard or used other visual (overhead)
_____ **Skipped step completely**

Step 2. State purpose of skill (Part II, Section A)

_____ Described why to use skill or how skill can be useful (e.g., to let partner know you are not ready or don't want to have sex)
_____ **Skipped step completely**

Draft: 10-26-93

CHAPTER NINE

Using Children as Change Agents to Increase Fruit and Vegetable Consumption Among Lower-Income African American Parents

Process Evaluation Results of the Bringing It Home Program

Marsha Davis, Tom Baranowski, Marilyn Hughes, Carla L. Warneke, Carl de Moor, and Rebecca M. Mullis

Increasing fruit, 100 percent juice, and vegetable intake (FJV) to five to nine servings per day is a national priority. Dietary factors, particularly insufficient consumption of FJV, have been associated with major types of cancer, several chronic diseases, and obesity (Block, Patterson, and Subar, 1992; Subar and others, 1994; Patterson and others, 1995; Steinmetz and Potter, 1996; McCrory and others, 1999; McCrory, Fuss, Saltzman, and Roberts, 2000; Li and others, 2000; Joshipura and others, 1999; Beilin, 1999; Gortmaker and others, 1999; Epstein and others, 2001). Lower-income African Americans consume less FJV than other Americans and are at greater risk of obesity and chronic disease (Patterson, Krebs-Smith, Pivonka, and Kessler, 1995; Li and others, 2000; Serdula and others, 1995; Dennison, Rockwell, and Baker, 1998). Yet few programs have been developed to increase FJV consumption in this high-risk, underserved population.

Bringing It Home was funded by the National Cancer Institute, grant R01 CA63578.

Traditionally, schools have been used as a channel to promote behavior change among children. Because adult family members control children's access to food in the home and can influence consumption, many school nutrition education programs have targeted the family for promoting dietary change among children (Resnicow and Robinson, 1997). These school-based efforts have been shown to affect dietary behaviors among elementary school children, but the extent to which children may in turn affect the dietary habits of their family has not been determined.

Using the child as a "health messenger" has been shown to be effective in a variety of health promotion efforts, including those concerned with hypertension and heart disease (Fors and others, 1989). Using children as change agents in a dietary program delivered through schools may be an effective strategy for promoting dietary change in their parents. The children can motivate their parents to make dietary changes through skills learned at school, and parents and children can work together to adapt the information to their own family life.

Design of the Bringing It Home Program

The goal of Bringing It Home was to build upon this parent-child dynamic to promote increased FJV consumption in lower-income African American parents of fourth-grade school children (Davis, Baranowski, and others, forthcoming). Bringing It Home was implemented in a southeastern, urban, inner-city school system. Ninety-eight percent of the students were African American, most of whom came from families that, compared with national norms, faced socioeconomic disadvantage. Ninety percent of the students participated in the free or reduced-price meal program.

Based on a community participatory approach (Israel, Schulz, Parker, and Becker, 1998), we conducted a series of focus groups to guide intervention development. Four schools in the participating school district served as developmental schools. Parents within those schools were recruited to participate in focus groups. Two types of focus groups were conducted with African American parents of fourth-grade students. Ten focus groups (with twelve to fifteen parents in each group) were conducted to explore behavior patterns of FJV consumption, and six focus groups (each consisting of twelve to fifteen parents) were conducted to obtain information related directly to the intervention structure and delivery (Davis, Hughes, and others, forthcoming).

The intervention was based on social cognitive theory (SCT) (Bandura, 1986), and it integrated the sociocultural context of African American families with the SCT individual and socioenvironmental levels for behavior change (Stokols, 1996; Resnicow, Baranowski, Ahluwalia, and Braithwaite, 1999). Guided by the formative evaluation results and theoretical framework, we translated these messages into an intervention to ensure that the materials would capture the attention of both parents and children, were integrated across the intervention components, and were culturally appropriate.

Reading was not the most favored learning activity in these families; the communication medium they preferred was videotapes. A random survey of a hundred parents in the school district found that over 98 percent of the families had VCRs in their homes and 100 percent had access to a VCR through their child's school, a community center, or a relative's home. This finding made the option of a video-based intervention viable.

The intervention was delivered to the fourth grade over a seven-month period (October–April). For parents, the intervention consisted of videotapes with corresponding magazines, a calendar, tailored letters mailed to the home, and telephone calls to encourage them to participate in each of the intervention components. A curriculum to give the children skills to encourage their parents to eat more FJV was delivered at school by the project staff.

Curriculum

The Bringing It Home curriculum contained two thirty-minute classroom sessions each month. Because of the efficacy nature of the trial, project staff members assisted regular classroom teachers in delivering the sessions. Teachers from each intervention school attended a one-day training workshop. During the training, teachers viewed all the parent materials, participated in a session-by-session review of the curriculum, and practiced presenting a curriculum session, as well as preparing an FJV recipe.

During each month of the Bringing It Home program, the fourth-grade curriculum was focused on eating FJV for a specific meal or snack, or it was focused on FJV behavior—such as shopping for FJV. The sessions were experiential and emphasized skills for encouraging parents to eat FJV, for overcoming barriers to eating FJV, for asking parents to have FJV in the home, and for preparing FJV recipes in class. Home activities for each child to complete with his or her parents included keeping diaries to track FJV consumption, encouraging each other to eat FJV for meals and snacks, preparing FJV recipes at home, watching the videotapes, reading the magazines, and setting goals with parents to eat more FJV.

Calendar

The calendar highlighted program events, including receipt of the monthly mailing, curriculum activities, and encouragement calls. Each month, a seasonal fruit or vegetable was promoted through a colorful photograph or recipe, and purchase, storage, and preparation tips were given. Written reminders to the parents were placed throughout the calendar month, telling them to watch the videos, make FJV recipes, and eat FJV. Additional messages targeted the children by suggesting specific activities they could participate in to assist their parents in the consumption of more FJV.

Videos and Magazines

Parents received one video per month for a total of seven throughout the intervention period. They received three core videos at the beginning (introductory), two videos at the midpoint (booster), and two videos at the end of the intervention period (maintenance). These videos followed a family documentary style—showing a child and parent making changes to eat more FJV, children giving guidance to parents for eating more FJV, and FJV recipe preparation, as well as demonstrating skills for increasing the consumption of FJV.

For the two booster and two maintenance videotapes, parents chose from a library of twelve videos in three categories: cooking and shopping advice, saving time and money, and health benefits. In the monthly encouragement telephone call, parents were asked to select the library tape they would like to receive. If a parent was not reached, a video was chosen based on responses in the baseline survey. The videos varied in content and method of presentation. Some of the videos used humor or musical entertainment to educate, whereas others appealed to a deeper cultural structure (Resnicow, Baranowski, Ahluwalia, and Braithwaite, 1999), such as African American family values, traditional recipes, spiritual connections, the building of a stronger generation for the children, and culturally relevant role models. All the videos featured nationally and locally famous African Americans talking about their favorite FJV and the importance of eating FJV.

Consistent throughout the videos were messages about ways to increase FJV availability and accessibility, fast and easy preparation methods, and the buying and storing of FJV. The magazines elaborated in print form the messages and recipes shown in the video. Each included interactive parent-child activities, such as games to identify favorite FJV to have at home.

Tailored Letters

Personalized letters were sent to parents monthly. Each letter contained a message suggesting an FJV behavior at the meal or snack emphasized that month in the curriculum. The message was tailored to the parents' reported usual consumption pattern for that meal or snack and their FJV preferences. FJV preferences were assessed at baseline, and the usual meal or snack FJV behaviors were assessed during the monthly encouragement calls. Messages were developed to suggest the easiest FJV behavior to change in light of usual practices.

Encouragement Calls

Parents were telephoned each month during the intervention and asked whether or not they had watched the video, read the magazine, completed the home curriculum activities with their child, or made any of the FJV recipes for that month. If parents had not participated in an intervention component, they were given motivational messages to do so. If they had participated, they were encouraged to continue participation and to adopt the intervention messages.

The effectiveness of the intervention was tested in a group-randomized trial wherein twenty-two schools were pair-matched in terms of size, mobility rate, and participation in the free or reduced-price meal program, and they were randomly assigned to a treatment or control condition. Parental FJV intake was measured pre- and postintervention with a food frequency questionnaire (FFQ) and one twenty-four-hour dietary recall (24H) over the telephone. Parents' body mass index (BMI) was calculated from their self-reported height and weight.

Because the school was the unit of randomization, mixed-model regression procedures were used to adjust for the potential correlation of measurements within the school. Using SAS PROC MIXED (SAS Institute, 1997), analyses of the outcome measures were conducted by regressing the postintervention FJV measures on treatment group and baseline measures, with the school modeled as a random effect nested within the treatment group and the treatment group modeled as a fixed effect.

The results indicated that the intervention group consumed 1.16 total FJV servings more than the control group (p = .0001), as measured by FFQ, and it consumed 1.33 total FJV servings more when measured by 24H (p = .0001). The intervention effect was 1.75 servings among those with a BMI greater than or equal to 25 (p = .04). The average postintervention self-reported weight among the intervention group was 3.6 pounds less than that of the control group (p = .05). For those with a BMI greater than or equal to 25, the difference was 5.0 pounds (p = .03) (Davis, Baranowski, and others, forthcoming).

These outcome results suggest that with the strategy of using children as change agents, the program demonstrated significant and substantial changes in FJV consumption. Finding ways to help people eat more FJV offers the potential for the prevention of cancer, cardiovascular disease, and other chronic health problems through the increased consumption of phytochemicals. Bringing It Home was more effective among those who were overweight and wished to achieve weight loss. This research suggests that increased FJV may also help prevent chronic disease through the enhanced control of body weight.

Given the complexities of implementing community-based studies—such as Bringing It Home—as well as the multiple components that encompassed the intervention, rigorous process evaluation was needed to elucidate the results of the outcome evaluation. It needed to provide information on how many individuals were reached and the various levels of participation in the intervention, measuring how well each of the components of the intervention was implemented and providing directions for increasing program efficiency and effectiveness. The remainder of this chapter outlines the model that guided the process evaluation measures used in Bringing It Home, highlights the results of the process evaluation, and provides direction for future process evaluation efforts.

Process Evaluation Methods

The process evaluation methods used in Bringing it Home were based on a mediating model for process evaluation that was proposed by Baranowski and Stables (2000). This model posits that for a program to result in behavior change, certain processes must occur. The function of process evaluation is to measure each of these components: (1) the recruitment and maintenance of participants, (2) the context within which the program functions, (3) the resources available to the program and the participants, (4) implementation of the program, (5) the receipt of materials by the target population, (6) the barriers to implementing the program, (7) the initial use of the program activities, (8) the continued use of the program, and (9) contamination of the treatment and control groups.

Both quantitative and qualitative methodologies were employed to answer each process evaluation question. Table 9.1 denotes the types of measures and methods used to address each of the process evaluation components.

Key informant interviews and focus groups with school leaders, teachers, and parents were conducted prior to implementation development and delivery to determine strategies for recruitment and maintenance, to assess contextual factors in the environment that could influence intervention delivery, to develop salient intervention messages, and to ensure that the intervention was culturally appropriate.

The quality of delivery of the intervention was assessed by measures collected by teacher questionnaires, staff field notes, direct observation, and telephone interviews of parents. Each measure was pretested prior to use.

TABLE 9.1. PROCESS EVALUATION QUESTIONS AND METHODOLOGIES USED.

Component of Process Evaluation	Measures and Methods
Recruitment of schools and participants	• Types of messages employed to attain participation • Number of potential participants obtained from school/class rosters
Maintenance of participants	• Types of messages employed to maintain participation • Number of participants who continued monthly by telephone survey • Differences among maintained sample, recruited sample, and population
Aspects of the environment on the intervention	• Types of contextual factors from community assessment, observation, and field notes
Resources	• Types of resources from community assessment, observation, and field notes
Implementation of the program: extent to which program was implemented as planned	• Level of teacher ability and motivation to deliver the curriculum • Quality and number of classroom sessions held as measured by classroom observation
Reach: extent to which the program was received by the target group	• Number of parents receiving each of the intervention components as measured by monthly telephone calls and postintervention telephone survey and focus groups
Exposure: extent to which participants viewed/read the materials that reached them	• For each classroom component, how much of each component was preferred by the child • For each parent component, how much of each activity was liked as reported by the parents during the monthly telephone calls and postintervention focus groups
Initial use	• Number and type of classroom activities conducted as measured by classroom observation • Number and type of intervention activity completed by parents as reported in monthly telephone calls, completed forms returned to school by the child, postintervention surveys and focus groups
Continued use	Throughout the seven-month intervention: • Number and type of classroom activities conducted as measured by classroom observation • Number and type of intervention activity completed by parents as reported in monthly telephone calls, completed forms returned to school by the child, postintervention surveys and focus groups
Barriers and facilitators	• Types of barriers and facilitators, as observed by project staff, reported by parents during monthly telephone calls, and reported by teachers and parents in postintervention focus groups
Contamination	• Numbers and types of competing programs reaching participants, as measured by observation of the schools and postintervention focus groups of parents and teachers and postintervention telephone calls of treatment and control parents

The level of preparation needed to conduct the major tasks of the curriculum and the motivation to influence dietary changes in students and their parents were asked of teachers following teacher training. After the intervention, all teachers (n = 48) were given a questionnaire that asked them open-ended questions about what they thought were the best and worst characteristics of the program, how they would incorporate the curriculum into their classroom, and what changes they would make.

To determine the extent to which the curriculum was implemented as planned, every curriculum session was observed. Five raters used an observation form that listed the sequential tasks identified from the curriculum. The observer recorded whether or not each task was performed, and the curriculum tasks were coded into categories that reflected the specific purpose of that task: (1) procedure (distribution of materials), (2) FJV preparation and consumption in class, and then student modeling, (3) participatory learning, (4) encouragement of parents to participate in each of the intervention components (by having them watch the videotapes, complete the FJV diary, prepare recipes, read the magazines, and participate in the calendar activities), (5) rewards for the successful completion of tasks (social incentives), (6) problem solving, and (7) teacher modeling. Two project staff members coded curriculum tasks independently and a consensus was reached in cases of inconsistent categorization.

To determine the reach and receptivity of each of the parental intervention components and the initial and continued use of program materials, parents were telephoned monthly during the intervention by evaluation staff members and were asked whether or not they had participated in that month's intervention activities. In addition, at the end of the program, parents were surveyed by telephone and were asked about their participation in the program, how the program influenced their FJV intake, and the influence of their child on making dietary changes, and they were asked to give suggestions for program improvement. Children were asked to bring back to school completed parent-child FJV activity diaries.

Six postintervention focus groups—with twelve to fifteen parents in each—were held to gather qualitative data about program impact and receptivity. Questions were asked about each component of the intervention, which components were most influential in promoting dietary change, and the role of the child in parental participation and behavior change.

Observations were made monthly in all fourth-grade classrooms in the control schools to ascertain if programs similar to Bringing It Home were being implemented. In addition, on the postintervention survey, parents in the control schools were asked if they had received any videotapes about eating fruit and vegetables or if they had participated in any nutrition programs.

Results

Recruitment of Schools and Participants

Recruitment messages, gleaned from the key informant interviews, focus groups, and field notes, built upon the mission of the school to increase family involvement and improve the nutritional status of students. Messages to the parents were built upon a deep cultural structure, as they were concerned with the family unit working together, the health benefits of FJV, parents' being role models to their children, generational ties, and the idea of longing for the past and the way "we were meant to eat."

Twenty-two schools that met the criterion for inclusion—having enrolled at least forty fourth-grade students—were asked to participate in the program. No school refused participation in the program. In August 1998, 1,855 fourth-grade students were enrolled in the twenty-two study schools. Consent forms were received from 1,577 (85.0 percent) of their parents. Of those, 1,535 (97.3 percent) agreed to participate. During the data collection period (August–September 1998), baseline FFQ survey data were collected for 825 parents. Of those for whom data were not collected, 349 (23 percent) had disconnected telephone numbers, 298 (19 percent) had working numbers but were not reached after an average of twenty attempts, and sixty-three (4 percent) declined the interview. We were not able to gather data to indicate if there were any differences between those who were reached for baseline data collection and those who were not.

Maintenance of Schools and Participants

Messages from Bringing It Home to schools to encourage their participation in the program built upon the commitment of the schools to the study, the visibility of the program in the schools and community, and the schools' mission to increase parental involvement in the schools. The schools' messages to the parents emphasized the benefit of the program to their families, their commitment to the child's education, and their continued contact with parents throughout the program, as well as monthly educational extenders, and monthly family recognition at each school.

No school withdrew from the program. Parental postintervention data were collected during May–June 1999. By May 1999, fifty-four parents (7 percent) who had completed the baseline survey no longer had a child who attended a study school, and one declined further participation in the study. Of the 770 families remaining in the study, 634 (82.3 percent) completed the postintervention FFQ survey. Of those not contacted, 103 (13 percent) had disconnected phone numbers, twenty-six (3 percent) could not be contacted after a mean of twenty-five attempts, seven (1 percent) refused, and nineteen (2 percent) had incomplete data. The study cohort consisted of 615 parents, yielding an overall retention rate of 75 percent.

There were no significant differences between those who remained in the cohort and those who did not, with regard to the study condition, school membership, marital status, the percentage working full-time, relationship to the child, parents' age, the number of children in the household, or the baseline values of FJV intake or BMI. A significantly higher percentage of those who had an education past high school (40 percent versus 28 percent, p = .002) and more televisions in the home (3.1 versus 2.4, p = .01) remained in the cohort.

Effect of Environmental Factors on the Intervention

Based on the analyses of the field notes and focus groups with teachers and other school leaders, the most potent factors in the environment that facilitated implementation of the program were that (1) the mission and delivery of Bringing It Home built upon the existing school infrastructure of family involvement, (2) students received recognition for their involvement, and (3) the school, as a delivery channel, was important, because of the trust that had already been established between the school and the community.

Resources

A major source of resources for the program came from the grant funding. However, contributions from the community were also invaluable assets. Principals and key school leaders served as proponents of the program, which likely led to the schools' adoption of the program and the increased participation of parents in the program. Community business leaders donated resources, such as movie tickets, cookbooks, and hotel stays, which were used as incentives for motivating parental participation in the program. Community and school leaders, local newscasters, politicians, and entertainers donated their time, being filmed for the videotapes and serving as advocates for the program.

Implementation and Reach of the Program

All of the teachers attended teacher training, and immediately following the training, about half of the teachers said they needed more self-preparation before conducting specific curriculum tasks, such as guiding role-plays, completing the FJV diary, and preparing FJV recipes in class. Over 70 percent were prepared after training to remind their students to encourage their parents to participate in the parental intervention—by watching the videotapes, reading the magazines, completing the parent-child goal setting activity, and so forth. Eighty-four percent of the teachers reported that they were very supportive of the program and 96 percent reported a high level of school administration support.

For the classroom sessions, data were analyzed from the observation forms. All classroom sessions were implemented (n = 519) and all were observed by trained evaluation staff members. Just over 41 percent of the classes were implemented primarily by the classroom teacher and 58.2 percent were implemented primarily by the Bringing It Home staff. Individual items within common categories were summed across sessions to identify the number of tasks throughout the curriculum, and proportions of tasks completed within each category were computed within each session and were averaged across sessions.

Table 9.2 presents the mean proportion completed for each task by classroom teacher and program staff member. The majority of the tasks were implemented at a high level of fidelity (less than 80 percent), with problem solving and teacher modeling behaviors being lower. There were no significant differences between the mean proportion implemented primarily by classroom teachers and those implemented by program staff members.

At the end of Bringing It Home, teachers reported liking best the hands-on activities for students and the contact between parents, teachers, students, and the program staff, as well as the enthusiasm and support of the program staff, the incorporation of math, language, values, and art in each of the sessions, the hands-on activities—especially the FJV preparation, and the focus on child and parent nutrition and health. The weaknesses noted were those related to the amount of time needed for preparation and teaching, the length of the sessions, and the necessity to follow the specific curriculum components as written.

Reach

Table 9.3 outlines the month-by-month receipt of each of the parent intervention materials as reported in the monthly telephone calls. Approximately 76 percent of the intervention cohort were reached each month by the telephone survey that

TABLE 9.2.   BRINGING IT HOME CLASSROOM OBSERVATIONS.

Type of Curriculum Task	Mean Proportion Completed
Procedural	98.7
FJV preparation	97.8
Student modeling	96.6
Participatory learning	93.4
Encouraging parent to participate in intervention activities	91.4
Rewards	89.6
Problem solving	75.9
Teacher modeling	66.5

TABLE 9.3. REACH AND USE OF PARENT INTERVENTION MATERIALS AS ASSESSED MONTHLY BY TELEPHONE SURVEY.

	Oct	Nov	Dec	Jan	Feb	Mar	Apr	Mean
Contacted for encouragement call	75.4%	76.5%	69.6%	77.8%	72.7%	82.6%	76.8%	75.9%
Video								
Received video	92.3	94.2	95.6	93.0	95.3	95.0	91.6	93.9
Parent watched video	71.1	52.6	59.5	50.9	57.1	55.2	58.7	57.9
Child watched video	67.6	51.7	56.9	48.1	54.7	54.3	55.8	55.6
Made recipes presented in video	29.9	21.8	38.5	23.6	30.5	27.0	29.6	28.7
Magazine								
Received magazine	75.1	65.6	73.0	71.1	69.0	67.8	70.2	70.3
Read magazine	80.0	70.1	79.9	79.0	80.3	75.0	76.6	76.8
Did magazine activity with child	83.1	46.9	59.7	55.6	57.8	54.3	57.6	59.3
Parent filled out pledge in magazine	69.9	44.2	59.1	56.2	59.9	60.4	58.2	58.3
Child filled out pledge in magazine	74.7	54.4	63.8	62.3	69.4	64.0	63.3	64.6
Made recipes presented in magazine	24.7	28.6	53.0	40.1	40.8	34.1	42.4	37.7
Tailored Letter								
Received tailored letter	NA*	74.1	78.9	82.5	82.2	86.8	84.0	81.4
Tried letter suggestion	NA*	74.1	69.6	49.5	63.4	60.0	61.4	63.0
Calendar								
Received calendar	97.5	NA*	NA*	NA*	NA*	NA*	NA*	NA*
Made calendar recipe	23.1	27.7	37.7	40.4	39.9	31.0	44.9	34.9
School to Home Materials								
Received FJV diaries	81.4	87.1	NA*	77.2	79.3	79.3	79.1	80.6
Parent used FJV diary	85.0	83.1	NA*	88.1	88.2	83.9	89.3	86.2
Child used FJV diary	100.0	93.3	NA*	96.0	93.5	96.9	95.5	95.9
Received school recipes	NA*	62.1	70.1	61.0	60.1	60.7	59.1	62.2
Parent made school recipes	NA*	29.0	47.1	31.6	30.5	30.6	31.6	33.4

*No activity for that month

assessed receipt of the intervention materials. Nearly every parent (97 percent) reported receiving a videotape each month. Of the videos chosen by parents, 40 percent of the videos sent were from the cooking and shopping advice category, 36 percent were from the health benefits category, and 24 percent were from the saving time and money category.

Just over 85 percent reported receiving the magazine and tailored letter each month. This was consistent throughout the intervention period: October through April. Receipt of materials that the children were supposed to bring home from school was lower (80 percent for the FJV diary and 65 percent for the recipes) but was also consistent throughout the intervention.

Exposure and Initial and Continued Use

Patterns of use throughout the intervention as reported by parents from the encouragement calls are shown in Table 9.3. Although receipt of the intervention materials was consistent over the intervention period and initial use was fairly high, the use of some of the materials waned over the seven months of intervention. In the first month of the intervention, over 71 percent of parents reported watching the video, with 80 percent reading the magazine, 83 percent completing the FJV diary, 23 percent making the calendar recipe, and 65 percent reading the tailored letters.

Over time, a little over half of the parents tried the tailored behavior change suggestion in the letter and read the magazine throughout the seven months. Doing the magazine activity with their child dropped from 62 percent at the beginning of the intervention to 40 percent at the end of the intervention. Continued viewing of the parent video leveled at around 50 percent after the first video. FJV diary completion remained fairly high among the parents and children. Preparing recipes from the video, magazine, calendar, and school was consistently low throughout the intervention (ranging from a mean of 27 to 53 percent).

In interpreting these results, it is important to recognize potential sample bias. For any given month, 17 to 30 percent of the participants were not contacted, and it is likely that those not contacted may differ in their use of intervention materials compared with those contacted. It is also important to note that the data is self-reported and therefore poses validity and reliability concerns. For example, the magazine and tailored letter were in the same package, so there should not be any differences in the reporting of receipt of the two. However, it is possible that parents are more likely to recall receipt of the most preferred or most easily recognized intervention piece.

The use of intervention materials, based on the number of forms returned to school, indicates that approximately 40 percent of the parents watched the videos, 40 percent of the parents completed the FJV diaries, 42 percent of the children watched the videos, and 38 percent of the parents completed other activities, such as reading the magazine, making the calendar recipe, and goal setting. The return rates were much higher at the beginning of the intervention period (59 percent) and dropped throughout the seven months, with a low of 26 percent in the final month of the intervention.

These numbers denote substantially lower use than those reported in the monthly telephone calls. Whether this discrepancy indicates a reporting bias or a difference in use is unknown. Most likely, the differences are due to the sample bias that was introduced by the low return rates, as well as the extra respondent burden of having the child or parent return the process evaluation.

Use measured by telephone survey after the intervention indicated that 67 percent of the parents reported watching all the videotapes and 30 percent reported watching some. Fifty percent reported reading all the magazines and 40 percent reported reading some. Seventy percent reported reading all the letters and 23 percent reported reading some. Eighty-seven percent reported making all or some of the recipes. Sixty-five percent reported keeping all of the FJV diaries and 24 percent reported keeping some of the diaries. Eighty four percent of the parents felt that as a result of the program they were eating more FJV than before and 88 percent said that their child was eating more FJV. The two biggest factors in having more FJV in the diet were that more FJV were in the home and more FJV were eaten as snacks. Over 88 percent of the parents said their child had a great deal of influence on making changes to eat more FJV.

In the postintervention focus groups, parents reported that the videotapes were the most enjoyed and persuasive method of communicating. Calendars were second in terms of motivating parents to eat FJV and make FJV recipes. Critical to the impact of the letters was that each was personalized and tailored with explicit FJV behavior change suggestions. The magazines were reported as the least effective resource for behavior change, primarily because parents identified reading as a least favored activity. Every parent reported preparing some of the recipes. Most parents could not recall the source of the recipe (curriculum, magazine, video, or calendar) and would have preferred a central place where all recipes could be located. The monthly encouragement calls were a program component the parents said could be eliminated; they described the calls as being more annoying than motivational.

All the parents in the focus groups said that their child's involvement in the program was the major influence on their participation and behavior change. Typical comments by parents were, "Well, I kept at it because my son and I are really close, and anything that he is excited about I try my best to be 100 percent involved in," "I did it because of my child, and I want him to be healthy and eat more fruits and vegetables," and "Since he was part of this program and excited about it, I was going to be."

The child served as an encourager, a reminder, and an information resource for the family. Parents expressed it this way: "My child would not let me forget," or "My child, he runs to the mailbox—'Grandma, Grandma, Bringing It Home has sent you something,' and he comes in with the letter, opens it, and says 'Let's see what's in it,' and then we'd watch the tape and read the letter." Parents emphasized that it was important that the program be a part of their child's school, providing them with the impetus to participate in their child's education.

Barriers and Facilitators

Barriers to using the intervention materials, as reported by parents in the postintervention survey and focus groups, were primarily lack of time, lack of resources, and lack of access to FJV in stores. The motivation for making nutrition changes was relatively low, given the other competing priorities of a family living in poverty.

Responses from the teacher questionnaires indicate that the major barriers to implementing the curriculum included limited classroom management, competing academic programs, the demands of the climate of school accountability for raising achievement test scores, the need for more training to implement a behaviorally based nutrition curriculum, and the perceived teachers' limitations to seeing themselves as influential in changing child and parent eating habits.

Factors in the environment that proved challenging for the program were those that are endemic to urban, inner-city schools. The curriculum placed high demands on the classroom teachers for learning new skills, for class preparation, and for implementation time. The staff provided extra support beyond the training to help teachers gain the necessary skills to implement the curriculum activities. However, with the current movement toward standardized academic achievement testing in the interest of ensuring accountability for school performance, nutrition education was given lower priority in the classroom. Therefore, had it not been for the program staff members present in the classroom or teaching the curriculum, it is likely that the teachers would not have devoted enough class time to be instrumental in producing dietary behavior change.

However, the school environment was very supportive of the presence of the program and promoted the program as well as parental involvement in the community. Facilitators at the parent level, as measured in the telephone survey and the postintervention focus groups, were committed to the program because of their child's involvement at school, their desire to be role models for their child, their health concerns, and the program's method of delivery—mailing the materials to their home, which enabled them to participate with their child on their own time rather than having to attend activities outside the home.

Contamination

There were no competing nutrition programs in the control schools. Topics of nutrition were covered in the general health curriculum but not at a level comparable to Bringing It Home. Nor had the emphasis been on family involvement in the child's nutrition. No control parent reported receiving any videotapes, magazines, or tailored letters during the period of intervention.

Lessons Learned About Process Evaluation

This section highlights five lessons learned from the process evaluation efforts in Bringing It Home.

LESSON 1. *Incorporate process evaluation into planning and outcomes evaluation activities by using a guiding framework.*

Process evaluation should not be viewed as a unique component of program evaluation, unconnected with planning and outcome evaluation. When guided by an evaluation and intervention framework, questions can be focused and resources for data collection can be conserved. For example, in Bringing It Home, in the formative assessment phase, we asked questions to ascertain what messages would be important for increasing FJV intake and we used them in the intervention development. In the process evaluation, we asked specifically if the messages were received and acted upon. In the outcomes evaluation, the behavior was measured. Together, these data complete the cycle of program development through to program evaluation.

LESSON 2. *Process evaluation should be thorough and should assess multiple components.*

Process evaluation should be more than "count" data. Program monitoring, quality assurance, and quality control are only part of the functions of process evaluation. It is not enough to know, for example, *how many* program events were planned and held, although this is important data. When process evaluation can collect data beyond count data, such as the data for recruitment, exposure, dose, and fidelity, this data can be used for explaining program outcomes, for creating a model of the pathways of change of the program, and for program improvement. Evaluators must move beyond simple documentation of delivery in order to understand how the programs are working. Following a model of process evaluation as proposed by Baranowski and Stables, which we did in Bringing It Home, is important for understanding how and why health behavior programs succeed or not.

Using the data from Bringing It Home, we can categorize which components of the curriculum were delivered, explain why some of the intervention materials were not used, and, in future intervention programs, modify components accordingly to maximize behavior change. We capitalized on the variability in use to make inferences about the effectiveness of program components. Using children as change agents in the program appears to be a well-received and effective means of targeting parental FJV change. Watching videotapes and completing

FJV diaries were components that were used more than making recipes or reading informational material. These results can be used in the design and delivery of future programs.

LESSON 3. *Use both quantitative and qualitative methods.*

It is important to balance the breadth of obtaining quantitative data in process evaluation efforts with the depth of qualitative data. In Bringing It Home, both methods were useful in combination to provide a full interpretation of the data. The rich detail of words spoken by the participants in the focus groups—in answering questions as to why they participated in the program, what they found most motivating and helpful in the program for changing behavior, and what behaviors they changed—added much to the numerical data on participation and outcomes.

LESSON 4. *There remains a need for more methodological research in process evaluation.*

Multiple measures for process evaluation—surveys, focus groups, direct observations, and returned material—were used in Bringing It Home. These different methods, although generally yielding convergent information, may not be equally valid or reliable (Resnicow and others, 1998). Different methodologies should be explored in order to gather the most sound process evaluation while minimizing the burden on respondents and staff members.

LESSON 5. *Collect process evaluation data throughout the program.*

In understanding the pathways to behavior change, it is important to track process evaluation over the course of the program. If the time course of program indicators can be made and linked to behavior change, then the components of process evaluation can be related to mediating variables and outcomes. These data would provide a greater foundation upon which to design and implement successful health promotion programs.

Conclusions

The most salient process evaluation components were measured throughout the entire intervention period and the results present a pattern consistent with that of the outcome findings. The program was integrated well into the school's existing infrastructure and environment, the curriculum was implemented with fidelity, the participants received and used the program materials, and FJV consumption increased among the parents and the children.

Following a model for process evaluation, evaluation measures were obtained on every component of the intervention. A combination of quantitative and qualitative methods was used, imparting greater depth and clarity to the data. Process evaluation data were obtained at the individual and group level. Contextual data regarding the setting of intervention delivery were also collected. Together, these data provide an understanding of how well each of the program components was used and received, how well the program was implemented, and what worked and did not work in the program and why, as well as the direction needed for future program modification.

There are limitations to the methods and data in this study. Whereas assessment of the classroom curriculum implementation was observational, all the information from participants was self-reported. Observed exposure and use were not obtained.

The resources available to the program allowed for extensive and rigorous process data collection. The methods used required multiple instruments and questioning routes for focus groups to be developed, for the staff to be trained, and for numerous staff members to collect the data. Without those resources, the process evaluation would be much more limited in scope.

References

Bandura, A. *Social Foundations of Thought and Action: A Social Cognitive Theory. Prentice Hall Series in Social Learning Theory.* Englewood Cliffs, N.J.: Prentice Hall, 1986.

Baranowski, T., and Stables, G. "Process Evaluations of the 5-a-Day Projects." *Health Education and Behavior,* 2000, *27*(2), 157–166.

Beilin, L. J. 1999. "Lifestyle and Hypertension: An Overview." *Clinical and Experimental Hypertension,* 1999, *21*(5–6), 749–762.

Block, G., Patterson, B., and Subar, A. "Fruit, Vegetables and Cancer Prevention: A Review of the Epidemiologic Evidence." *Nutrition and Cancer,* 1992, *18*(1), 1–29.

Davis, M., Baranowski, T., and others. "Increasing Fruit and Vegetable Consumption in Parents Using Children as Change Agents: The 'Bringing It Home' Program." *American Journal of Public Health,* forthcoming.

Davis, M., Hughes, M., and others. "The 'Bringing It Home' Program: Formative Assessment Results." *Journal of Cancer Education,* forthcoming.

Dennison, B. A., Rockwell, H. L., and Baker, S. L. "Fruit and Vegetable Intake in Young Children." *Journal of the American College of Nutrition,* 1998, *17*(4), 371–378.

Epstein, L. H., and others. "Increasing Fruit and Vegetable Intake and Decreasing Fat and Sugar Intake in Families at Risk for Childhood Obesity." *Obesity Research,* 2001, *9*(3), 171–178.

Fors, S. W., and others. "Evaluation of a Diffusion Strategy for School-Based Hypertension Education." *Health Education Quarterly*, 1989, *16*(2), 255–261.

Gortmaker, S. L., and others. "Reducing Obesity via a School-Based Interdisciplinary Intervention Among Youth: Planet Health." *Archives of Pediatric and Adolescent Medicine*, 1999, *153*(4), 409–418.

Israel, B., Schulz, A., Parker, E. A., and Becker, A. "Review of Community-Based Research: Assessing Partnership Approaches to Improve Public Health." *Annual Review of Public Health*, 1998, *19*, 173–202.

Joshipura, K. J., and others. "Fruit and Vegetable Intake in Relation to Risk of Ischemic Stroke." *Jama*, 1999, *282*(13), 1233–1239.

Li, R., and others. "Trends in Fruit and Vegetable Consumption Among Adults in Sixteen U.S. States: Behavioral Risk Factor Surveillance System, 1990–1996." *American Journal of Public Health*, 2000, *90*(5), 777–781.

McCrory, M. A., Fuss, P. J., Saltzman, E., and Roberts, S. B. "Dietary Determinants of Energy Intake and Weight Regulation in Healthy Adults." *Journal of Nutrition*, 2000, *130* (supp. 2S), 276S–279S.

McCrory, M. A., and others. "Dietary Variety Within Food Groups: Association with Energy Intake and Body Fatness in Men and Women." *American Journal of Clinical Nutrition*, 1999, *69*(3), 440–447.

Patterson, B., Krebs-Smith, S., Pivonka, E., and Kessler, R. "Fruit and Vegetable Intake in the United States: The Baseline Survey of the 5-a-Day for Better Health Program." *American Journal of Health Promotion*, 1995, *9*(5), 352–360.

Resnicow, K., and Robinson, T. N. "School-Based Cardiovascular Disease Prevention Studies: Review and Synthesis." *Annals of Epidemiology*, 1997, *7*(S7), 14–31.

Resnicow, K., Baranowski, T., Ahluwalia, J. S., and Braithwaite, R. L. "Cultural Sensitivity in Public Health: Defined and Demystified." *Ethnicity and Disease*, 1999, *9*, 10–21.

Resnicow, K., and others. "How Best to Measure Implementation of School Health Curricula: A Comparison of Three Measures." *Health Education Research*, 1998, *13*(2), 239–250.

SAS Institute. *SAS/STAT Software: Changes and Enhancements, Through Release 6.12*. Cary, N.Y.: SAS Institute, Inc., 1997.

Serdula, M. K., and others. "Fruit and Vegetable Intake Among Adults in Sixteen States: Results of a Brief Telephone Survey." *American Journal of Public Health*, 1995, *85*(2), 236–239.

Steinmetz, K. A., and Potter, J. D. "Vegetables, Fruit, and Cancer Prevention: A Review." *Journal of the American Dietetic Association*, 1996, *96*, 1027–1039.

Stokols, D. "Translating Social Ecological Theory into Guidelines for Community Health Promotion." *American Journal of Health Promotion*, 1996, *10*(4), 282–298.

Subar, A. F., and others. "U.S. Dietary Patterns Associated with Fat Intake: The 1987 National Health Interview Survey." *American Journal of Public Health*, 1994, *84*(3), 359–366.

CHAPTER TEN

Lessons Learned from the Pathways Process Evaluation

Allan Steckler, Becky Ethelbah, Catherine Jane Martin, Dawn D. Stewart, Marla Nahmabin Pardilla, Joel Gittelsohn, Elaine J. Stone, David C. Fenn, Mary Smyth, and Maihan B. Vu

Obesity is a risk factor for both heart disease and type 2 diabetes (Welty, 1991). The prevalence of obesity among American Indians is higher than it is in the general U.S. population. One study reported that approximately 33.7 percent of American Indian adult males (aged eighteen and over) and 40.3 percent of American Indian adult females in the same age group are obese, compared with rates of 24.1 percent of adult males and 25.0 percent of adult females overall in the United States (Brousard and others, 1991). American Indian preschoolers and adolescents are more overweight than the general U.S. population in the same age groups. Studies suggest that obese children are more likely to be obese in adulthood than are children who are not obese (Brousard and others, 1991).

The authors would like to express their deepest appreciation and sincere thanks to the students, parents, leaders, school staff and administration, and American Indian communities in the following locations: Gila River Indian Community (Akimel O'odham), Tohono O'odham Nation, Navajo Nation (Dine), Oglala Sioux Tribe (Oglala Lakota), Rosebud Sioux Tribe (Sicangu Lakota), San Carlos Apache Tribe (Dee'), White Mountain Apache Tribe (Ndee'), and to all the staff members who assisted in the development, implementation, and evaluation of the Pathways study.

Funded by grants HL-50867, HL-50869, HL-50905, HL-50885, and HL-50907 from the National Heart, Lung, and Blood Institute, National Institutes of Health.

We would also like to acknowledge the many contributions to the Pathways process evaluation made by Margaret V. Thorley, Kelly O'Keefe, and Sarah L. Merkle.

In 1987, the National Heart, Lung, and Blood Institute (NHLBI) funded the first school-based, multicentered randomized trial, the Child and Adolescent Trial for Cardiovascular Health (CATCH). The multilevel intervention components were food service, physical education, classroom curricula, and family. The objectives of CATCH were to direct cardiovascular risk behaviors toward lower dietary intake of fat and sodium, increased levels of physical activity, and abstention from tobacco use. These behavior changes were, in turn, expected to lead to improved blood concentrations of lipids, decreased blood pressure, and increased physical fitness. The study was implemented in four regional sites across the United States in ninety-six elementary schools (Perry and others, 1990). The importance of process evaluation, especially in studies with multiple levels of intervention and measurement, was demonstrated in this study (Perry and others, 1997).

The second multicenter, school-based trial supported by the NHLBI was Pathways. This was also a large-scale, multisite study testing a school-based health promotion intervention designed to lower the percentage of body fat in American Indian elementary school children. The design and methods used in the Pathways study have been previously described (Caballaro and others, 1998).

Description of the Pathways Program

The Pathways intervention design was closely modeled on that of CATCH, but Pathways adapted its approaches as needed to be appropriate for Indian students and schools. The Pathways intervention also drew from previous school-based interventions designed specifically for American Indians, such as the Checkerboard Cardiovascular Curriculum, the Southwest Cardiovascular Curriculum, and Pathways to Health, as well as from the findings of an extensive formative assessment of the Pathways communities and schools (Gittelsohn and others, 2000). The Pathways interventions were based on social learning theory, which applies a multilevel strategy involving individual behavior change and environmental modifications to support changes in individual behavior (Baranowski, Perry, and Parcel, 1997).

Pathways included four intervention components designed to address both the behavioral and environmental factors related to students' dietary and physical activity patterns. The components were (1) a culturally appropriate classroom curriculum designed to promote healthy eating behaviors and increased physical activity, encouraging daily five-minute exercise breaks in the regular classroom, (2) a physical activity component aimed at maximizing energy expenditure during physical education classes and outside of PE class during exercise breaks, (3) a food service intervention intended to reduce the amount of fat in school meals by changing or enhancing food service staff skills in planning, purchasing, preparing, and serving lower-fat meals, and (4) a family program involving take-home *family action packs* linked to the classroom curriculum, as well as several school-based family events each year that would encourage parents to promote reduced-fat meals and exercise (Caballaro and others, 1998). Through these four components, Pathways attempted to increase student knowledge and self-efficacy about physical activity and food choices as well as change the school environment in order to provide more opportunities for exercise and more healthy food choices.

The final results of the Pathways trial found no difference in the average percentage of body fat or body mass index between the intervention and control students. However, the project was successful in lowering fat and saturated fat in food served in intervention school cafeterias. Also, although not statistically significant, there was a trend toward higher activity levels among intervention students, compared with the activity levels of students in control schools. Finally, there were significant, positive effects on intervention students' knowledge, attitudes, and self-reported behaviors concerning physical activity and nutrition.

Pathways included an extensive process evaluation component (Helitzer and others, 1999). Process evaluation is considered particularly important for projects that employ multiple interventions in order to document and assess the effects of each component (McGraw and others, 1994; Viadro, Earp, and Altpeter, 1997). The uses of process evaluation include documenting exposure to interventions, demonstrating degree of adherence to intervention protocols, providing data on environmental forces that affect interventions, informing outcome findings, and conducting quality assurance (Israel and others, 1995; Bartholomew, Parcel, Kok, and Gottlieb, 2001).

Baranowski and Stables (2000) suggest that program implementation consists of two main components: *fidelity* and *dose*. Fidelity is the quality of delivery and dose is the number or amount of units delivered or provided. Assessing fidelity and dose is a test of internal validity—that is, the implementation of the interventions as planned (Baranowski and Stables, 2000; Basch and others, 1985). *Reach,* another important process evaluation component, is defined as the degree to which the program contacted or was received by the targeted group (Baranowski and Stables, 2000). It is suggested in the literature that data concerning all three of these process evaluation measures be collected for as many intervention components as is practical in any given health promotion program (Baranowski and Stables, 2000).

This chapter summarizes the process evaluation design, methods, and results for the three years (1997–1999) during which the Pathways trial was implemented. In addition, lessons learned about process evaluation from this experience are presented.

Process Evaluation Methods

As shown in Table 10.1, a total of twenty instruments were used to collect process evaluation data for Pathways (Helitzer and others, 1999). The fourth column of Table 10.1 indicates the process evaluation component that each instrument was designed to measure. Several different types of process data were collected for each intervention, as described in the next section.

TABLE 10.1.   PROCESS EVALUATION MEASURES.

Intervention	Data Collection Forms	When Collected	Process Evaluation Component
Curriculum	1. Classroom teacher training attendance log	At each training session	Reach
	2. Training evaluation form	At each training session	Dose and Fidelity
	3. Family pack challenge return log	End of each semester	Dose and Fidelity
	4. Classroom teacher/curriculum checklist and interview	End of each semester	Dose and Fidelity
Physical Activity	5. PE teacher training attendance log	At each training event	Reach
	6. Training evaluation form	At each training event	Dose and Fidelity
	7. Physical education calendar	End of each semester	Dose
	8. PE mentor visit summary form	2 times in fall; 3 times in spring	Fidelity
	9. PE teacher checklist and interview	End of each semester	Fidelity
Food Service	10. Food service personnel training attendance log	At each training event	Reach
	11. Food service training evaluation form	At each training event	Dose and Fidelity
	12. Food service kitchen contact form	2 times in fall 3 times in spring	Dose and Fidelity
	13. Food service manager interview	End of each semester	Fidelity
	14. School lunch checklist	End of each semester	Fidelity
Family	Family events:		
	15. Registration form	At each family event	Reach
	16. Student evaluation form	"	Fidelity
	17. Adult evaluation form	"	Fidelity
	18. Field notes form	"	Fidelity
Student Exposure	19. Student exposure questionnaire	End of each year	Dose
Administration	20. Principal Interview	End of each semester	Fidelity

Classroom Curriculum

Four types of process data were collected for the classroom curriculum intervention component. Classroom teacher training occurred each year at the beginning of each semester. Teachers' attendance at each training session was recorded (reach). In addition, each teacher completed a brief evaluation of the training program (dose and fidelity). During the curriculum training, each teacher received a checklist that contained each unit and each lesson. The teachers filled out this form during the time they were teaching the Pathways curriculum. When students and their parents completed an activity at home, the students brought back to their teacher a signed Family Pack Return Card. These cards were used to document the number of activities completed at home (dose). At the end of each semester, a process evaluation staff person visited teachers, reviewed the checklist with them, and conducted a brief interview (dose and fidelity).

Physical Activity

Five types of process data were collected for the physical activity component of the Pathways intervention. At each physical activity training session, teacher attendance was recorded (reach), and the teachers completed a brief evaluation (dose and fidelity). Each physical education teacher completed a PE calendar each month during the three years of Pathways (dose). The calendars noted when PE was taught, how many students participated, and what activity or lesson from the Pathways physical education curriculum was used.

Physical education teachers were visited periodically by a mentor. The mentors were qualified physical education instructors hired and trained by the project to provide consultation to Pathways physical education teachers. Twice in the fall semesters, and three times in the spring semesters, PE mentors completed a brief form that indicated the purpose of their visit to each school, what lessons they had supported, demonstrated, or explained, and what their observations were concerning how the Pathways program was being implemented in the school (fidelity). The final process evaluation data collection for physical activity was an end-of-semester checklist and interview completed by the process evaluation staff with each physical education teacher. During this in-person interview, each teacher was asked to check those Pathways physical activities that had been taught that semester. In addition, the teachers were asked open-ended questions about how each lesson had been received by the students and about any problems they had in teaching any of the activities, and they were asked to give their overall comments about the Pathways physical activity curriculum (dose and fidelity).

Food Service

Process evaluation of the food service intervention involved the use of five data collection methods. Training of food service staff members was conducted at the beginning of each semester. Attendance at the training session by food service workers was recorded (reach), and each attendee completed a brief evaluation of each training session (dose and fidelity). Each Pathways site, as part of their research team, employed a nutritionist (called a food service coordinator), who periodically visited each intervention school cafeteria kitchen. At least twice during the fall semesters, and three times during the spring semesters, the coordinators completed a Food Service Kitchen Contact Form (dose and fidelity). On this form, the coordinators indicated the primary purpose of their visit, what guidelines they had explained, demonstrated, or supported, and what guidelines they had observed being carried out by the food service staff. If food service staff members were implementing a guideline incorrectly, this was also noted on the form. They also wrote their overall impressions of how the food service component of Pathways was going in that school.

At the end of each semester, a Pathways process evaluation staff member conducted a structured interview with the food service manager of each intervention school. In this interview, food service managers were asked to indicate which of the food service guidelines they had implemented, which guidelines they were not able to implement that semester, and any problems they had experienced in trying to implement the Pathways food service guidelines (fidelity). The process evaluation staff person ate lunch in the school cafeteria and completed a school lunch checklist on the day they conducted the food service manager interviews (fidelity).

Family

The goal of the process evaluation for the family intervention was to document how many family members of Pathways students attended each family event. To accomplish this, four data collection forms were used. At each family event the number of family members of Pathways students attending an event was logged (reach). In addition to attendance, each adult and each Pathways student completed a brief written evaluation of each family event (fidelity). A field notes form was developed to allow project staff members to record their observations of a family event (fidelity). The process evaluation staff members had been trained in what to observe and how to record their qualitative observations.

Students

At the end of each of the three school years of the Pathways study, students in both the intervention schools and the control schools completed a brief, in-class questionnaire concerning their perceived exposure to the Pathways interventions. Typical questions included: "Did you take short exercise breaks in class every week?" "Did your family go to family events at school about exercise?" and "Did you make and eat low-fat snacks in class?" The items were scored on a 0–1 scale, with 1 being the "exposed" value for all items. These questionnaire items measured the students' perceived exposure to the Pathways interventions (dose).

School Administrators

At the end of each semester during the three years of implementation of the Pathways program, a brief interview was conducted with each intervention school principal. The interview usually took fifteen to twenty minutes and asked the principal for his or her observations about how Pathways was going in the school, as well as asking what benefits Pathways had brought to the school and what (if any) problems the school had experienced as a result of Pathways (fidelity).

Summary of Process Evaluation Results

The following is a brief summary of the main process evaluation findings.

Results for Classroom Curriculum

Training. The attendance of teachers at the curriculum sessions was 95.6 percent during the third grade, 98.0 percent during the fourth grade, and 92.0 percent during the fifth grade. The teachers' evaluation of the curriculum training suggests that most of the teachers thought that they had learned why children needed to learn about nutrition and physical activity, what the purpose of each lesson in the Pathways curriculum was, what should be emphasized in each activity, how to coordinate teaching the curriculum with other Pathways programs, such as physical activity and food service, and what specific terms were used in the lessons.

Curriculum Implementation. On average, across all of the classrooms in the Pathways schools, over 90 percent of the Pathways curriculum lessons were successfully taught in the third, fourth, and fifth grades. Each year's curriculum also included suggested family activities. Throughout the curriculum, students took home family action packs, which were ideas for activities that families could do together to help improve nutrition and physical activity. Students were asked to return a card signed by their parents indicating completion of each activity. Overall, the rate of return for these cards ranged from a high of 63.2 percent in the fall of the third grade to a low of 39.8 percent in the spring of the fourth grade. The decline in returns of cards was significant over the three years of the project (Chi-square = 77.78, df = 2, $p < .005$), indicating a likely low dose for parents with regard to the family action packs.

Teachers' Comments About the Curriculum. In the analysis of the qualitative interview data with teachers for all three of the project years, five main themes were found: (1) the teachers reported that they could integrate the Pathways curriculum with other subjects, (2) snack preparation and taste testing were favorite activities of students, (3) active games included within the curriculum lessons each year were popular with students and teachers, (4) for many teachers, it took more time to teach the classroom curriculum than they had planned, and (5) teachers thought that the students benefited from the curriculum, and a number of teachers indicated that they would continue using it.

Results for Physical Activity

Training. At the physical education training sessions, there was 100 percent attendance of teachers in each of the three project years. The training sessions were successful in helping the teachers understand (1) the need for the Pathways physical activity program, (2) the goal of three to five PE classes per week, (3) the cultural significance of the American Indian games that were part of the physical education curriculum, (4) what to emphasize in the PE curriculum, and (5) the importance of daily recess.

Implementation of the Physical Education Curriculum. The goal for the intervention schools was to have teachers deliver the Pathways physical education curriculum for thirty minutes at least three times per week, or ninety minutes per week. Although the minimum goal was to teach physical activity three times per week, the schools were encouraged to teach it five times per week. In analyzing the physical activity process data, a key component of dose was the duration and number of days per week of physical education classes. We examined whether schools met the minimum of offering physical education three times per week and the extent to which they offered it five times per week.

All of the schools were able to teach physical education for thirty minutes whenever it was taught. In the third grade, the average number of minutes of physical education was 32.5, in the fourth grade, it was 32.9, and in the fifth grade, it was 33.2.

The second column of Table 10.2 shows the average number of days that physical education was taught in the third, fourth, and fifth grades of the Pathways

TABLE 10.2. MINIMUM AND MAXIMUM TOTAL NUMBER OF PE DAYS AS A PERCENTAGE OF ALL SCHOOL DAYS, BY GRADE.

Grade	No. of PE Days	Minimum Expected Days of PE		Maximum Encouraged Days of PE	
		Expected No. of Days	Percentage	Possible No. of Days	Percentage
Third	70.8	87.4	81.0	145.7	48.6
Fourth	87.9	88.6	99.2	146.6	60.0
Fifth	88.5	87.1	101.6	145.5	60.8
Total	82.4	87.7	93.9*	145.98	56.5**

*Chi-square = 3.18, df = 2, p = n.s.
** Chi-square = 84.33, df = 2, p < .005

intervention schools. The third column of this table indicates the expected number of days of physical education if the schools had taught it three times per week. The expected number of days has been adjusted for holidays and schoolwide events during which physical education could not have been taught. For instance, in the third grade, on average, the schools taught 70.8 days of physical education. If they had taught it every possible day, three times per week, they would have taught physical education for 87.4 days. Therefore, on average, physical education was taught on 81 percent of the days available for it. This table suggests that the teaching of physical activity at least three times per week increased from 81 percent of the available days in the third grade to 99.2 percent in the fourth grade and to 101.6 percent in the fifth grade.

PE Teachers' Comments About the Physical Education Curriculum. During all three years of the study, PE teachers indicated their positive reaction to the physical education curriculum. One teacher remarked that "the curriculum is laid out very well and it is good to work with." Another PE teacher said, "The activities really help the students, with fitness and learning, to listen and pay attention." In addition, several teachers spoke of how Pathways PE meshed well with their current PE curriculum. The few negative comments from some fifth-grade teachers concerned the perception that the games were no longer challenging for the students and that some students seemed to be bored.

Food Service Intervention Results

Training. As with the other interventions, there was good attendance at the food service trainings. During the third-grade attendance, it was 92.9 percent, during the fourth-grade attendance, it was 95.5 percent, and during the fifth-grade attendance, it was 166.7 percent. (Attendance was greater than 100 percent because schools sometimes sent more food service workers to the training than was required.) Evaluation of the food service training consisted of open-ended questions to which the food service workers were asked to give written responses. They were asked the questions "What did you like best about the training?" and "What did you like least about the training?" and then they were asked to write their "general comments."

Across all three years of the Pathways project, the food service staff members gave very positive reviews of the food service training. For instance, after the first training, one participant wrote, "I found everything educational and fun." Other attendees commented that "the whole training was all very good, no weak points." Another recurring theme was a desire to have more training.

Implementation of the Behavioral Guidelines. For the food service intervention, there were nine primary and four secondary (for a total of thirteen) behavioral guidelines that school food service personnel were trained to implement (Snyder and others, 1999). Table 10.3 lists each of the food service behavioral guidelines and the percentage of times they were observed being correctly implemented during the third-, fourth-, and fifth-grade interventions. The food service coordinators did an observation of a lunch preparation and service at least twice each fall semester and three times each spring semester. The coordinators noted whether (1) a particular guideline was being implemented that day (for example, no cheese was being served) and (2) if the guideline was being implemented correctly. The percentages shown in Table 10.3 are the number of times each guideline was observed being correctly implemented, divided by the total number of observations of each guideline for each of the three grades. (If a particular guideline was not observed on a given day, it is not counted in the denominator.)

The Pathways food service intervention group determined a specific goal for each guideline. These goals are shown in the second column of Table 10.3. As shown in Table 10.3, on average, the percentage of food service behavioral guidelines being implemented increased from 51.5 percent during the third grade to 80.6 percent during the fourth grade and to 87.5 percent during the fifth grade. Although not statistically significant, there was a trend of increasing implementation of the food service guidelines from third to fourth to fifth grades.

Family Intervention Results

The family events were designed to reach parents and other adult family members with the Pathways message, which states the benefits to both children and

TABLE 10.3. PERCENTAGE OF VISITS WHERE FOOD SERVICE GUIDELINES WERE FOLLOWED, BY GRADE.

		3rd Grade	4th Grade	5th Grade	Total
Number of Visits		134	306	237	677
Guideline	Goal	Percentage	Percentage	Percentage	Percentage
1. Offered only 1% or skim milk	90	24.6	64.7	71.8	60.5
2. Drained and rinsed ground meat	90	79.7	92.0	97.5	91.5
3. Used low-fat vendor entrees	80	37.3	86.6	82.4	75.4
4. Used low-fat salad dressing	80	36.2	80.0	91.9	75.5
5. Used low-fat cheese	80	39.3	62.2	71.8	61.0
6. Prep/serve breads w/o added fat	90	60.2	82.6	94.7	82.4
7. Prep/serve pasta w/ little/no fat	90	57.6	86.2	93.2	83.0
8. Prepare gravy with no fat	90	54.5	80.9	93.8	80.2
9. Prep/serve hot vegetables w/o fat	90	81.9	91.4	95.7	91.0
10. No fats on serving line	90	72.4	93.8	98.7	91.3
11. Offered choices of fruits and vegetables	75	37.5	58.4	69.7	58.2
12. No seconds of entrees	80	36.9	72.1	79.6	67.8
13. Offered required amount of menu items	90	**	93.9	97.3	95.4
Mean percentage	85.8	51.5	80.6	87.5	77.9
Number of guidelines meeting or exceeding goal		0/12	6/13	9/13*	

*Chi-square = 5.00, df = 2, p = n.s.
**Not measured

adults of eating lower-fat foods and getting regular physical activity. The events were held at the Pathways participating schools during the school day—in the late afternoon or during the early evening. The events were designed to be participatory, interesting, skills-oriented, and fun for students and their parents. There were four family events held during the third grade, three during the fourth grade, and two during the fifth grade.

Attendance at Family Events. Across the three years of the Pathways project, on average, 58 percent of the Pathways students attended each family event. Student attendance was 45.5 percent in the third grade, 67.3 percent in the fourth grade, and 66.3 percent in the fifth grade (an increase that was statistically significant). The main purpose of the family events was to reach parents and adult relatives with the Pathways message. The goal was to have one parent, guardian, or other adult relative attend for each Pathways student. In the third grade, the ratio of adults to the total number of Pathways students attending was 0.45, in the fourth grade it was 0.41, and in the fifth grade it increased to 0.63 (an increase that was not statistically significant). Over the three years of the Pathways project, the average overall adult attendance ratio was 0.47.

Comments Made by Adults About the Family Events. Adults who attended the family events were asked to complete a brief written evaluation form. When asked to comment on how worthwhile the family events were for them, adults overwhelmingly gave positive responses for all three years. Parents said that it was time that the family spent together, the activities were fun, they liked and were surprised by the tastiness of the low-fat foods, and they felt that they had learned what they could do at home to prepare low-fat meals and to boost their physical activity.

Perceived Student Exposure Results

In each year, there was a significant difference between intervention and control students' perceived exposure to the Pathways interventions. For instance, in the third grade, the least square mean was 0.71 for the intervention group, and it was 0.45 for the control group ($p < 0.0001$). Clearly, the intervention students perceived themselves to have been exposed to Pathways-type interventions to a much greater extent than the students in the control schools had been.

School Administrators' Results

From the third-grade end-of-semester interviews with principals and the observations made during site visits, it was clear that the amount of administrators' involvement with Pathways varied widely across schools and sites. Some administrators were familiar with how the Pathways interventions were progressing in their schools and some were unaware. Largely, principals noted that the feedback they had received from classroom teachers and students about the curriculum was very positive. The only negative comment heard from principals during the third grade concerning the curriculum was that it "takes too much time."

At the end of the fourth-grade interviews, principals responded positively to Pathways and its four intervention components. For instance, one principal remarked that "curriculum teachers are doing great, they love it," and another principal said, "PE, [it is] a more active curriculum—[I] can see a difference." Principals commented on how Pathways had raised awareness and influenced behavior among teachers and students in their schools.

At the end of the fifth grade, principals were interviewed one final time. Overall, the principals continued to be positive about Pathways. The most frequently mentioned effect of Pathways was changes in the food served in the school cafeteria. Principals noted that healthier meals were being served as a result of Pathways. Some principals said that as a result of Pathways, their physical education program was improved, and it was mentioned that one PE program was created where none had existed before. When asked what problems their school has had with Pathways, the principals commented about the time it took to complete all the data collection forms, the difficulty of finding time to schedule and fit in all the Pathways activities, and, particularly, the difficulty of fitting the Pathways curriculum into an already full curriculum.

Lessons Learned About Process Evaluation

This final section presents eight lessons learned about process evaluation from the Pathways study.

LESSON 1. *Determine the appropriate process evaluation components early in the study.*

Process evaluation is not a singular concept; rather, it has multiple components. For instance, Baranowski and Stables (2000) suggest the following possible components of process evaluation: fidelity, dose, reach, exposure, recruitment, maintenance, context, and resources.

When planning a process evaluation, researchers should think through which components of process evaluation are the most important to assess for their study. In Pathways, this was not done. The consequence was that when it came time to write up the results, it was somewhat awkward and difficult to link the measures used in the Pathways process evaluation to the components. For instance, as suggested in Table 10.1, dose and fidelity measures tended to be hard to separate from each other.

The reason this occurred concerns the development of process evaluation as a recognized, legitimate component of intervention research. The Pathways process evaluation was originally designed around 1993–94 (Helitzer and others, 1999), six years before the publication of the Baranowski and Stables (2000) seminal article. Although there had been prior studies—such as CATCH and

Working Well—that had extensive process evaluations, the detailed conceptual development of the process evaluation components, as described by Baranowski and Stables (2000), is relatively new.

LESSON 2. *Use process evaluation data for quality control of the intervention.*

Quality control of an intervention occurs when implementation-monitoring data are collected, analyzed, and reported to the intervention staff. The purpose is to help ensure that the intervention is implemented according to the planned reach, dose, and fidelity. Quality control is only effective when the results are available in a timely way so that adjustments in implementation can be made before the end of the study.

We successfully used the Pathways process evaluation data for intervention monitoring and quality control purposes. Most of the process evaluation data were collected at the end of each semester. The data were quickly analyzed in about four to six weeks. The results were given to the intervention committee, the measurement committee, and the project steering committee. Incipient implementation problems were highlighted by the process evaluation staff and were thus brought to the attention of those conducting the interventions at the study sites. For example, by the end of the third grade, it appeared that the physical education intervention program was not being implemented at an adequate dose level at a number of the study schools; that is, it was being implemented fewer than three times per week at some of them. Based on these early findings, the next year, additional training was provided to the physical education mentors, who were instructed to work more frequently with the school physical education teachers to ensure greater implementation of the physical education curriculum.

LESSON 3. *Collect process evaluation data from control groups.*

One of the primary purposes of process evaluation is to be able to help explain a project's final outcomes. This is particularly true when there is little or no difference in results between the experimental and control conditions. When this is the case, it is important to know whether the intervention was fully implemented in the intervention group. It is also important to know whether some type of similar intervention occurred in the control group. If it did, then it is possible that the lack of difference between the two groups was due to equivalent interventions in each group.

As previously noted, the Pathways results showed no difference in body mass index or physical activity between the intervention and control groups. Because process evaluation data were collected only on the intervention schools, we are not able to say whether any interventions or secular trends that might have occurred in the control schools contributed to this lack of difference.

In planning the Pathways process evaluation, we decided to focus almost all of our process evaluation resources on the intervention schools. In fact, the only process evaluation data collected from control schools were the end-of-year student exposure data.

We made the decision to focus on the intervention schools (versus the control schools) for two reasons. The first reason was limited resources. Given the resources available for process evaluation, we decided that it would be better to get more data and more in-depth data from all the intervention schools than it would be to get less data and less in-depth data from both the intervention schools and the control schools.

The second reason concerns the problem of collecting data about a "negative"; that is, how do we collect process evaluation data when the control schools do not offer something that is parallel to the interventions in the experimental schools? What do we observe? What questions do we ask? What do we measure in a control classroom that does not offer a curriculum that covers nutrition and physical activity? In retrospect, however, we could have collected some minimum process data from the control schools.

LESSON 4. *Assessment of implementation fidelity remains problematic for process evaluation.*

Resnicow and others (1998) rigorously compared three methods of measuring teacher fidelity to a nutrition curriculum. They concluded that classroom observation by trained observers produced the most valid results, in-person, structured interviews done soon after the teacher had completed teaching the curriculum produced the second-best results, and questionnaires completed by the teacher and then mailed to the researchers produced the least satisfactory results.

Although classroom observations of program implementation is the "gold standard" for assessing implementation fidelity, it is not always feasible, because of the personnel and travel costs involved for large-scale studies conducted in rural, remote areas. In fact, this is the reason we chose to use in-person interviews at the end of each semester for the Pathways process evaluation. Resnicow and others (1998) found acceptable correlations between in-person interviews and observations, which suggests that end-of-semester interviews with program implementers, especially where prompts such as a curriculum or a structured interview guide are used, can produce valid implementation fidelity measures.

However, recall bias is a problem when using interviews that occur long after the intervention has been completed. In Pathways, when classroom teachers, physical education teachers, and food service managers were trained concerning the intervention, they also received an orientation to the process evaluation, including the end-of-semester interviews. Classroom teachers were given a copy of the structured questionnaire during training and were asked to fill it out as they completed each lesson. We found that some teachers conscientiously followed the requested procedure and some did not. For those who did not, a process evaluation staff person conducted an interview with the teacher and asked her to recall the various lessons, how she had taught them, and what the students' reaction had been. This interview was conducted at the end of the semester. The actual teaching of the curriculum took place weeks earlier during the semester, which raised the possibility of teacher recall bias.

All of this suggests that valid and reliable measures of implementation fidelity remain problematic for process evaluation. This is an evaluation component that warrants further methodological development.

LESSON 5. *Plan for ongoing training of process evaluation field staff.*

In Pathways, a process evaluation data collection field staff member was employed by each field center. In three of the sites, the person hired was an American Indian. Over the three years of the intervention, two of the American Indian process evaluation site staff members left the project and were replaced with new personnel: one American Indian and one non–American Indian.

Field staff members were trained at the beginning of each of the three intervention years. In addition, there were monthly conference calls that included the four field site staff members and the coordinator of the process evaluation. Also, process evaluation staff members from the project coordinating center made on-site consultative visits each year with the local site staff when they were collecting the end-of-semester process evaluation data.

Extensive training, continuous consultation, and technical assistance were necessary because of the complexity of the process evaluation design; that is, there were twenty different process evaluation data collection instruments for which each field staff person was responsible. Not only were there a large number of instruments, but most of the instruments included both quantitative and qualitative data, requiring field staff to be skilled in collecting both types of data.

The field staff found that it was important to establish frequent and friendly working relationships with school personnel because school staff members were then more likely to be open and honest in answering qualitative questions, as opposed to telling the field staff members what they thought they wanted to hear.

LESSON 6. *Include process evaluation in planning a project's total respondent burden.*

As mentioned, twenty different process evaluation instruments were used in Pathways. Each instrument required some type of action or response from school personnel. Even though we designed the process evaluation data collection methods to be as brief as possible in order to minimize the response burden on the school staff, there was still a high total respondent burden.

The process evaluation was only a small part of all of the measures used in Pathways. Students filled out end-of-year questionnaires, they were weighed, their height was measured, the percentage of their body fat was measured, and they wore motion sensors to measure movement. Data were collected about school cafeteria menus and observations were conducted of students' eating patterns in the cafeteria. At the end of each school year, a number of interviews were conducted with school personnel for purposes of assessing the school climate.

Due to their commitment to Pathways, all schools completed the three-year involvement; however, there was a high respondent burden on school staff members, who were already very busy. Therefore, in planning any school-based intervention research project, the respondent burden for process evaluation needs to be carefully considered in relation to the total respondent burden for the overall project.

LESSON 7. *Determine school-related issues that might affect process evaluation.*

Pathways was conducted with schools on American Indian reservations that were primarily located in rural and somewhat remote areas. To reach their schools, some students often had to ride the school bus for over an hour. Because of their large service areas, some of the schools were both boarding and day schools. The long distance from home to school and the fact that some students were boarders may have been barriers to both student and parent participation in school events. The process evaluation focused on school-based activities and did not attempt to collect data concerning the home-based activities that were recommended to parents and students through the family events and family action packs. Therefore, we had no information about how the family events and action packs were used, if at all, by parents and students at home. The process evaluation could have done some type of home-based data collection, which would have helped us understand how the Pathways interventions affected families.

LESSON 8. *Process evaluation can help show the pattern of adoption of intervention components.*

In Pathways, for instance, the physical education and food service interventions showed gains over time—that is, there was an increase in implementation from the third to the fourth to the fifth grade. In other words, school interventions, and perhaps interventions in other settings, do not launch at full steam; they take time to build up to full implementation, and process evaluation can help elucidate patterns of change over time.

References

Baranowski, T., and Stables, G. "Process Evaluations of the 5-a-Day Projects." *Health Education and Behavior*, 2000, *27*, 157–166.

Baranowski, T., Perry, C. L., and Parcel, G. S. "How Individuals, Environments, and Health Behavior Interact: Social Cognitive Theory." In K. Glanz, F. M. Lewis, and B. K. Rimer (eds.), *Health Behavior and Health Education: Theory, Research, and Practice.* (2nd ed.) San Francisco: Jossey-Bass, 1997.

Bartholomew, L. K., Parcel, G. S., Kok, G., and Gottlieb, N. H. *Intervention Mapping: Designing Theory and Evidence-Based Health Promotion Programs.* Mountain View, Calif.: Mayfield, 2001.

Basch, C. E., and others. "Avoiding Type III Errors in Health Education Program Evaluations: A Case Study." *Health Education Quarterly*, 1985, *12*, 315–331.

Brousard, B. A., and others. "Prevalence of Obesity in American Indians and Alaska Natives." *American Journal of Clinical Nutrition*, 1991, *53* (supp. 6), 1535S–1542S.

Caballaro B., and others. "Pathways: A School-Based Program for the Primary Prevention of Obesity in American Indian Children." *Journal of Nutritional Biochemistry*, 1998, *9*, 535–543.

Gittelsohn, J., and others. "Food Perceptions and Dietary Behavior of American-Indian Children, Their Caregivers, and Educators: Formative Assessment Findings from Pathways." *Journal of Nutrition Education*, 2000, *32*(1), 2–13.

Helitzer D., and others. "Process Evaluation in a Multisite Obesity Primary Prevention Trial for Native American School Children." *American Journal of Clinical Nutrition*, 1999, *69* (supp.), 816S–824S.

Israel, B. A., and others. "Evaluation of Health Education Programs: Current Assessment and Future Directions." *Health Education Quarterly*, 1995, *22*, 364–389.

McGraw S. A., and others. "An Overview of Process Evaluation on CATCH: The Child and Adolescent Trial for Cardiovascular Health." *Health Education Quarterly*, 1994, *25* (supp.), S5–26.

Perry, C. L., and others. "School-Based Cardiovascular Health Promotion: The Child and Adolescent Trial for Cardiovascular Health (CATCH)." *Journal of School Health*, 1990, *60*, 406–413.

Perry C. L., and others. "The Child and Adolescent Trial for Cardiovascular Health (CATCH): Intervention, Implementation, and Feasibility for Elementary Schools in the United States." *Health Education and Behavior*, 1997, *24*, 716–735.

Snyder, P., and others. "The Pathways Study: A Model for Lowering the Fat in School Meals." *American Journal of Clinical Nutrition*, 1999, *69*, 810S–815S.

Viadro, C. I., Earp, J., and Altpeter, M. "Designing a Process Evaluation for a Comprehensive Breast Cancer Screening Intervention: Challenges and Opportunities." *Evaluation and Program Planning*, 1997, *20*, 237–249.

Welty, T. "Health Implications of Obesity in American Indians and Alaska Natives." *American Journal of Clinical Nutrition*, 1991, *53*, 116S–120S.

APPENDIX A: FOURTH-GRADE KITCHEN CONTACT FORM.

To be completed by Pathways staff:	
School ID: _____	Form Code: **KC4**
Version: **A** Grade: **4**	Seq. #: _____

Fourth-Grade Kitchen Contact Form
Site:_____
School:_____
Date:_____
Time of Arrival in Kitchen:_____
Time of Departure from Kitchen:_____

A. Pathways staff

	Name	Title
A1	_____	_____
A2	_____	_____
A3	_____	_____
A4	_____	_____

B. Food service staff contacted (List all that apply)

		Name
B1	Food Service Director	_____
B2	Cook Manager	_____
B3	Cook	_____
B4	Other kitchen staff	_____

C. Type of visit (Check all that apply)
C1   ❑   Visit to kitchen
C2   ❑   Visit to Food Service Director
C3   ❑   Other—Please specify: _____

D. Focus of contact (Check all that apply)
D1   ❑   Implemented Pathways Food Service Guidelines* (See below for directions)
    —
D2   ❑   Reinforced/follow-up on implementation of Pathways Food Service
         Guidelines** #__ __ __ __ __ __ __ __ __ __ __ __ __ __ __
D3   ❑   Met briefly with food service staff
D4   ❑   Helped serve breakfast
D5   ❑   Observed school breakfast
D6   ❑   Ate breakfast
D7   ❑   Helped serve lunch
D8   ❑   Observed school lunch
D9   ❑   Ate lunch
D10 ❑   Helped prepare school meal
D11 ❑   Coordinated curriculum or family food service activities
D12 ❑   Met with Administrators
D13 ❑   Other—Please specify: _____

If any food preparation or meal serving was observed, please complete the following pages.

*Refer to the following pages for guidelines and specific activity codes. For example, if Guideline #1 was imple-
  mented (Offer Lower-Fat Milk), write "1D" to indicate offered 1% milk, or "1E" to indicate offered skim milk.
**Indicate number of guideline. Specific activity codes are not necessary.
May 1, 1998   Process Evaluation KCF.4: Food Service Kitchen Contact Form

APPENDIX A: (CONTINUED)

Pathways Behavioral Guidelines Evaluation

Directions:

If you **observed** the Pathways Food Service behavioral guideline being implemented as stated:
Check yes (1) if guideline was implemented
Check no (2) if guideline was not being implemented
Check no opportunity (3) if no opportunity to observe whether the guideline was implemented or not

Guideline #1: Offer Lower-Fat Milk (skim, 1%)		1-YES	2-NO	3-No Opportunity
1A	Offered no whole milk	1❑	2❑	3❑
1B	Offered no 2% milk	1❑	2❑	3❑
1C	Offered no 1 1/2% milk	1❑	2❑	3❑
1D	Offered 1% milk	1❑	2❑	3❑
1E	Offered skim milk	1❑	2❑	3❑
1F	Offered other milk	1❑	2❑	3❑
1G	List other milk(s): _____			

Guideline #2: Drain and Rinse Ground Meat		1-YES	2-NO	3-No Opportunity
2A	Drained fat from cooked ground meat	1❑	2❑	3❑
2B	Rinsed cooked ground meat with hot water and drained again	1❑	2❑	3❑

Guideline #3: Purchase Lower-Fat Vendor Products		1-YES	2-NO	3-No Opportunity
3A	Used lower-fat entrees that meet the Pathways nutrition guidelines	1❑	2❑	3❑
3B	List specific product(s): _____			
3C	Used low- or non-fat salad dressings that meet the Pathways nutrition guidelines	1❑	2❑	3❑
3D	List specific dressing(s): _____			
3E	Offered no high-fat salad dressing	1❑	2❑	3❑

Guideline #4: Use Low-Fat Cheese		1-YES	2-NO	3-No Opportunity
4A	Used lower-fat cheeses that meet the Pathways nutrition guidelines	1❑	2❑	3❑
4B	List specific cheese(s): _____			
4C	Offered no high-fat cheese	1❑	2❑	3❑

Guideline #5: Use Less or No Butter and Other Fats*		1-YES	2-NO	3-No Opportunity
5A	Served breads (including rolls, muffins, and biscuits) with no added butter to top of hot breads from the oven	1❑	2❑	3❑
5B	Served breads on the serving line with no butter or other fats*	1❑	2❑	3❑
5C	Cooked spaghetti, macaroni, noodles, or rice in water with little or no fat*	1❑	2❑	3❑
5D	Served spaghetti, macaroni, noodles, or rice with no added fat*	1❑	2❑	3❑
5E	Prepared gravy with no fat*	1❑	2❑	3❑
5F	Prepared vegetables with no added fat*	1❑	2❑	3❑
5G	Served vegetables with no added fat*	1❑	2❑	3❑

*Fat includes butter, margarine, lard, meat drippings, regular cheese sauce, regular sour cream, regular shortening, and vegetable oil.

May 1, 1998   Process Evaluation KCF.4: Food Service Kitchen Contact Form

(Continued)

APPENDIX A: FOURTH-GRADE KITCHEN CONTACT FORM. (CONTINUED)

Guideline #6: Remove Butter and Other Fats from the Serving Line	1-YES	2-NO	3-No Opportunity
6A	Offered no butter, margarine, or other fats on the serving line	1❑	2❑	3❑

Guideline #7: Offer Choices of Fruits and Vegetables	1-YES	2-NO	3- No Opportunity
7A	Offered two or more fruits	1❑	2❑	3❑
7B	List fruits: _____			
7C	Offered two or more vegetables	1❑	2❑	3❑
7D	List vegetables: _____			

Guideline #8: Serving Seconds (Check Seconds Offered)	1-YES	2-NO	3-No Opportunity
8A	Offered no seconds of entree	1❑	2❑	3❑
8B	Offered seconds of fruit	1❑	2❑	3❑
8C	Offered seconds of vegetable	1❑	2❑	3❑
8D	Offered seconds of bread	1❑	2❑	3❑

Guideline #9: Portion Size	1-YES	2-NO	3-No Opportunity
9A	Used standard serving utensils	1❑	2❑	3❑
	If no, list foods: _____			
9B	Used standard serving utensils correctly	1❑	2❑	3❑
9C	Offered required amount of menu items	1❑	2❑	3❑
	If no, list foods: _____			

List follow-up actions needed:

1)_____

2)_____

3)_____

List Breakfast Served:

_____

_____

_____

List Lunch Served:

_____

_____

_____

_____

General Comments:

_____

_____

PART FOUR

National or State Process Evaluation Efforts

In the final section of this book are three chapters on process evaluation that represent variation in scope (national versus statewide efforts), variation in the target population (program evaluation staff members, health professionals, and the general public), and variation in subject matter (the development of a statewide tracking system, a focus on the process of conducting an evaluation with the Indian Health Service, and the evaluation of a national media campaign). However much the content varies from one chapter to the next, each chapter facilitates an understanding of the complexity and challenges of designing and implementing large-scale process evaluation efforts.

In Chapter Eleven, Blaine, Guire, and Forster highlight the development and testing associated with a program monitoring tool—the Statewide Tobacco Endowment Process Evaluation System (STEPES)—designed to evaluate a statewide tobacco control program. Each chapter preceding Chapter Eleven acknowledges the depth and complexity of the data required to conduct a comprehensive process evaluation effort, yet, in each of these chapters, there is little focus on the tracking systems required to maintain the data effectively and to ensure that the data are usable on a timely basis. Moreover, while it has been emphasized that having trained personnel available to work on process evaluation is essential (see Chapter One), it is equally important to have the technology and resources to collect and maintain data effectively. Many projects continue to build systems for each new process evaluation effort. Using STEPES, Blaine, Guire, and Forster offer some practical advice for creating, pretesting, and evaluating process tracking systems that are relevant for many projects and studies.

What is unique about STEPES is that it is a custom-designed program monitoring and reporting database system that records both descriptive and qualitative program-level data. This database tool was created for practitioners who have limited (if any) experience with computers. Four sample form layouts (and related databases) are shared with readers: the Contact Entry Form, the Event Entry Form, the Meeting Entry Form, and the Quarterly Report Entry Form. The authors describe how local practitioners enter program information into STEPES, transfer the data to a central, integrated, and searchable master database, and use queries to generate user-specific reports that provide descriptive and summary information. To create this system, the authors explain how the developers of STEPES engaged in a utilization-focused evaluation with principal end users (state health department staff members and local tobacco control practitioners). The formative evolution followed two parallel tracks of database design and creation and content development. The thoughtful development and testing process is clearly articulated in this chapter, including information for creating reports, user manuals, and the alpha testing process.

We encourage all readers to carefully consider the cautions and wise advice offered in this chapter, which also emphasizes that the next generation of database monitoring systems will be Web-based, bringing additional security and privacy considerations that are beyond those chronicled in this chapter.

In Chapter Twelve, Crump and Letourneau broaden the scope of process evaluation conducted at a local or statewide level, to include a national focus. A collaborative evaluation effort between the authors, who are located at the Injury Prevention Center at the University of North Carolina, Chapel Hill, and the program staff at the Indian Health Service (IHS) Injury Prevention Program (IPP) has been under way since 1997. Crump and Letourneau detail the relationship that formed between these organizations, and they describe the program stage of development assessment (PSDA) tool and its role in the process evaluation of the IHS area IPPs. This tool is consistent with principles of empowerment and utilization-focused evaluation, and it serves as a best practice guide for the IHS area IPPs.

Several indicators are listed for each evaluation component in the PSDA tool: (1) mission/vision, (2) resource allocation/accounting, (3) management support, (4) staffing, (5) training, (6) partnerships/collaborations, (7) needs assessment/ defined service populations, (8) surveillance data collection, (9) program planning and implementation, (10) marketing/advocacy, (11) evaluation/reporting, and (12) technical assistance/building tribal capacity. Crump and Letourneau describe reports generated for each of the twelve IPPs in the IHS that received feedback using the PSDA tool, the rating scale used by evaluators to give feedback to the IPPs on each indicator, and the process used by evaluators to share these process evaluation results.

The authors critically evaluate the strengths and limitations of conducting a comprehensive evaluation that includes empowerment principles. Staff time to prepare information, conduct the evaluation, and get involved in the iterative process required to conduct a participatory evaluation effort is substantial. In addition, the authors consider the bias that might be introduced with external evaluators who are not familiar with the context in which these programs are implemented. Implications for future process evaluation efforts and research on the PSDA tool are suggested. This chapter is unique in its detailing of both the process of implementing this tool and the critical evaluation of the usefulness of the process evaluation tool as it is applied to a national-level IPP that is sponsored by the IHS.

In Chapter Thirteen, the final chapter in this section of the book, Daniel, Prue, and Volansky present process evaluation results from the Centers for Disease Control and Prevention-sponsored national folic acid media campaign. The National Council of Folic Acid was formed in 1997 and its mission is to reduce the number of neural tube defect-affected pregnancies by recommending that women of childbearing age consume 400 mcg of folic acid daily. A national public education media campaign was developed using the CDCynergy health communication planning framework. Key communication objectives for the campaign were to increase awareness (1) about folic acid, (2) that folic acid reduces the risk of birth defects, and (3) that folic acid should be taken before pregnancy. Multiple communication channels, including mass-reach media (TV and radio) and interpersonal channels, such as group presentations and counseling, were used.

Process evaluation of the national folic acid media campaign included the monitoring of media coverage, content analysis of news media, the monitoring of nonmedia activities, the use of media and nonmedia measures to create exposure indices, and the tracking of women's recall of the campaign. Both qualitative and quantitative methods for assessing these process variables were used. Readers who are involved in measuring the effects of media campaigns will be introduced to a number of unique strategies for operationalizing the data collected in this project, especially the detailed description of the development and evaluation of exposure indices.

Daniel, Prue, and Volansky provide a description of the process evaluation associated with a government-sponsored national media campaign, they provide unique insights into the complexity and challenges of working with multiple partners/agencies to create new measures and data collection tools that can be adapted at multiple localities, and they shed light on the resources required to conduct an evaluation of this magnitude. A theme brought out in this chapter and echoed throughout the book is the concern about collecting too much data and then not making use of all the data that are collected. A thoughtful planning process that helps prioritize key process evaluation questions (see Chapter One) appears to be critical to avoiding this issue.

CHAPTER ELEVEN

STEPES: The Development and Testing of a Database Program Monitoring Tool

Therese M. Blaine, D. Knight Guire, and Jean Forster

The public health community frequently extols the importance of monitoring and process evaluation to help explain behavior change outcomes, identify best practices, and improve program delivery. Yet the appeal for good evaluation methods and monitoring systems is only occasionally accompanied by examples of technology-based data collection tools. This is surprising, given the significant role that computer technology plays in our information age.

The speed and accuracy of data processing, exchange, and management hold immense opportunity for the field of public health (Friede, Blum, and McDonald, 1995). The cost and complexity of government- and foundation-funded community-based interventions, in combination with advances in computer and Internet technology, demand shifts in how we monitor and assess programs. Funding agencies expect timely and meaningful evaluations that facilitate quality improvement that is simultaneous with program delivery. New advances in technology-driven information management systems limit the use of

The study discussed in this chapter was funded from 1999 to 2002 by the Centers for Disease Control and Prevention, grant U48 CCU 513331. The authors gratefully acknowledge their collaborators at the Minnesota Department of Health, Tobacco Control Section, as well as local public health practitioners in Minnesota, for their contributions to the development and implementation of the STEPES tool. The authors also note the significant effort of Margo Rowe, cocreator of STEPES, and the intellectual contributions of Marsha Davis and Laura Ehrlich.

paper-driven program reporting. Although the inherent value of narrative documentation remains, its usefulness is seriously diminished because it lacks the capability for database manipulation, electronic transfer, and quick synthesis.

Public health funding agencies, managers, and practitioners expect management information systems (MIS) in the health arena to match the quality of the MIS technology they encounter in other facets of their lives—for example, on-line purchasing or banking ("Information Needs and Uses . . .", 2000). This expectation, along with a growing emphasis on outcomes accountability, opens the door for the development of comprehensive program monitoring and evaluation database systems (Fiene, 1988; Telleen, 1999). Database systems can facilitate consistent data collection and produce standardized data. Information inside a master database can be easily and quickly synthesized and used for a variety of evaluation purposes.

Health promotion interventions and individual health assessments using stand-alone or Web-based databases are frequently employed in school and clinic settings (Safran and others, 1994; Skinner, Siegfried, Kegler, and Strecher, 1993; Paperny, 1997; Hall, forthcoming). However, examples of computer technology used for program monitoring and evaluation purposes are less common. One example of a program monitoring and evaluation database system is that of the National Tobacco Control Program (NTCP), called NTCPChronicle. Created by the CDC, NTCPChronicle is used for monitoring and evaluating state programs funded by the CDC (Petersen and Babb, 2001). As of 2001, in the field of tobacco prevention, several state health departments, including those of California, Florida, Massachusetts, Minnesota, North Carolina, Oregon, and Washington, use stand-alone or Web-based database systems to collect and process information for monitoring and evaluation (Augustyniak, 2000; Celebucki, Biener, and Koh, 1998). Discussions with the creators and users of these database systems indicate that the complexity, content, and sophistication of these databases vary widely. Notably, discussions of the development, implementation, and testing of computerized program monitoring database systems is scant in the current published literature. Stand-alone and Web-based database systems for program monitoring and evaluation will soon be commonplace in the public health arena.

Description of the Overall Evaluation Program

Many states have implemented comprehensive, statewide tobacco control programs with tobacco tax proceeds or tobacco industry settlement funds (National Association of County and City Health Officials, 2001). These initiatives face challenges in developing systems to collect program data, hindering states' ability to link local-level efforts to intermediate and long-term outcomes (Habicht, Victoria, and Vaughan, 1999). With money from the state's settlement with the tobacco industry, the 1999 Minnesota legislature created the Tobacco Prevention and Local Public Health Endowment funds, which are being used to implement a comprehensive statewide tobacco control program. Using interest from the endowments, the Minnesota Department of Health (MDH) awarded competitive grants to community public health agencies and to local and statewide tobacco control organizations. The legislated goal of these grants is to achieve a 30 percent reduction in youth tobacco use by 2005.

Several evaluation methods and research teams are studying the short-term, intermediate, and long-term effects of the MDH Youth Tobacco Prevention Initiative. The component of the overall evaluation program described here is called STEPES—the Statewide Tobacco Endowment Process Evaluation Study. Funded by a grant from the CDC, the chief goal of the collaboration between the University of Minnesota (UM), Twin Cities, researchers and the MDH staff is to develop and implement a computerized process for monitoring local tobacco control programs—one that collects and reports on information specific to tobacco prevention and control. The aim of this chapter is to provide future public health managers and practitioners with a detailed review of how this system was developed, implemented, and tested. It is our hope that a discussion of the strengths and limitations of the system, as well as lessons learned, will inspire the creation of enhanced variants of this system that will address a host of public health issues and programs.

What Is STEPES?

STEPES is a custom-designed program monitoring and reporting database system that records descriptive and qualitative program-level data. Although the information entered into STEPES can aid the process evaluation of a local program, STEPES was designed to answer the question What are we doing? rather than How well are we doing it?

Created by using FileMaker Pro 5, Developer's Version (FileMaker, Inc., 1998), the STEPES runtime version is distributed on a compact disk, and it executes on both Macintosh and PC Windows operating systems. A runtime version is a desktop executable file that can operate without the installation of a base FileMaker Pro software application. User-friendly functions include navigation buttons and import and export scripts for easy data transfer. The database tool was built for practitioners with limited to no experience with computers. Throughout this chapter, public health staff members at county health service agencies and nonprofit health organizations who enter data into STEPES are generally referred to as "grantees."

STEPES has four layout forms into which grantees can enter data. The forms are: (1) the Contact Entry Form, which is like an electronic directory where substantive contacts with community members and groups are recorded, (2) the Event Entry Form, which is used by grantees to record details about tobacco control events and their interpretation of an event's impact on program goals, (3) the Meeting Entry Form, which is where grantees record information about meetings of their coalitions, allowing them to track the planning and implementation actions of their organization, and (4) the Quarterly Report Entry Form, which is where grantees report on their program's assets and barriers, identify technical assistance needs, and document progress on intermediate outcomes. The four layouts are constructed as individual databases. The layouts mostly contain fields with predetermined sets of options in pull-down lists. Each form also contains free text, binary, calculation, and editable menu fields.

Once local practitioners enter program information into STEPES, the information is transferred quarterly via diskettes—in this case to the UM project staff members, who then download the data into a searchable, integrated master database file. Data from community-based efforts can be sorted and compared on a wide variety of variables. Moreover, a master database user can write queries that will generate user-specific reports that provide descriptive and summary information for reporting, planning, or evaluation purposes.

Program Monitoring and Evaluation Functions

At this point, it is important to clarify what STEPES is and what it is not. STEPES is a program reporting and monitoring tool. Using STEPES, MDH grant managers can determine if activities executed by a grantee match contract duties. Local practitioners entering program information into STEPES can use the tool's preformatted report forms to evaluate their own progress toward meeting program goals and to make summary reports of their activities for supervisors or local boards. Stakeholders can query the STEPES master database to obtain summative information about the type, focus, and amount of tobacco prevention activity occurring in a particular city, county, or region—or statewide.

But STEPES cannot function as the sole process evaluation instrument for individual programs. Whereas the tool does require data entry regarding common process evaluation measures, such as participation levels and target audience, the design of the tool limits its capacity to request the type of data necessary to evaluate the content and quality of discrete activities. Process evaluation issues—such as whether a unique project or event has met content and dose goals or whether it has maintained implementation fidelity—are idiosyncratic and thus difficult to measure with a standardized tool. Information captured by STEPES cannot answer standard process evaluation questions, such as, Was this training delivered as planned? or How effective was the program in reaching its target audience? Answers to these important process evaluation questions are typically obtained in other ways.

Even so, STEPES performs useful evaluation functions. It can serve as a meta-process evaluation tool. For example, in the aggregate, information stored in the STEPES master database can help policymakers determine if the local component of Minnesota's Youth Tobacco Prevention Initiative was implemented as planned and whether it reached the intended audiences (see Table 11.1). Moreover, STEPES was designed to collect information about the vast array of independent variables contributing to Minnesota's tobacco prevention initiative. Subsequently, researchers can use program-level data collected by STEPES for summative evaluation purposes and to help explain changes in behavior outcomes, including the dependent variable—youth tobacco use.

Formative Development Process

The concept of utilization, both of an evaluation tool and of the information it collects, is critical to system design and development (Patton, 1997). To explore this concept, developers of STEPES engaged in an iterative process with the principal STEPES users: the MDH staff and local tobacco control practitioners. The eight-month-long process included focus groups, key informant interviews, regular meetings, e-mails, phone calls, and repeated document reviews.

The next section of this chapter expands on how we employed the principle of utilization throughout the development process, and the section following reviews the process of identifying the needs of those who entered program information into STEPES (grantees) and the needs of the end users of the information generated (grantees, grant managers, and policymakers), and it reviews the principles that guided the STEPES content and design specifications. Key questions that have guided this exploration include: Is STEPES easy to use? Does it enhance reporting? Does it improve communications between local practitioners and MDH? and Will the information captured by the tool and stored in the master database be easily accessible and useful to stakeholders?

STEPES's formative evolution followed two parallel tracks: (1) database design and creation and (2) content development. We will discuss these tracks separately, even though, for the most part, their development occurred simultaneously. In

TABLE 11.1. POTENTIAL USES OF STEPES.

STEPES Users	Potential Data Uses	Examples of Questions Data Collected by STEPES Can Answer
Local health practitioner/grantees	Event documentation Program reporting Quality improvement Communication Progress assessment	How many young people planned and participated in program activities over the past quarter? How many events reached targeted audiences? To what extent is a given collaborator or sector involved in the program? How many program events and/or meetings had focus X? How has my assessment of the program's strengths and weaknesses changed over time? What types of program activities are most likely to be covered by local print media?
State health department staff	Program monitoring Technical assistance Grant management Report writing Program evaluation Program planning Resource allocation	Do program activities match grantee contract duties? Which coalitions were most active during period X? Is region Y more likely than the rest of the state to focus on secondhand smoke? Are particular program assets and barriers tied to geographic region, program focus, or stage of coalition development? During the past year, how many grantees identified the need for X type of technical assistance? What percentage of programs introduced policy measures to city councils in Quarter 4?
Policymakers	Decision making Policy analysis Resource allocation Program planning Summative evaluation	What percentage of programs focus on youth tobacco access? Secondhand smoke? What type of coalitions are most likely to achieve policy goals? What are the characteristics of the most active coalitions? programs? Did the local component of the statewide tobacco initiative meet identified goals and objectives? Did activity levels meet expectations? Across the state, how many events targeted a given population at risk?
Researchers	Summative evaluation Covariate analysis	Does a community's exposure to messages about the risks of secondhand smoke, as measured by the number of secondhand smoke related events recorded in the Event form, predict the likelihood of local-level policy development pertaining to indoor smoking bans? Is intensity of local tobacco prevention activity associated with changes in tobacco-related behaviors and attitudes?

fact, throughout the development phase of STEPES, the tracks merged more often than they diverged. Even so, each track of STEPES's creation presented distinct issues and was driven by slightly different goals.

Database Planning and Development

Why is a tool like STEPES needed? What niche could it fill? To answer these questions, researchers conducted four focus groups, two involving MDH staff members who provide technical assistance to grantees, and two involving local public health practitioners. These discussions indicated that existing paper-driven program-monitoring systems and reporting tools were not very efficient, effective, or useful. Grant managers generally developed reporting systems to meet individual management styles, and grantees were frustrated by the amount of time they spent writing lengthy narratives to document their quarterly progress. Program-level data provided to the state were not always consistent across programs and were not easily synthesized or analyzed because the information was imbedded in tables and narratives. Nearly all the focus group participants agreed that the ideal system would be paperless, with entry forms containing mostly categorical and preformatted selections—which describes a computerized database. Only a few participants expressed hesitation about a computerized system. Mostly, those who were wary questioned whether or not a nonnarrative reporting format could accurately capture the subtleties of their programs.

Satisfied that a computerized database tool could fill an important void, developers began to identify the users of STEPES and their values regarding program tracking and monitoring. Practitioners in county and city health departments would be the largest group using the STEPES software. In focus groups, developers asked them such questions as, What is it about the process of reporting information to the state that is most important to you? and How could a computerized reporting tool help you do your work? Responses from participants indicated that they were proud of their efforts and would value a reporting mechanism that could accurately report their work to funding agencies. Practitioners also expressed a high level of frustration about the time and effort invested in completing progress reports, claiming that it is wasteful because the information provided is not in a format useful to grant managers or policymakers. Finally, participants wanted a reporting system that was easy to use. Overall, local health practitioners valued their time and efforts and wanted any new system to facilitate quick and accurate reporting.

MDH grant managers and decision makers were identified as the other main group using the STEPES system. When asked in focus groups what they desired in a computerized reporting system, time was the prominent factor discussed.

MDH staff members wanted a system that would minimize grantee reporting time and facilitate more effective and efficient grant management. Grant managers also expressed a strong need for a flexible and accessible master database. They wanted to easily manipulate local-level information for program monitoring and report generation.

The focus groups and key informant interviews brought to the surface two main findings regarding the computerized information management system: (1) the system needed to be time-efficient and easy to use and (2) the data it captured must be useful to grantees, grant managers, and policymakers. Noting these chief concerns, developers created initial designs for a flexible database system with four data entry layouts that match the primary elements of health practitioner effort: (1) making community contacts, (2) documenting meetings, (3) planning and implementing activities, and (4) reporting on coalition progress. Information must be standardized to achieve the goal of easily accessed and synthesized data. Subsequently, most entry fields were made categorical in nature. A significant portion of qualitative information typically collected through text narratives was forced into single-choice fields with a list of prefixed options. For clearly subjective information, such as progress toward goals or level of coalition empowerment, Likert scales were developed.

At the stage of choosing a platform and database software, the conversations between the UM staff members and their MDH partners focused on grantee access to technology and cost. Originally, MDH had hoped STEPES would be developed for the Internet and the World Wide Web. However, budget constraints, coupled with uncertainties about who would house and maintain the Internet server, persuaded the STEPES staff to build and release the first version of the tool on compact disk.

Content Planning and Development

To ensure that the monitoring system could effectively capture the breadth and depth of local tobacco prevention activities, experienced local tobacco practitioners, state tobacco prevention specialists, and tobacco prevention researchers provided feedback on STEPES content.

When STEPES was originally conceived, its primary function was to capture information that could report on the big picture or provide a "script of all that is being done in a region or in the state as a whole" (quoted from staff focus group, Minnesota Department of Health, Mar. 9, 2000). Developers initially hoped that the tool's design would be flexible enough to give grantees some capacity to conduct process evaluation of their unique programs. However, the lack of uniformity in local-level programs poses multiple challenges to using a standardized tool for individual program measurement.

Although focus group participants and key informants demanded that the tool collect only useful information, given the variety of groups using the system and the potential uses of the information generated, utility was conditional, based on the user. Based on potential user requests, STEPES evolved from a program-tracking tool (that would record information about program inputs and outputs—such as meetings and events—into a formal reporting mechanism. During the design phase, grantees expressed the desire to use the tool to communicate with MDH staff members about issues germane to the progress of their programs. Likewise, MDH staff members wanted to use program data captured by STEPES to augment normal information channels for grant management.

STEPES Data Entry and Report Forms

The Event Entry Form (see Figure 11.1) contains fields that document an event type, purpose, focus, desired intermediate outcome, targeted audience, key collaborators, and media coverage. The form's layout is designed to lead the user through a quasi-logic model, where they are forced to think through the intent, focus, and desired outcome of an activity rather than just document that an activity occurred. The forced choice fields (where practitioners must select an option from a predetermined list) may seem limiting; however, by exposing grantees to types, purposes of events, and target audiences that they may not regularly consider, these lists could expand their work scope.

The Quarterly Report Entry Form (see Figure 11.2) and the Progress Assessment Form (see Figure 11.3) were designed to replace the standard periodic reporting between grantees and grantors. These forms are also meant to elicit reflections that may result in program improvement and course corrections. Program managers enter opinions and subjective information about progress toward program goals. Fields on the quarterly report form include (1) check boxes, where obstacles and barriers are identified, (2) text boxes, where program details can be discussed, (3) matrices, where progress toward policy development and local enforcement actions are recorded, and (4) a series of Likert scales, where grantees can quickly record their sentiments on issues ranging from the quality of their coalition to the state of relations with the MDH staff. As shown in Figure 11.3, the Progress Assessment Form contains nine "agree"-"disagree" statements that assess members' perceived coalition progress.

The Contact Entry Form (see Figure 11.4) and the Meeting Entry Form (see Figure 11.5) are intended to aid the local practitioner with program coordination and coalition management. They are less essential to the goals of overall program monitoring.

Sixteen preformatted report forms accompany the entry forms. One of the goals of STEPES was to create a system that allowed grantees to have easy and

FIGURE 11.1. EVENT ENTRY FORM.

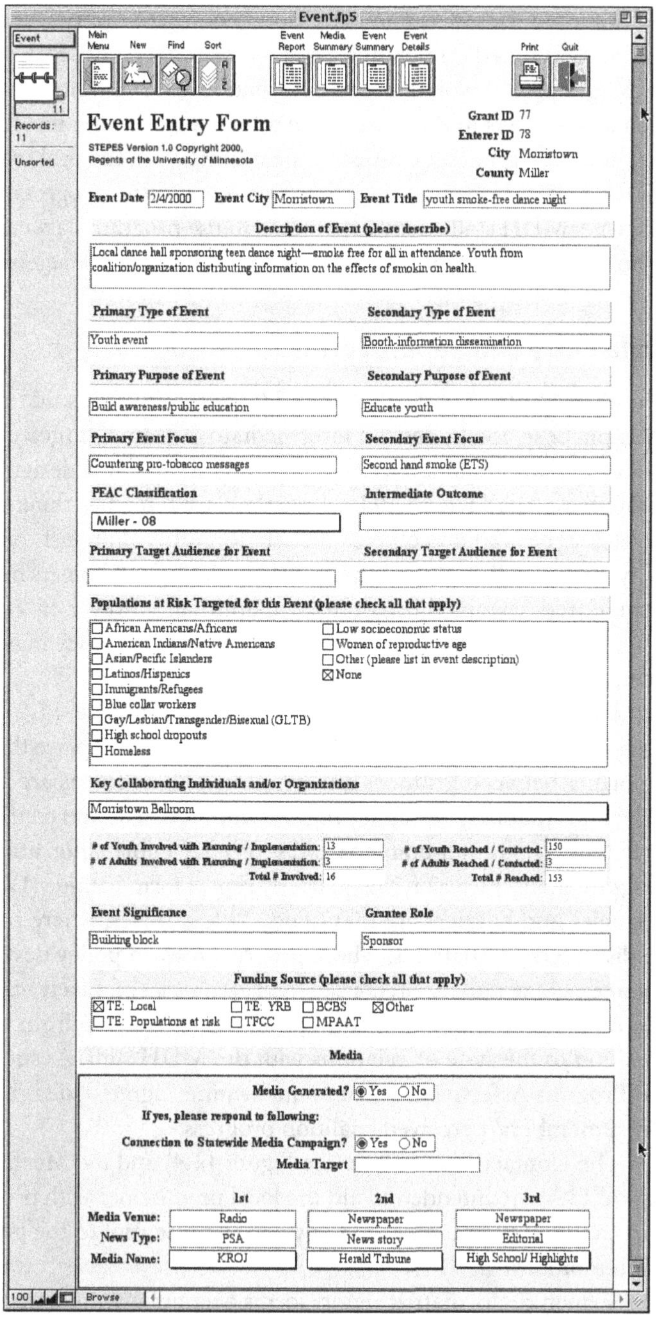

Event.fp5

Event | Records: 11 | Unsorted

Main Menu | New | Find | Sort | Event Report | Media Summary | Event Summary | Event Details | Print | Quit

Event Entry Form

STEPES Version 1.0 Copyright 2000, Regents of the University of Minnesota

Grant ID 77
Enterer ID 78
City Morristown
County Miller

Event Date 2/4/2000 **Event City** Morristown **Event Title** youth smoke-free dance night

Description of Event (please describe)

Local dance hall sponsoring teen dance night—smoke free for all in attendance. Youth from coalition/organization distributing information on the effects of smokin on health.

Primary Type of Event: Youth event
Secondary Type of Event: Booth-information dissemination

Primary Purpose of Event: Build awareness/public education
Secondary Purpose of Event: Educate youth

Primary Event Focus: Countering pro-tobacco messages
Secondary Event Focus: Second hand smoke (ETS)

PEAC Classification: Miller - 08
Intermediate Outcome:

Primary Target Audience for Event:
Secondary Target Audience for Event:

Populations at Risk Targeted for this Event (please check all that apply)

- ☐ African Americans/Africans
- ☐ American Indians/Native Americans
- ☐ Asian/Pacific Islanders
- ☐ Latinos/Hispanics
- ☐ Immigrants/Refugees
- ☐ Blue collar workers
- ☐ Gay/Lesbian/Transgender/Bisexual (GLTB)
- ☐ High school dropouts
- ☐ Homeless
- ☐ Low socioeconomic status
- ☐ Women of reproductive age
- ☐ Other (please list in event description)
- ☒ None

Key Collaborating Individuals and/or Organizations: Morristown Ballroom

# of Youth Involved with Planning / Implementation: 13
# of Adults Involved with Planning / Implementation: 3
Total # Involved: 16

# of Youth Reached / Contacted: 150
# of Adults Reached / Contacted: 3
Total # Reached: 153

Event Significance: Building block
Grantee Role: Sponsor

Funding Source (please check all that apply)

☒ TE: Local ☐ TE: YRB ☐ BCBS ☒ Other
☐ TE: Populations at risk ☐ TFCC ☐ MPAAT

Media

Media Generated? ◉ Yes ○ No

If yes, please respond to following:

Connection to Statewide Media Campaign? ◉ Yes ○ No

Media Target

	1st	2nd	3rd
Media Venue:	Radio	Newspaper	Newspaper
News Type:	PSA	News story	Editorial
Media Name:	KROJ	Herald Tribune	High School/ Highlights

100 | Browse

FIGURE 11.2. QUARTERLY REPORT ENTRY FORM.

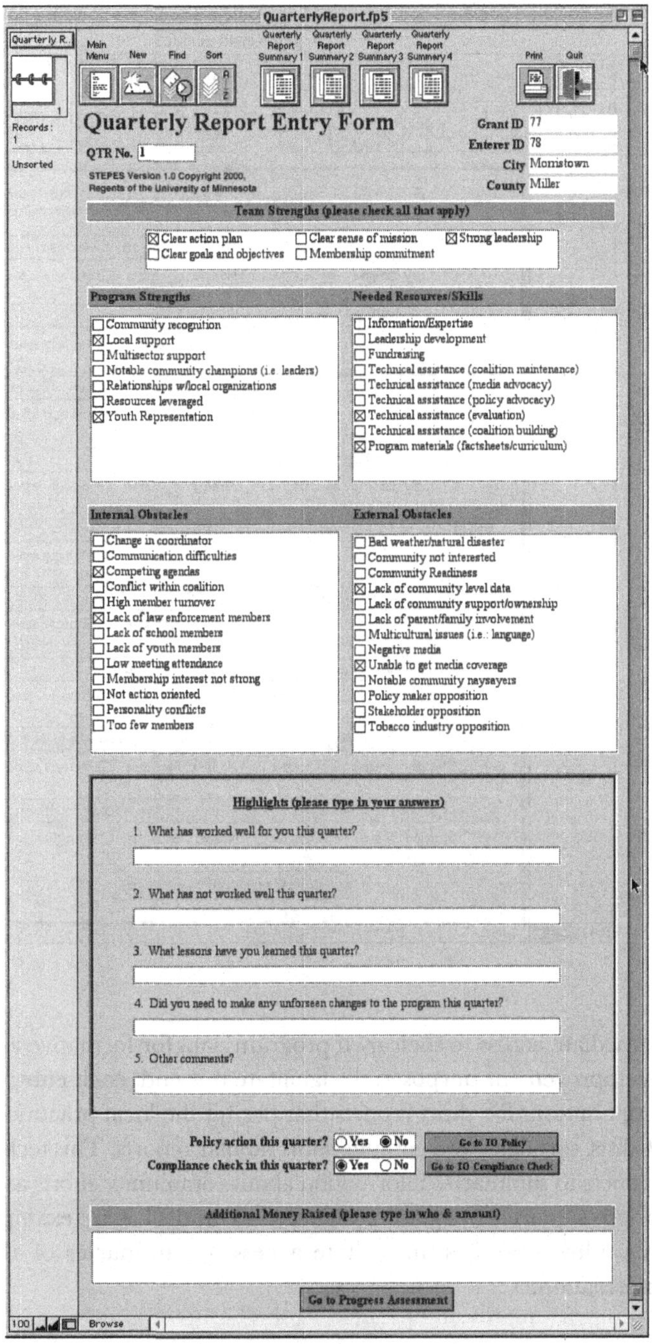
QuarterlyReport.fp5

Quarterly R...

Records: 1

Unsorted

Main Menu | New | Find | Sort | Quarterly Report Summary 1 | Quarterly Report Summary 2 | Quarterly Report Summary 3 | Quarterly Report Summary 4 | Print | Quit

Quarterly Report Entry Form

QTR No. 1

STEPES Version 1.0 Copyright 2000, Regents of the University of Minnesota

Grant ID 77

Enterer ID 78

City Morristown

County Miller

Team Strengths (please check all that apply)

- ☒ Clear action plan
- ☐ Clear sense of mission
- ☒ Strong leadership
- ☐ Clear goals and objectives
- ☐ Membership commitment

Program Strengths

- ☐ Community recognition
- ☒ Local support
- ☐ Multisector support
- ☐ Notable community champions (i.e. leaders)
- ☐ Relationships w/local organizations
- ☐ Resources leveraged
- ☒ Youth Representation

Needed Resources/Skills

- ☐ Information/Expertise
- ☐ Leadership development
- ☐ Fundraising
- ☐ Technical assistance (coalition maintenance)
- ☐ Technical assistance (media advocacy)
- ☐ Technical assistance (policy advocacy)
- ☒ Technical assistance (evaluation)
- ☐ Technical assistance (coalition building)
- ☒ Program materials (factsheets/curriculum)

Internal Obstacles

- ☐ Change in coordinator
- ☐ Communication difficulties
- ☒ Competing agendas
- ☐ Conflict within coalition
- ☐ High member turnover
- ☒ Lack of law enforcement members
- ☐ Lack of school members
- ☐ Lack of youth members
- ☐ Low meeting attendance
- ☐ Membership interest not strong
- ☐ Not action oriented
- ☐ Personality conflicts
- ☐ Too few members

External Obstacles

- ☐ Bad weather/natural disaster
- ☐ Community not interested
- ☐ Community Readiness
- ☒ Lack of community level data
- ☐ Lack of community support/ownership
- ☐ Lack of parent/family involvement
- ☐ Multicultural issues (i.e.: language)
- ☐ Negative media
- ☒ Unable to get media coverage
- ☐ Notable community naysayers
- ☐ Policy maker opposition
- ☐ Stakeholder opposition
- ☐ Tobacco industry opposition

Highlights (please type in your answers)

1. What has worked well for you this quarter?
2. What has not worked well this quarter?
3. What lessons have you learned this quarter?
4. Did you need to make any unforseen changes to the program this quarter?
5. Other comments?

Policy action this quarter? ○ Yes ◉ No [Go to 10 Policy]

Compliance check in this quarter? ◉ Yes ○ No [Go to 10 Compliance Check]

Additional Money Raised (please type in who & amount)

[Go to Progress Assessment]

100 Browse

FIGURE 11.3. PROGRESS ASSESSMENT FORM.

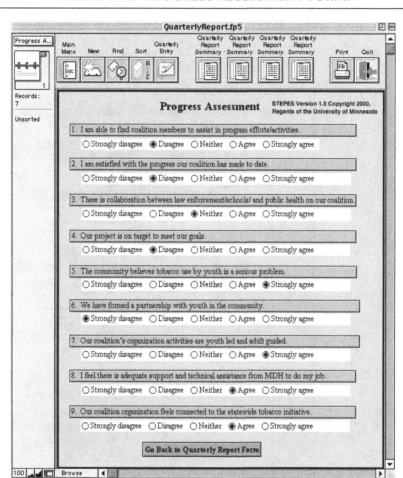

immediate access to their own program data for formative evaluation and quality improvement purposes. To facilitate this end, each entry form contains four script buttons for short reports that permit the local practitioner to easily generate lists, sort data, and compile short tabular reports. This technology allows practitioners to summarize information about community efforts and monitor program progress quarter by quarter. Figures 11.6 and 11.7 are examples of report forms that allow grantees immediate access to summaries of their own program information.

FIGURE 11.4. CONTACT ENTRY FORM.

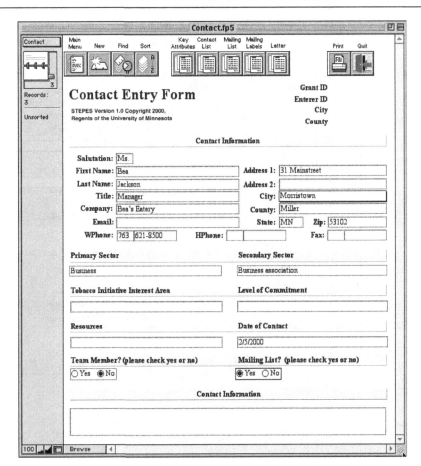

STEPES User Manual

Like most tools, STEPES is accompanied by instructions. The unique nature of STEPES and its standardized layouts for qualitative and subjective data made it critical that information be consistently documented. Multiple rounds of feedback were necessary to achieve agreement on fields and forced-choice definitions. In addition, because database technology was new to many grantees, explicit instructions were written to lead the user through every step, including installation, data entry, report making, and data exporting. The seventy-page STEPES user manual took several months of concentrated effort to write and edit.

FIGURE 11.5. MEETING ENTRY FORM.

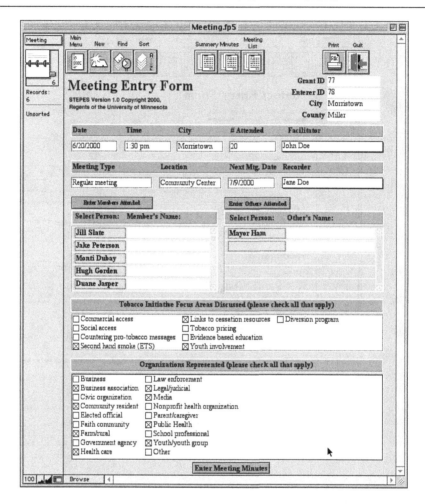

Alpha Testing: The Final Formative Development Phase

The final phase in the formative development of STEPES was an alpha testing period. Several months prior to a wide release of STEPES, the software underwent scrutiny by approximately twenty-five test users. The first set of fourteen test subjects (six local public health practitioners and eight MDH personnel) participated in a pilot test in which initial studies on the usability, validity, and feasibility of the tool were conducted. Results of an interrater test during the pilot session indicated a high degree of agreement between participants' choices on selected

FIGURE 11.6. EVENT REPORT.

Event Report

STEPES Version 1.0 Copyright 2000,
Regents of the University of Minnesota

Reporting period: _____ to _____
First sort query: _____
Second sort query: _____

Pages: 1

Script:
[Continue]
[Cancel]

Event Date	Event Title	Primary Type of Event	Primary Event Focus	Grantee Role	Media Generated
2/4/2000	Youth smoke free dance night	Youth event	Countering pro-tobacco messages	Sponsor	● Yes ○ No
4/5/2000	WoodsFest 2000	Booth-information dissemination	Second hand smoke (ETS)	Coordinator	● Yes ○ No
8/3/2000	ETS and You presentation	School event/after school	Second hand smoke (ETS)	Coordinator	● Yes ○ No
9/3/2000	City Council Day	City council/committee meeting	Countering pro-tobacco messages	Coordinator	● Yes ○ No
2/8/2000	Diversion for our town	Presentation	Diversion program	Coordinator	○ Yes ● No
8/9/2000	Smoke-free Message	Mass mailing	Second hand smoke (ETS)	Coordinator	● Yes ○ No
9/3/2000	Austin Community Celebration	Community celebration/parade	Links to cessation resources	Supporting/Participant	● Yes ○ No
4/7/2000	Healthy hearts	Faith community	Second hand smoke (ETS)	Coordinator	○ Yes ● No
1/3/2000	Compliance Checks	Enforcement	Commercial access	Monitor	○ Yes ● No
6/9/2000	School assessment	School assessment	Evidence-based education	Coordinator	● Yes ○ No

Total Events: 10

fields. In addition to the pilot test, a rough cut of the software and an accompanying rough draft of the user manual were distributed to several key informants, who agreed to install the system on their computers and test the system's key functions, including data entry, report generation, and printing. This pilot test and field trial uncovered multiple problems with the tool's content (flaws and omissions) and software (programming glitches). In spite of repeated tests by developers, the practitioners, who actually used the tool for its intended purpose, were best at identifying critical defects within the system. The value of the alpha testing phase to STEPES's ultimate usability cannot be overstated.

Training on How to Use the Tool

Ideally, all grantees using STEPES would be given a six- to eight-hour training session, during which they would have the opportunity to receive hands-on instruction in a computer lab. However, budget and geographic constraints limited

FIGURE 11.7. SUMMARY OF MEETINGS.

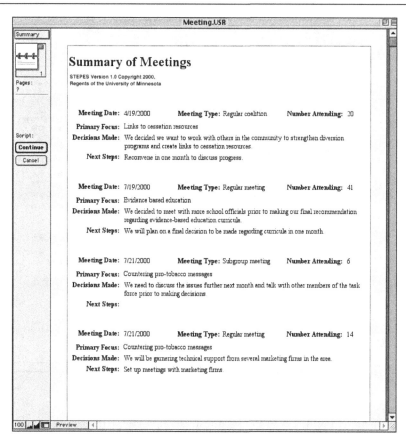

the feasibility of this option. Most grantees were trained via video teleconference, with the software developers located at a central site and grantees gathered in various computer labs throughout the state. Follow-up hands-on training was offered to grantees at three regional sites. STEPES training covered various topics, including installing the software on computer systems, entering data, navigating between layouts, generating reports, and transmitting data to the administrators of the STEPES master database. The training also reviewed STEPES content information. Developers provided the rationale for data entry layouts, field types, and field and menu contents. Instructions were provided on how to make determinations about activities that did and did not warrant documentation and how to use the STEPES user manual as a reference for definitions of field and menu options. Additional training and ongoing technical support is available from the university-based coordinator and the MDH staff.

Expertise Involved in STEPES Development

A computerized program monitoring/process evaluation tool of this scope cannot be created in a vacuum. However, involving a large number of people in the formative process will inevitably multiply the number of requests for system revisions and will cause delays in development. In spite of this, we and the developers of a similar system found that involving a host of key players throughout the creation process is politically expedient and cost-effective, and it ultimately enhances the tool's utility (Hardin and Reis, 1997).

Many players shaped STEPES software design and content. The UM team involved two investigators, a project director, a coordinator, and two computer programmers. Key collaborators at MDH included two program evaluation staff members and a tobacco control manager. In addition, approximately ten grant managers with expertise in tobacco control as well as many local health practitioners provided feedback on the system. The scope of skills and knowledge employed in the development and implementation of STEPES was expansive. Expertise was necessary in evaluation methods, research design, tobacco prevention programming and implementation, focus group facilitation, questionnaire design, management information systems, interviewing, software development, computer programming, grant management, manual writing, technical editing, graphic design, medium production, and law. This program monitoring software was developed in approximately one year on a budget of about $75,000, whereas it is estimated that a similar system, developed with Web-based software for Internet use, would have cost at least twice that amount.

Evaluation of the STEPES Tool

Why evaluate STEPES? Computerized, standardized program monitoring and management information systems like STEPES are proliferating across the country. However, staffing and resource constraints in state agencies make it unlikely that newly developed systems are undergoing extensive methods testing. Nevertheless, questions regarding the usability, validity, and reliability of these data collection tools must be examined. A series of methods tests on STEPES has the potential to provide valuable information to public and nonprofit agencies interested in using similar technology-based systems for monitoring and evaluating major public health initiatives.

At a more pragmatic level, the UM developers wanted to know if STEPES was actually doing what it was designed to do. The evaluation explores this question from the perspective of two user groups: the local health practitioner and the state health department staff. From each viewpoint, the evaluation tests STEPES's performance regarding the reliability and usefulness of program data collected (content) and the functionality of the software tool (product). Some of our key evaluation questions were:

- Is the STEPES tool collecting valid program-level data in a reliable manner?
- Is a standardized data collection instrument flexible and robust enough to capture the scope and diversity of local programs?
- Can STEPES data produce meaningful summaries of programs that are useful to local practitioners, grant managers, and legislators?
- Does this database instrument provide the level of accountability and quality assurance necessary for a state agency to successfully monitor a locally implemented statewide initiative?
- Is STEPES software easy to install and use?
- Is it efficient, reliable, adaptable, robust, and maintainable for the software administrators, the grantees, and the state health department?
- Is the system being used correctly and consistently, and if not, can the barriers to accurate and reliable use be overcome?

When analyzing the STEPES tool in terms of content or "the actual data being collected," questions of validity, reliability, and usability are explored. Results of our methods study design will gauge whether STEPES (1) generates accurate, complete, consistent, and useful program-level data, (2) improves program quality, (3) enhances communications between local practitioners and state health department staff members, and (4) increases the efficiency of grantee reporting.

To test STEPES's functionality, our evaluation focused on external software quality characteristics—in other words, those most apparent to the various users. We employed several commonly accepted criteria to measure the quality of the STEPES software, including (1) usability (is the software user-friendly, is it easy to install, can the end user successfully use the program after adequate training, and are most end users able to use the system with minimal ongoing technical assistance?), (2) understandability (do the software's navigation functions and internal scripts make sense to the user, and is the format of the data entry layouts logical?), and (3) accuracy (does the software perform the job it was created for, and in the particular case of STEPES, is it meeting a variety of users' program recording and monitoring needs?).

Issues pertaining to the quality of the system's code and integrity were primarily tested in the alpha development stage, prior to the launch of the beta version of the software. Although this discussion does not explore computer code testing, its importance to producing quality software cannot be overstated. For a thorough discussion of the issue, see Steve McConnell's *Code Complete* (1993).

Methods Study Design and Results

Sample group selection. For our methods study, a study sample of twenty participants was selected from the entire population of grantees using STEPES (approximately 120). Criteria for inclusion in the study included (1) proximity within 150 miles of the Twin Cities metro area, (2) computer hardware and software configurations that would accommodate STEPES software use and data transfer, and (3) representation by populations-at-risk programs. All MDH grantees that met these requirements ($n = 32$) received a letter from UM researchers requesting their participation in the study. From this group, twenty MDH grantees then signed consent forms agreeing to comply with validity and reliability tests required by researchers. In exchange for participation, study participants received earlier access to the STEPES program, more extensive hands-on training, direct user support from the developers, and opportunities to provide feedback to developers on how the STEPES tool should be improved.

Reliability and usability studies. Once the beta version of STEPES was ready to be released, the tool's formal evaluation began. Two studies were conducted during the training session for the STEPES study sample, and the key aim of these initial studies was to identify problems with the content and product that would impede reliable and effective use of the STEPES tool. After developers reviewed the study results, appropriate changes were made to the beta version of STEPES and the user manual. By releasing the beta version of STEPES to study participants prior to a wide-scale release to all MDH grantees, developers had useful preliminary data regarding the tool's correctness, usability, robustness, and reliability.

First, we conducted an interrater reliability study to determine the likelihood that a diverse group of local-level practitioners using STEPES would choose the same predetermined menu items selected by UM researchers to describe two single events. Results from a comparison of sixteen records found that on the five primary fields tested, practitioner selections matched the researchers' selections 84 percent of the time on the first scenario and 85 percent of the time on the second scenario. The high degree of concordance among choices indicated that in a controlled environment, the STEPES tool can capture accurate and reliable data from a variety of enterers.

Second, at the end of the training session, study participants completed a survey about their initial impressions of STEPES. The questionnaire measured user judgment regarding the four key evaluation constructs previously noted. Responses indicated that 95 percent of the sample group found that STEPES provided enough choices to accurately describe grant activities, 100 percent thought that STEPES would save them time, 97 percent thought that STEPES would improve communications with grant managers, and 71 percent reported that by using the tool the quality of their work improved. In general, 90 percent of the participants found STEPES software simple to learn and use.

After the first quarter, evaluation data were collected from a sample of grantees and members of the original research group to obtain their feedback regarding one-quarter of STEPES's use. The results of this user survey indicated that 85 percent of the respondents (n = 40) agreed that STEPES made it easy to communicate grant activities, and 75 percent agreed that STEPES improved their ability to track their progress on grants and report them to grant managers.

Following two-quarters of STEPES's use, an intrarater reliability test was conducted with fourteen participants. The purpose of this test was to determine if a grantee who had recorded an event into STEPES at point one would, after hearing his or her narrative description of the event, choose the same menu choices for key fields at point two. In most cases, at least two weeks had passed between data entry points. This study's goal was to provide information about the capacity of STEPES to facilitate reliable and consistent data entry over time on the six variables considered most important to MDH. For the fourteen study participants, the average percentage of agreement on the selected fields was 69 percent (with a range of 43 to 93 percent). We acknowledge that kappa values would be the best test of agreement between respondents; however, the small sample size and the low number of observations limits the capacity of a kappa value to indicate intrarater reliability.

Approximately six months after STEPES's release, researchers conducted a structured dialogue with MDH grant managers. The meeting's key aim was to determine if STEPES was enhancing the grant's management functions and improving communications between local practitioners and the MDH staff. Feedback suggested that several important changes were necessary in the reports available to the MDH staff. Limited access to the master database was forcing MDH grant managers to use hard copies of preformatted reports specifically designed for the health practitioner. Also, grant managers wanted to efficiently match grantee activities with contract deliverables. To accommodate these needs, the STEPES master database underwent several revisions, making it relational and more usable. The process of creating these desired changes tested the maintainability and flexibility of the software.

Lessons Learned About Process Evaluation

LESSON 1. *Manage expectations.*

Developers should take pains to make clear, from the initial stages of development and throughout implementation, what their tool can and cannot do. When introduced to potential stakeholders and users, a tool like STEPES can generate a great deal of enthusiasm. However, the onus is on developers to clarify—for everyone who will be using the system and the data it collects—that in reporting quicker and more easily, the system will not meet all process evaluation or grant management needs. A database reporting system can facilitate data transfer and enhance communications, but it cannot substitute for highly contextual information that is best captured by case studies and face-to-face communications.

LESSON 2. *At the beginning of the design process, clearly state the strengths and limitations of using a computerized data management tool for program reporting and evaluation purposes.*

A standardized data collection instrument can be used for evaluating individual programs only if those programs are implemented uniformly. In other words, programs must be executed with fidelity to the same method and must have similar target audiences and the same goals. As STEPES evolved, the developers made many efforts to clarify that STEPES recorded information that best served program tracking and monitoring rather than process evaluation purposes. Its intended use as a program monitoring tool was clearly stated in the STEPES user manual and during software training. Even so, the tool's name became associated with the acronym for the study that funded the development and testing of the tool—the Statewide Tobacco Endowment Process Evaluation Study. This misnomer has created confusion about the system's intended use and value.

LESSON 3. *Don't underestimate the technical expertise necessary to develop a quality software program.*

Neither the MDH nor the UM developers had previously undertaken the process of creating a computerized data management tool. In fact, software development was not in the collective expertise of either group. Indeed, the project encountered significant snags in the software development and computer programming arena. STEPES staff members felt confident about their expertise in process evaluation and tobacco prevention, but the gulf between that knowledge and the language of software development and programming was not anticipated. And the computer programming team hired to write STEPES lacked familiarity with public health concepts and practice. In addition, the highly iterative formative development process frustrated the programming team, as they repeatedly needed to rewrite computer code based on changes requested by both the UM staff members and their MDH partners. In hindsight, the content development team needed more computer savvy. A naive understanding of software technology and programming language undercuts database design possibilities and forces the system customer to work within the experience and knowledge parameters of the computer programming team. Ideally, before beginning a design process, content developers will go on-line to review a variety of data management systems and become familiar with the range of possibilities that current technology offers. Most important, computer programming should not commence until database content and layout specifications are finalized.

LESSON 4. *All databases within a system should be relational.*

The STEPES master database is built to be relational, whereas the runtime version of STEPES was not. This is a serious limitation of the runtime system. A relational database links information across different types of records, based on key fields, allowing data to be organized and analyzed in many meaningful combinations. It also limits the amount of redundant information that must be entered into discreet records by the user, saving time and effort as well as increasing the integrity of the data. The extra benefits and power that relational databases provide is substantial and far outweighs the additional time and financial resources needed to program a relational capacity into an existing database system.

LESSON 5. *Automated tools can lead to overcollection and overreporting of local-level data.*

When developing any process or tracking tool, it is critical to temper desires for information with the reality that scarce resources and time are available for local-level program documentation. With this in mind, STEPES developers aimed to clearly identify information needs and streamline priorities to avoid excessive data collection (Lytle and others, 1994). Nevertheless, our experience revealed that a heightened danger of overcollecting data exists when tools are automated. On-line data entry can create the illusion that documentation is less arduous, so that the evaluator or grantor is tempted to request more program information than is useful. The other face of the data overcollection dilemma is the potential for overreporting activities. When on-line entry is made quick and easy for practitioners, they may fall prey to using a monitoring tool as a means of "getting credit" for every aspect of a program, regardless of whether it meets the predetermined definition of a reportable event. Moreover, the potential for overreporting may be heightened by the various users and uses of information collected by a computerized database system. For example, although program information entered into STEPES can be aggregated for a summative evaluation of the local-level component of the statewide tobacco initiative, practitioner fears that data will be used to evaluate individual programs may invite inflated descriptions of program activity levels and successes (Cooley and Bickel, 1986).

LESSON 6. *Training practitioners on how to use a computerized monitoring system is costly and must be ongoing.*

Factors contributing to the cost and ongoing nature of software training include (1) the number and location of the system users, (2) the need for hands-on training, which may necessitate renting a centralized facility with ample computers, (3) staff time and resources for one-on-one tutorials, (4) the degree to which regular turnover of the staff entering data into the computerized system will create the demand for frequent and time-consuming one-on-one training sessions, and (5) the cost of developing and updating a user manual.

We found that initial software training takes several hours. A four- to five-hour session explores content issues pertaining to the information requested and covers the rudiments of data entry and system navigation. However, full use of a system's more sophisticated operations, including data sorting and customized report generation, often requires additional software training. Because scarce resources limited the amount of training available to practitioners using STEPES, only savvy computer users appear to have tapped STEPES's potential for improving program delivery and reporting to local stakeholders.

LESSON 7. *A reliable, customized program monitoring system demands a significant investment of time and money.*

As we discussed throughout this chapter, the development of a new software system can take up to a year. We have presented a detailed account of the staff and resource demands of the highly iterative content and system development process, but the ongoing costs of maintaining a computerized information system cannot be overlooked. State and nonprofit agencies deliberating the development of a database monitoring tool should also ponder the annual costs and staffing needs associated with the tool's use. Resource considerations include master database management, materials development (producing a user manual and burning CDs), initial and follow-up training sessions, provision of ongoing technical support, and server maintenance in the case of a Web-based application.

LESSON 8. *Carefully consider who will have access to the master database.*

When a wealth of descriptive data about a costly statewide program are available in a single master database, practical and ethical issues regarding data access and data misuse will surface. The potential for the misuse and abuse of program monitoring and evaluation data always exists (Stevens and Dial, 1994). Important questions must be considered, such as, Who will have access to the data and who will be responsible for managing, analyzing, and interpreting the data? Also, protocols must be established to ensure that data will be accessed and used appropriately, because the availability of a master database will provide the opportunity for diverse stakeholders to use the information to meet their own needs.

The following examples are hypothetical; however, the potential for any of them to occur poses a serious threat to the utility of a database program monitoring system, whether it is stand-alone or Web-based. First, individuals who are opposed to a particular program may be able to mine a master database for information that bolsters a particular policy position. Second, managers might be inclined to withhold access to the master database and only release information on a "need to know" basis. Although this "gatekeeping" behavior may seem antithetical to the purposes of a centralized information system, these actions are often based on rational self-interest to keep standard operating procedures intact (Buchanan, 1989). Third, with the desire to enhance accountability as a justification, agency managers may use a master database's vast array of descriptive program information to micromanage local-level initiatives. Fourth, because of the vast amount of information available in a master database, a data practices request served by an opponent could result in severe damage to a politically vulnerable policy or program.

LESSON 9. *Don't invest in a database monitoring system unless there is a commitment to use the data.*

Even when the goal of obtaining standardized, easily synthesized program-level data is met, the power of a master database and the data it holds is severely diminished by lack of use. Information in a master database can languish from excessive gatekeeping by managers, insufficient analysis and evaluation resources, and an unmotivated agency staff. An underused master database is no more valuable than paper reports filed in a desk drawer. To prevent underuse, a master database must be designed to be flexible and easily queried. Preformatted reports should be created with managers and stakeholders in mind. Finally, staff resources must be allocated for managing the master database, asking appropriate evaluation questions, analyzing the data, and writing meaningful reports.

Conclusion

STEPES's Strengths and Implementation Successes

STEPES is a successful first-generation, custom-designed, database-monitoring system for local-level tobacco prevention programs in the state of Minnesota. The tool met the key requirements of grant managers, local health practitioners, and stakeholders by capturing program-level data in a systematic, useful manner.

Approximately one hundred grantees use the system regularly as their primary reporting instrument for tobacco control activities.

By most evaluations, STEPES is a user-friendly system that requires minimal technical assistance. This is substantiated by the fact that we did not need to establish a hot line for grantees, as first anticipated. In fact, most end user inquiries come near quarterly report submission deadlines and are primarily regarding data transfer issues.

STEPES is a relatively low-cost system. Because STEPES was developed using FileMaker Pro 5, Developer's Version, which costs approximately five hundred dollars, the runtime version of STEPES could be installed on approximately a hundred computer systems at no additional cost. Only individuals who have access to the STEPES master database need to purchase and install the FileMaker Pro software package. Also, given the small amount of Random Access Memory (RAM) necessary to run STEPES, it is easily supported by older versions of common operating systems.

The STEPES master database serves as an archive for statewide tobacco prevention activities. The system allows grantees immediate access to their own program data for the purposes of report generation and program review. Access to the STEPES master database gives grant managers and decision makers the opportunity to summarize local-level data by grantee or region—or statewide. Summarized information can be easily downloaded into statistical or graphic software to generate pie charts, histograms, and tabular reports. Information in the STEPES master database can be manipulated and analyzed by MDH stakeholders for purposes of program planning, decision making, and resource allocation. Also, evaluation researchers are planning to use STEPES data to link short-term outcomes to changes in behavior outcomes.

The Limitations of STEPES

The Database. Budget constraints and questionable user access capability required STEPES to be released as a runtime user software package instead of as a Web version. This required grantees to have the capacity to install the software, and it required the STEPES support group to give technical support for problems that occurred on a variety of user software/hardware systems. To build the STEPES master database, periodic collection of data from all grantees is required. This is a tedious process. Grantees must generate STEPES export files, locate the export files on their systems, copy them to a diskette, and physically mail them to the university. Because of export file format limitations, e-mail was not used. However, these limitations can be eliminated and electronic mail transfer can be used if data files are condensed by using specialized software. The university receives approximately 120 diskettes each quarter, and the diskettes must be manually read and imported into the master database. New software was written to support this process. Additional efforts are required to coordinate the receipt and cleaning of all user data. A copy of the master database must also be delivered to the state health department at the end of each quarter in a timely fashion.

Another limitation of STEPES is that any software changes must be developed on a new copy of the entire user runtime version, which must then be distributed to each STEPES user. The user then has to un-install his or her previous version and install the new version of STEPES. This process works, but a Web-based version would eliminate this inconvenience.

The Content. STEPES is designed to collect program-level outputs, but, subsequently, a key criticism of the tool is that it does not allow for adequate documentation of the start-up or relationship-building phase of coalitions and programs. In spite of our intense formative development process, UM researchers and their MDH partners overlooked the need for STEPES to capture time-consuming coalition formation and activity planning processes. This limitation was most frustrating for local practitioners, who felt that a portion of their effort during their grant's first year was not sufficiently documented. A number of grantees used ad hoc adjustments to STEPES to document their formative efforts; however, the lack of uniformity in data entry makes the information less useful to stakeholders.

STEPES's design as a uniform data collection tool presented a significant challenge to determining field content. This challenge was magnified by the reality that the funding cycle of the researchers' grant from the CDC necessitated that formative work on the content of STEPES precede final refinement of the strategic plans and goals of the Minnesota Youth Tobacco Prevention Initiative. Consequently, the developers needed to make a number of assumptions about the program goals and implementation approaches of potential grantees. Entry form content and field design had to be flexible and robust enough to capture the breadth and depth of a wide variety of initiatives. As a result, we erred on the side of overcollecting program information. Any significant degree of imprecision about exactly what information needs to be documented results in too much data entry, thereby limiting the tool's usability, and it results in too much data, which limits the data's usefulness.

A final important limitation of STEPES is that it is difficult to ensure the quality of the program information entered into the system. Concerns about quality control are intrinsic to program reporting, regardless of whether it is aided by computer technology. Without an objective observer at every activity or meeting, the subjective nature of program reporting by grantees to grantors almost guarantees some level of self-reporting bias. This said, there are additional quality control problems a system like STEPES can compound. The first of these is keystroke error. For example, when a grantee quickly scrolls down a list of fifteen items to select an option from a prefixed field, it is likely that, occasionally, an unintended item will be selected. Second, because most information entered into STEPES is qualitative and subjective in nature, the developers determined that it was not reasonable or efficient to lead enterers through stepwise or branching questions to ensure enterer accuracy in approximately thirty-five fields per entry form. Third, there isn't a prompt in the runtime version of STEPES to warn a grantee against making a duplicate record. To rectify some of these quality control problems, the STEPES master database has been programmed to identify and eliminate a variety of data entry mistakes, such as duplicating records and making calculation and date errors.

Implications for Future Practice

The use of technology for program monitoring, data collection, and data transfer can only expand in the coming decade. The Internet holds immense capacity for knowledge-based information and communication systems. Technology will offer program managers and funders instant access to program-level data, and at the same time it will fuel expectations for higher levels of accountability between agencies funding programs and the practitioners who implement them. Opportunities abound, and so do challenges.

In the future, monitoring systems like STEPES will be developed nearly exclusively for the Web. Because Web-based programs require the coordination of several different software components, sophisticated planning, software development, and system management are critical. Security issues are of preeminent importance when information is entered via a Web-based platform. A system's Web-enabled version, as well as its network server, must be current with all security issues. This means that the network server must have *firewalls*—that is, network configurations and software defenses against the often-changing security threats that users face.

Contribution to Process Evaluation Literature

This review of the development and testing of the STEPES tool should provide health practitioners with a primer on the important issues to consider when developing or purchasing, and then implementing, a database-oriented program-monitoring tool. STEPES's value as a component of the overall evaluation of the MN Tobacco Control Initiative is less clear, as the results of initial behavior outcome studies are only now being analyzed. We have learned that database tools like STEPES can improve agency understanding of locally implemented programs and can enhance information management and stakeholder reporting.

References

Augustyniak, R. *Web-Based Solutions for Managing Florida's Tobacco-Free Partnerships.* Tallahassee: Florida State University, Florida Tobacco Control Clearinghouse, 2000.

Celebucki, C., Biener, L., and Koh, H. "Methods and Strategy for Evaluation— Massachusetts." American Cancer Society: *Journal of Cancer*, 1998, *83*(S12A), 2760–2765.

Cooley, W. M., and Bickel, W. E. *Decision-Oriented Educational Research.* Boston: Kluwer-Nijhoff, 1986.

Fiene, R. J. "Human Services Instrument-Based Program Monitoring and Indicator Systems." In B. Glastonbury and others (eds.), *Information Technology and the Human Services.* Chitchester, U.K.: Wiley, 1988.

FileMaker, Inc. FileMaker Pro 5, Developer's Version, 1997–1999. Santa Clara. Calif.: FileMaker, Inc., 1998. Software.

Friede, A., Blum, H. L., and McDonald, M. "Public Health Informatics: How Information-Age Technology Can Strengthen Public Health." *Annual Review of Public Health*, 1995, *16*, 239–252.

Habicht, J. P., Victoria, C. G., and Vaughan, J. P. "Evaluation Designs for Adequacy, Plausibility and Probability of Public Health Programme Performance and Impact." *International Journal of Epidemiology*, 1999, *28*, 10–18.

Hall, J. R., and others. "Challenges to Producing and Implementing the Consider This Web-Based Smoking Prevention and Cessation Program." *Electronic Journal of Communication*, forthcoming.

Hardin, P., and Reis, J. "Interactive Multimedia Software Design for TD Prevention Applications: Concepts, Process, and Evaluation." *Journal of Health Education and Behavior*, 1997, *24*(1), 35–53.

"Information Needs and Uses of the Public Health Workforce—Washington, 1997–1998." *Morbidity and Mortality Weekly Report*, 2000, *49*(6), 118–120.

Lytle, L. A., and others. "Challenges of Conducting Process Evaluation in a Multicenter Trial." *Health Education Quarterly*, 1994 (supp. 2), S129–S141.

McConnell, S. *Code Complete.* Redmond, Wash.: Microsoft Press, 1993.

National Association of County and City Health Officials. *Program and Funding Guidelines for Comprehensive Local Tobacco Control Programs.* Washington, D.C.: National Association of County and City Health Officials, Tobacco Prevention and Control Project, 2001.

Paperny, D.M.N. "Computerized Health Assessment and Education for Adolescent HIV and STD Prevention in Health Care Settings and Schools." *Journal of Health Education and Behavior*, 1997, *24*(1), 54–70.

Patton, M. Q. *Utilization Focused Evaluation.* (2nd ed.) Thousand Oaks, Calif.: Sage, 1997.

Petersen, L., and Babb, S. "Establishing a Web-Based Program Reporting System: Issues to Consider and Lessons Learned." Paper presented at the National Conference on Tobacco or Health, New Orleans, Nov. 2001.

Safran, C., and others. "Trends in Computer Applications in Medical Care." *MD Computing*, 1994, *11*(3), 155–159.

Skinner, C. S., Siegfried, J. C., Kegler, M. C., and Strecher, V. J. "The Potential of Computers in Patient Education." *Patient Education and Counseling*, 1993, *2*, 22–34.

Stevens, C. J., and Dial, M. "What Constitutes Misuse?" In C. J. Stevens and M. Dial (eds.), *Preventing the Misuse of Evaluation.* San Francisco: Jossey-Bass, 1994.

Telleen, S. "Developing a State Outcomes Monitoring System in Public Health Maternal and Child Health." *Journal of Medical Systems*, 1999, *23*(3), 227–238.

CHAPTER TWELVE

Developing a Process to Evaluate a National Injury Prevention Program

The Indian Health Service Injury Prevention Program

Carolyn E. Crump and Robert J. Letourneau

Evaluation and public health professionals have agreed that the participation of a diverse group of stakeholders is an important element in both evaluation and program planning (Learmonth, 2000; South and Tilford, 2000). There remains, however, a need to delineate methods that effectively use participatory inquiry and utilization-focused principles to conduct program evaluations that will increase program effectiveness (Fetterman, 1995; Kegler, Twiss, and Look, 2000; Milstein and Wetterhall, 2000; Smith, 1998). Faculty and staff members from the Injury Prevention (IP) Research Center at the University of North Carolina (UNC), Chapel Hill, have collaborated with the Injury Prevention Program (IPP) of the Indian Health Service (IHS) since 1997 to develop and implement a process evaluation for their IPPs. Process evaluations allow for a detailed explanation of how a program, organization, or relationship operates (Patton, 1990).

The IHS's national IPP is decentralized; therefore, the management and implementation of IP activities varies across the twelve IHS regional areas (see Figure 12.1), which are responsible for providing health care and IP services to American Indians and Alaskan Natives (Indian Health Service, 1998–1999). The program stage of development assessment (PSDA) process, developed by the UNC

The authors wish to acknowledge Alan Dellapenna Jr., deputy director of the Indian Health Service's Division of Environmental Health Services, and Richard Smith, who was manager of the Indian Health Service's Injury Prevention Program at the time this project was initiated, for their contribution to the development and implementation of the program stage of development assessment process.

FIGURE 12.1. INDIAN HEALTH SERVICE AREAS AND SERVICE POPULATION, 1998–1999.

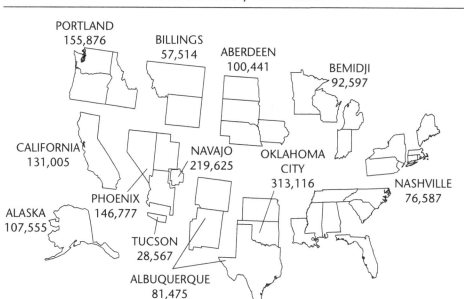

Source: Indian Health Service, 1998–1999.

faculty and staff to evaluate and provide feedback to IHS staff members to improve the effectiveness of their IPPs, has been completed in six of the twelve IHS areas. Thus, the process evaluation conducted for the IHS describes the extent to which each area IPP is operating in an effective manner and identifying the area program strengths and challenges (Patton, 1990). This chapter describes the development, pretest, implementation, and lessons learned from the implementation of the PSDA process. In addition, the evaluators will describe how the PSDA process is consistent with the principles of empowerment and utilization-focused evaluation (Fetterman, Kaftarian, and Wandersman, 1996; Patton, 1986), as well as with evaluability assessment (EA), which was popularized in the 1970s by Joseph Wholey and his colleagues at the Urban Institute (Smith, 1989).

Evaluation Frameworks

There are multiple frameworks and standards available to guide the design and implementation of a program evaluation (Centers for Disease Control and Prevention 1999; Chelimsky, 1997; Dale, 1998; Fetterman, 1997; House and Howe,

1999; Patton, 1990; Pawson and Tilley, 1997; World Health Organization, 1998). As emphasized by Fetterman, Kaftarian, and Wandersman (1996), a singular approach to evaluation is not responsive to the needs and demands of program staff members and participants, who often must deal with rapidly changing, highly unstable environments. Evaluation is applied research and, as such, struggles both to be useful and to address issues of validity, reliability, and generalizability, if appropriate (Learmonth, 2000; Patton, 1986). Standards of practice outlined in various frameworks remind evaluators of issues that should be considered, based on the evaluation approach selected, as they design an evaluation.

Chelimsky (1997) identifies three general evaluation approaches, which she categorizes as "accountability"—the measurement of results or efficiency, "knowledge"—the acquisition of a more profound understanding in some specific area or field, and "development"—the provision of evaluative help to strengthen institutions or programs, based on the purpose of the evaluation. She outlines for each evaluation approach the characteristics on nine dimensions: (1) purpose, (2) the need for implementation, (3) the user, (4) the role of the evaluator, (5) independence, (6) advocacy, (7) acceptability of approach by the client, (8) objectivity, and (9) the position under policy debate. The PSDA process is focused on program improvement, identified by Chelimsky's classification system as a developmental perspective rather than as an accountability assessment or a knowledge gain (Chelimsky, 1997; South and Tilford, 2000).

The evaluation developed by the external evaluators for the IHS needed to be realistic and relevant, and it needed to result in recommendations—generated by both the program staff members and the UNC external evaluators—that were appropriate and useful (Chelimsky, 1997; Patton, 1986). Therefore, an empowerment evaluation approach was used to guide the evaluation process developed for the IHS. Empowerment evaluation, also referred to as "participatory evaluation," is a collaborative process between program stakeholders and the evaluators, which depends on both qualitative and quantitative data (Fetterman, 1994). As outlined by Fetterman (1994), the main steps involved in an empowerment evaluation include (1) taking stock or determining where a program stands, including both strengths and weaknesses, (2) establishing goals and determining where the program should go in the future, with explicit emphasis on program improvement, (3) developing strategies and helping program staff members determine their own approaches to accomplish program goals and objectives, and (4) helping program staff members determine the type of evidence required to credibly document progress toward their goals. Whereas the external evaluators were responsible for the implementation of the evaluation developed for IHS, IPP staff members were involved in each step of the evaluation, thus following principles of empowerment evaluation and ensuring that the process evaluation results were relevant.

An empowerment evaluation approach also considers the context and developmental "life-cycle" of a program (Fetterman, 1995). Less developed programs should not be held to the same standards as mature programs; therefore, recommendations must be tailored to the appropriate program stage of development. The reason for using a participatory evaluation process is to understand the program from multiple stakeholder perspectives and to identify ways of improving the program (Fetterman, 1997). Involving program staff members in the evaluation process increases commitment to an ongoing process of reflection, learning, and program improvement.

The approach used to develop the PSDA process is also consistent with EA, the principles of which emphasize the need to understand the structure and functioning of a program before a summative evaluation may be conducted. The EA process may be used to conduct (1) a summative evaluation determining the program's effect, (2) a formative evaluation identifying what needs to be changed about a program to make it more effective, and (3) the defining of goals, objectives, activities, and resources needed to increase the effectiveness of a program.

Injury-Specific Program Guidelines

Best practices for preventing injuries have been identified and were used to guide the overall framework developed for the IHS evaluation (Berger and Mohan, 1996; Bonnie, Fulco, and Liverman, 1999; Christoffel and Gallagher, 1999; Christoffel and Teret, 1993; Rivara, Grossman, and Cummings, 1997a; Rivara, Grossman, and Cummings, 1997b). Guidelines suggesting best practices for community-based IP, published by the State and Territorial Injury Prevention Director's Association (STIPDA), identified five components for a model state IPP: (1) data collection and analysis, (2) program design, implementation, and evaluation, (3) coordination and collaboration, (4) technical support and training, and (5) public policy (Safe States Working Group, 1997). Criteria specific to each of these program components were identified and organized by three phases of program development. With these guidelines, STIPDA was emphasizing the developmental nature of state IPPs, indicating that Phase I programs were just getting started, Phase II programs have targeted programs but lack a comprehensive approach to injury prevention, and Phase III programs address the major causes of injury morbidity and mortality.

The PSDA process for the IHS was developed by the UNC faculty and staff as a best practices guide for IHS area IPPs. The IHS area assessment process and PSDA tool (see Appendix A) were used to evaluate each area IPP on twelve program components. The PSDA tool outlines criteria that describe a progressively more comprehensive area program to prevent injury-related mortality and morbidity.

The criteria used to identify the program stage of development (basic, intermediate, or comprehensive) was based on information provided to the evaluators, which was collected through small group interviews and reviewed by the IHS staff.

The Indian Health Service Injury Prevention Program

American Indians and Alaskan Natives have the highest unintentional injury and suicide rates and the second-highest homicide rates in the United States (Centers for Disease Control and Prevention, 2002). The relative risk of injury-related death is one and one-half to five times greater than national rates, depending on the IHS area and the cause of injury (Smith and Robertson, 2000). Figure 12.2 shows the ten leading causes of death among American Indians and Alaskan Natives at ages one through fifty-four from 1994 to 1998. Unintentional injuries—from motor vehicle crashes and other accidents—are the leading causes of death among American Indians and Alaskan Natives at ages one through thirty-four. Figure 12.3 highlights the injury death rates among American Indians and Alaskan Natives by age group from 1994 to 1998.

FIGURE 12.2. TEN LEADING CAUSES OF DEATH AMONG AMERICAN INDIANS AND ALASKAN NATIVES, 1994–1998.

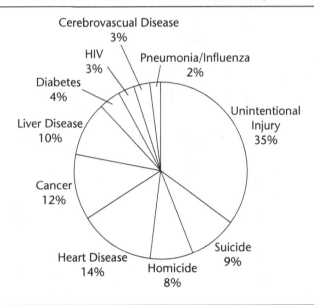

Source: Centers for Disease Control and Prevention, 2002.

FIGURE 12.3. TEN LEADING CAUSES OF INJURY DEATH AMONG AMERICAN INDIANS AND ALASKAN NATIVES BY AGE GROUP, 1994–1998.

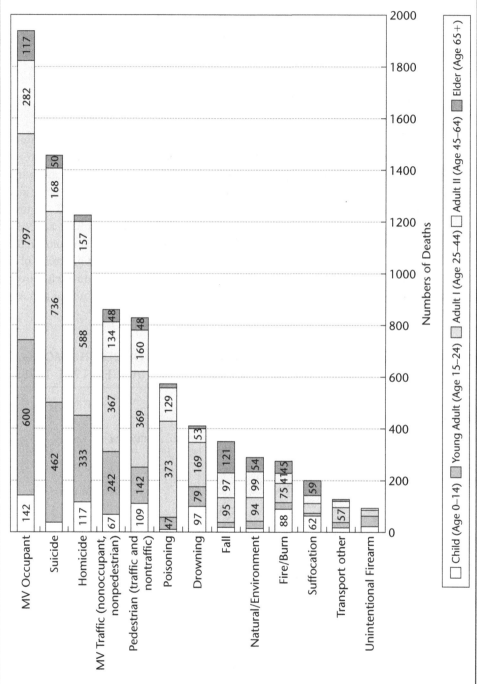

Source: Centers for Disease Control and Prevention, 2002.

The IHS is the principal federal health care provider and health advocate for American Indian and Alaskan Native people living in the United States. It currently provides health services to approximately 1.5 million American Indians and Alaskan Natives, who belong to more than 557 federally recognized tribes in thirty-five states. The IHS is divided into twelve service areas, with separate and distinct organizational structures and with varying numbers and sizes of federally recognized tribes being served. Most IHS service areas are divided into districts and are further divided into service units. The twelve IHS service areas are listed in Table 12.1.

The IHS IPP is located organizationally within the IHS Office of Public Health, Division of Environmental Health Services. An IPP manager is responsible for the management and direction of the national IHS IPP, and each of the twelve service areas has a designated area IP specialist. Each area's IPP is at a different level of maturity or development, and the formal training and experience of each area IP specialist is unique. In addition, the time allocated to IP by the local environmental health (EH) staff varies. District IP specialists are located in two IHS areas: Navajo and Phoenix. Through tribal self-governance initiatives, such as the Indian Self-Determination Act (Public Law 93–638 Amendment), some tribes or tribal organizations do not receive EH or IP services from IHS staff and have therefore hired additional IP specialists—as in, for example, the Alaska area. IHS area IP specialists devote between 10 and 90 percent of their time to injury prevention activities, with the balance of their time being allocated to providing other EH services. District and service unit EH staff members devote approximately 30 percent of their time to IP activities, although this varies by service unit and area. Additional IHS and tribal staff members—such as health educators, law enforcement officers, community health representatives, public health nurses, and other staff members—also contribute staff time to local IP activities.

The IHS IPP was initiated in the early 1970s, with a focus on community education. During the 1980s, it concentrated on building a federal infrastructure to support area and local IP efforts, using a public health approach and including local data collection to facilitate environmental hazard reduction. In the mid-1980s, the IHS IPP shifted its efforts to develop and implement local injury surveillance systems to track injuries among American Indians and Alaskan Natives (Smith and Robertson, 2000). In the late 1980s, the IHS IPP emphasized building the capacity of tribes and tribal organizations to prevent injuries through training, technical assistance, coalition building, and direct funding to tribes for IPPs. This led, in the early 1990s, to the IHS's development of a framework entitled the Complete Injury Prevention Program, which included the following six primary components: (1) epidemiology, (2) coalition development, (3) intervention activities, (4) advocacy, (5) marketing, and (6) evaluation (Smith and Robertson, 2000).

TABLE 12.1. STATE, SERVICE POPULATION, AND NUMBER OF TRIBES BY IHS AREA, 1998–1999.

IHS Area	State(s)	Service Population	Percentage of IHS Service Population	Number of Tribes or Tribal Entities
1. Aberdeen	ND, SD, IA, NE	100,441	6.6	12
2. Alaska	AK	107,555	7.1	13 corporations
3. Albuquerque	NM, CO	81,475	5.4	28
4. Bemidji	MN, MI, WI	92,597	6.1	34
5. Billings	MT, WY	57,514	3.8	8
6. California	CA	131,005	8.7	33
7. Nashville	ME, NY, MA, CT, RI, NJ, PA, IN, MI, TN, AK, TX, LA, MS, AL, SC, FL	76,587	5.1	32 (including urban)
8. Navajo	Parts of NM, AZ, UT	219,625	14.5	1
9. Oklahoma City	OK, KS	313,116	20.7	37
10. Phoenix	AZ, NV, UT	146,777	9.7	54
11. Portland	ID, OR, WA	155,876	10.3	42
12. Tucson	Southern AZ	28,567	1.9	2

Source: Indian Health Service, 1998–1999.

To further enhance local capacity, congressional funding in 1997 established the Tribal Injury Prevention Grants Program, which was designed to increase the tribal capacity to develop, implement, and evaluate IPPs. This grants program initially funded twelve tribes or tribal organizations at $25,000 per year for up to three years. In late 2000, the grants program funded twenty-five tribes or tribal organizations for up to five years, at $50,000 per year.

In 1997, the IHS IPP manager contacted faculty members at UNC for technical assistance to develop and implement an evaluation plan for the IHS IPP. The IHS IPP manager wanted to know how effective the area IPPs had been in reducing disability and death from unintentional injuries. The external evaluators suggested that prior to the design and conduct of an impact evaluation, it was important to know how and to what extent each area conducted IP activities. The extent of program delivery is not an organizational characteristic that can be assumed. A process evaluation is required if decision makers want to be confident about information from an impact evaluation (Scheirer, 1994). As suggested by the principles of EA, learning the history and current organization of the IHS IPP at the headquarters and at the area offices was a critical first step in the development of an assessment process that could be used to evaluate twelve separate IHS area IPPs located across the country (Smith, 1989).

Program Evaluation Focus, Approach, and Tools

The data collection methods and tools developed to assess IHS area IPPs were developed and pilot tested in two IHS areas: Oklahoma City and Navajo. Based on the IHS IPP scope of work and guidelines (Smith, 1994), and with input from most IHS area IP specialists, the evaluators defined twelve evaluation components to guide the assessment process (see Table 12.2).

The core component of this process evaluation approach is the PSDA tool, which was developed to summarize and interpret information collected about an area's IPP (see Appendix A). This tool was designed to describe the stage of development—basic, intermediate, or comprehensive—for each of the twelve evaluation components. In addition, the PSDA tool was developed to provide a consistent way to summarize IHS area IPP activities and their development across a wide range of programs.

To assess an area's IPP stage of development as being either basic, intermediate, or comprehensive, several indicators (three to six per component) are listed for each evaluation component in the PSDA tool. Review and input by IHS IPP staff members assisted in the identification of indicators and criteria for each evaluation component by program stage of development. The tool was developed to

TABLE 12.2.   DEFINITIONS AND INDICATORS FOR THE EVALUATION COMPONENTS IDENTIFIED IN THE PROGRAM STAGE OF DEVELOPMENT ASSESSMENT PROCESS.

Evaluation Component	Definition	Indicators
1. Mission/Vision	Describes the mission/vision and program planning process of the area's injury prevention program	• existence of an injury prevention program plan • process used to develop the plan • staff involved in developing the plan • extent to which the plan is disseminated • frequency of plan updates/reviews • the existence of long-range program planning
2. Resource Allocation/ Accounting	Describes resources used to support the area's injury prevention program	• amount, types, and sources of funding used for area-wide injury prevention activities • funding allocation methods used to disburse funds within the area • spending authority/autonomy for program staff • number and types of external funding sources used for program activities
3. Management Support	Describes the management support provided to support the area's injury prevention program	• amount and types of support provided by management (IHS and tribal) to the injury prevention program • extent to which the area's injury prevention program staff have authority and freedom (e.g., autonomy) to develop and implement the injury program • extent to which injury prevention performance standards are used to measure support for the area's injury prevention program
4. Staffing/Roles and Responsibilities	Indicates the staff roles and responsibilities that support the area's injury prevention program	• existence of injury prevention program-specific job descriptions • extent to which area-level staff are responsible for conducting injury prevention activities • extent to which district injury prevention positions and service unit staff are filled and are responsible for conducting injury prevention activities • extent to which district and service unit environmental health staff fulfill injury prevention program roles and responsibilities

TABLE 12.2. (CONTINUED)

Evaluation Component	Definition	Indicators
5. Training	Describes the training activities conducted and supported by an area's injury prevention program	• training levels of staff involved in the injury prevention program • number and types of training activities conducted within an area • extent of tribal involvement/ participation in area injury prevention training activities • extent to which training activities are reflected in the area's injury prevention program budget
6. Partnerships/ Collaboration	Describes the collaborative relationships developed to support an area's injury prevention program	• existing partnerships supporting the injury prevention program • extent, quality, and results of existing partnerships and collaboration • frequency and content of collaboration with developed partnerships • extent to which partnerships and/or coalitions have been formed with tribes
7. Needs Assessment/ Defined Service Population	Describes assessment of needs used to guide an area's injury prevention program	• extent to which and for what purposes needs assessments are collected • extent to which tribes/communities are involved in identifying injury prevention needs • how needs assessment data are used for program planning, implementation, and evaluation
8. Surveillance Data Collection	Describes the data collection systems used to guide an area's injury prevention program	• types of injury surveillance data collected • sources of injury data used • extent to which data are disseminated • quality of injury data surveillance systems • the use of advanced injury surveillance data collection technology

(Continued)

TABLE 12.2. DEFINITIONS AND INDICATORS FOR THE EVALUATION COMPONENTS IDENTIFIED IN THE PROGRAM STAGE OF DEVELOPMENT ASSESSMENT PROCESS. (CONTINUED)

Evaluation Component	Definition	Indicators
9. Injury Program Planning and Implementation	Describes the types of interventions conducted by an area's injury prevention program	• planning processes used to develop injury programs • staff/personnel involved with implementing injury programs • extent to which tribal members are involved in developing and implementing programs • types of injury prevention interventions implemented • extent to which monitoring and support is provided for injury prevention programs
10. Marketing/ Advocacy	Describes marketing/ advocacy activities to support components of an area's injury prevention program	• types of marketing materials developed • staff involvement in marketing and advocating for the injury prevention program • use of media to promote awareness of the burden of injury and the area's injury prevention program efforts • overall awareness of the burden of injury
11. Evaluation/ Reporting	Describes the reporting and evaluation activities conducted as part of the area's injury prevention program	• types of evaluations conducted • frequency of conducting evaluations • staff involved in conducting evaluations • extent to which evaluation results are reported and used
12. Technical Assistance/ Building Tribal Capacity	Describes technical assistance activities of an area's injury prevention program	• training provided to and received by tribal members • technical assistance provided to tribes in securing injury prevention program funding • involvement of tribal members in identifying tribal injury prevention needs • extent to which tribes are involved with injury prevention program planning, implementation, and evaluation • extent to which partnerships and collaborations have been formed with tribes for program planning, implementation, and evaluation

be general enough so that it could be used to guide the process evaluation conducted in each of the twelve IHS area programs. Therefore, expert knowledge related to each component is required to effectively apply the tool to each area's program. The tool provides specific criteria or standards that allow for the objective identification of the stage of development of an area's IPP. To apply the tool effectively, expert opinion is required to balance the extent to which each area meets criteria described for each component with unique contextual factors specific to each area.

The twelve evaluation components identified by UNC faculty and staff members and the IHS staff to guide the PSDA process are listed in Table 12.2. The evaluation components provide a framework that is used to guide the development of an IHS area's IPP.

The first four evaluation components serve as the foundation for an overall IPP. These components should be developed first for the remaining components to be effective. For example, without a guiding mission or vision, or a planning process for an area's IPP, only limited success is expected in the other evaluation components. The resource allocation and accounting component is important for an overall program because, with minimal funding, the ability of an area's IPP to implement interventions that will prevent injuries in tribal communities will be limited. Similarly, without adequate management support at the area or tribal level, an area's programs can be derailed. Management support may be demonstrated in multiple ways, such as by providing an adequate budget or by assuming specific responsibility for the program budget that supports IP activities and staff members. Finally, staffing roles and responsibilities, or the degree to which IPP staff members are supported (both philosophically and financially) to perform IPP responsibilities (as primary or collateral duties), also influences the effectiveness of an IPP. Without dedicated staff time to develop and implement targeted IP interventions, the interventions implemented may primarily be "off the shelf" programs that may not be appropriately tailored to the needs or issues of the intended service population or target audience.

The next five evaluation components are focused on the intended target audience and describe actions required to support the design and implementation of comprehensive IP interventions. For example, once staff positions are available, training in effective program development, implementation, and evaluation is critical. Through training, program staff members learn how to collect needs assessment and surveillance data and how to use that information to design, select, and evaluate effective interventions. The partnerships and collaboration component emphasizes that IP activities are multifaceted and involve multiple partners. In an era of diminished resources, an effective way to meet program objectives is to nurture partnerships, and staff members conducting IP activities should seek to involve diverse partnerships for developing, implementing, and evaluating IP interventions. Needs assessment, defined service population, and surveillance data collection relate to the need for appropriate and reliable local data to better tailor the IP interventions. These data are important in shaping perceptions (knowledge, attitudes, and beliefs) about injury problems, in categorizing the injuries addressed (as intentional or unintentional), in denoting causes of the injuries addressed (such as auto accidents, fires, and falls), and in indicating types of interventions selected (multiple versus single-focus, or behavioral, environmental, or policy change), as part of an area's IPP planning and implementation.

The remaining three components represent the more advanced focus of IPPs that have solid staffing and experience and therefore effective program activities. An emphasis on program evaluation and reporting is required so that the effectiveness of IP interventions is adequately documented and assessed and results are easily disseminated through routine reports. The marketing and advocacy of IP activities is also important, particularly for educating community members and tribal decision makers and policymakers about the scope, impact, cost, and social consequences of preventable injuries—especially considering that the health care resources of many tribes and tribal organizations are limited. Technical assistance/building of tribal capacity is an important component to measure because tribal self-governance has increased in recent years, meaning that tribes and tribal organizations have requested and been given direct control of federally allocated resources for medical and public health care services rather than being provided resources and services by the IHS staff. Therefore, IHS programs designed to enhance capacity are desired.

Considered together, these twelve evaluation components guided the evaluation of the IHS IPP and may be used to further enhance the IHS IPP activities. The process evaluation data collected about each of these twelve components are useful for evaluating programs in complex systems like those expected in area programs (Scheirer, 1994). These twelve components may be modified or updated as appropriate to support the continued improvement of the program evaluation process.

The Program Stage of Development Assessment Process

The procedures used to conduct the process evaluation of the IHS area IPPs are detailed in the program stage of development assessment process, which includes three steps: (1) preparing for the area site visit, (2) conducting the area site visit, and (3) completing post–site visit follow-up activities. Although it is intended that site visits be similar in format, each visit has unique aspects. Challenges to uniformity of experience among site visits include (1) geographic barriers to travel, (2) prohibitive travel costs, and (3) difficulties in scheduling dates so as to include all possible site visit participants.

Preparing for an Area Site Visit

To prepare for an area site visit, it is necessary to identify dates, times, and specific locations of site visit meetings and field visits. Four to six months before a site visit is held, the evaluators seek approval for the month during which the visit will take place and begin planning for the visit by talking with the area IP specialist. Approximately ten weeks prior to a site visit, a formal request is made for documents describing the area's program emphasis, staffing, and tribes served, as well as specific programmatic information about an area's IPP. These typically include the number and types of IP training activities that have been conducted in the area for the past ten years and, if available, a summary of local injury surveillance data. Along with the request for documents, the evaluators describe in a cover letter the PSDA process and ask that the area IP specialist distribute an introduction letter, a two-page list of general site visit questions, the PSDA tool, and a PSDA worksheet to all area, district, service unit, and tribal staff members participating in the site visit. Prior to the site visit, the evaluators review the background information submitted by the area IP specialist and prepare additional site visit questions.

Conducting an Area Site Visit

During the site visit, the evaluators facilitate individual and group meetings with IHS area, district, and service unit staff members, with the group meetings lasting an average of four to six hours and focusing on the twelve program components included in the PSDA process. At the end of a meeting, the evaluators collect the completed PSDA worksheets, on which staff members are required to record their perceptions of the program stage of development (basic, intermediate, and comprehensive) for each evaluation component. The worksheet also requests information about the contextual factors that should be considered when determining the area's program stage of development. In addition to the formal meetings with the IHS staff, the evaluators visit tribal project staff members and interview tribal IP practitioners and partners (for example, local IP coalition members).

Post–Site Visit Activities

After a site visit, the evaluators review additional documents and interview notes describing the area's IPP. Based on this information, the evaluators describe the structure and function of the area IPP and identify important contextual factors that may have an impact on an area's program. A draft evaluation report is submitted to the area IP specialist, who often distributes the draft report to other area IPP staff members. Area IPP staff members are encouraged to carefully review the draft report prior to conducting a conference call with the external evaluators. As Hendricks (1994) states, the draft report is especially valuable because it will be reviewed by program staff members, who have an opportunity to provide additional data to clarify issues discussed in the written report. Sensitive issues that may not have received enough attention during the site visit may be mentioned in the draft report to generate specific discussion about the issues. The follow-up telephone call provides an opportunity for staff members to clarify or correct sections or statements in the report. The review process provides for focused dialogue and reflective deliberation, which is an important component of participatory evaluation processes (House and Howe, 1999). The final report is distributed to the area IP specialist and the IHS headquarters IPP staff, and a formal summary presentation of the findings is made at the semiannual IHS IPP meeting. Table 12.3 lists the post–site visit steps needed to complete the PSDA.

TABLE 12.3.   POST–SITE VISIT STEPS TO COMPLETE THE PROGRAM STAGE OF DEVELOPMENT ASSESSMENT PROCESS.

1. Summarize site visit interviews and observations by evaluation component.
2. Organize and summarize injury prevention program documents by evaluation component.
3. Review program stage of development worksheets completed by staff.
4. Identify and interpret the extent to which program indicators for each evaluation component were a part of an area's injury prevention program.
5. Identify the program stage of development (basic, intermediate, comprehensive) for each evaluation component (using the program stage of development assessment tool).
6. Justify the stage of development rating and describe contextual factors related to each evaluation component.
7. Identify recommendations and suggested resources to assist the area's injury program staff in moving to the next stage of program development for each evaluation component.
8. Send draft area evaluation report to area injury prevention specialist for review.
9. Conduct conference call with area injury prevention specialist to collect feedback on draft area evaluation report.
10. Revise area evaluation report, write executive summary, and distribute final copy of area evaluation report to the IHS area injury prevention specialist and IHS headquarters staff.

The results of the area IP PSDA process are summarized in an evaluation report that includes seven separate sections (see Table 12.4). For each of the twelve evaluation components discussed in the program evaluation report, an overall stage of development rating is provided. These ratings are based on the indicators detailed for each evaluation component in the PSDA tool. The process used to determine an evaluation component's rating is based on (1) site visit interviews, (2) site visit observations, (3) document reviews, (4) input collected from area, district, service unit, and tribal IP personnel during and after a site visit (for example, contextual factors and the stage of development worksheet), and (5) the experiences and expertise of the evaluators. The information gleaned from those sources is reviewed and considered independently by the two evaluators and is then discussed until consensus is reached for each evaluation component rating.

Recommendations provided in the program evaluation report are based on best practices for program development and implementation and the evaluators' experience with public health and IP initiatives. Recommendations are also based on the evaluators' understanding of the IHS and tribal organizational structure, as well as on Native American beliefs and cultural characteristics. Recommendations for each of the twelve evaluation components are designed to assist area IPP staff members in overcoming barriers to program development and improving the indicators of each evaluation component. For example, some common

TABLE 12.4.   SECTIONS INCLUDED IN THE STAGE OF DEVELOPMENT ASSESSMENT PROCESS EVALUATION REPORT.

1. Executive Summary (approximately 5–7 pages)

2. Area Background and Organizational Structure (approximately 3 pages)

3. Summary of Area Program Evaluation Process (approximately 2 pages)

4. Program Stage of Development for Each Evaluation Component (approximately 50–60 pages)
     Review of Indicators
     Overall Rating
     Justification and Contextual Factors
     Recommendations
     Resources

5. Summary Profile of Area Evaluation Component Ratings

6. References

7. Appendices
     Site Visit Summary
     Site Visit Questions
     Program Stage of Development Assessment Tool
     Program Stage of Development Assessment Worksheet
     Site Visit Introduction Letter

recommendations based on six area evaluations completed to-date include (1) developing more formal and regular program planning processes, (2) developing more structured funding allocation mechanisms for the distribution of area IPP funds for local district, service unit, or tribal IP interventions, and (3) increasing the extent to which IPP activities are evaluated. Whenever possible within the recommendations section, specific references are made to IHS area, district, service unit, and tribal best practices and are discussed during the site visit. In addition, resources—such as books, articles, and Web sites—to guide area staff in completing recommendations are provided in the report.

Lessons Learned About Process Evaluation

The evaluators have identified ten lessons learned from the process evaluation developed and implemented for the IHS area IPPs. The lessons learned are organized into the following three categories: (1) the benefits and process of empowerment evaluation (for example, how to involve program staff members in the evaluation), (2) the value of comprehensive data collection, and (3) the benefits of evaluators' multiple perspectives and skills.

LESSON 1. *Involving staff in identifying evaluation criteria increases the relevance and acceptance of the program assessment process.*

As Fetterman (1994) notes, there are an endless number of components that may be rated or considered in a process evaluation. A strength of this evaluation was the collaboration with IHS staff members to identify relevant evaluation components used to guide the area assessment process (Smith, 1998). This was clearly the case, as the evaluation components and criteria by which a program's stage of development are rated (basic, intermediate, and comprehensive) were universally accepted by the staff in each area. Synergy was gained through collaboration between the external evaluators, who have content expertise in IP and evaluation methods, and the IHS staff members responsible for the development and implementation of the IHS IPP. Using the twelve evaluation components included in the PSDA process enabled the evaluators to determine the organizational capacity of each IHS area IPP to deliver effective IP interventions. In addition, the PSDA tool is being used by several IHS area, district, service unit, and tribal staff members as a program planning tool.

LESSON 2. *Written materials and worksheets describing the evaluation process assist in involving program staff members in the PSDA process.*

The use of the PSDA tool and worksheets facilitated the involvement of IHS and tribal staff members in the evaluation process used to evaluate an area's IPP.

Asking area staff members to refer to the tool to identify the stage at which their IPP had developed allowed them the opportunity to understand and experience the assessment method being used by the evaluators. Second, this process allowed area staff members to think critically about the documents and materials provided to the evaluators and to prompt IPP staff members to refer the evaluators to additional documents or materials that would be useful to them when rating the area's program stage of development. Third, the worksheet provided area staff members with the opportunity to identify and discuss contextual factors—such as the special circumstances or barriers they face—that the evaluators should consider when rating the area's program stage of development for each of the twelve evaluation components.

LESSON 3. *Those involved in the site visit gain from their participation an understanding of comprehensive IPPs.*

IHS and tribal staff members' participation in the assessment process was important to their understanding of the assessment process. Several staff members indicated that participating in the evaluation process afforded them a unique opportunity to critically examine their program efforts and to apply the concepts guiding the assessment process to improve their program activities. Especially for staff members with less experience, the focus group discussions provided an educational opportunity, as IHS and tribal staff members increased their knowledge of the IP field and the history of IP activities conducted in their area. During the evaluation process, staff members had an opportunity to hear their colleagues' opinions and ideas about the area's IPP, which is an important element of empowerment evaluation (Fetterman, 1997). Another positive outcome of the site visit interview process was that staff members' commitment to a program may be increased when they are asked their opinions. The focus group type of interviews conducted during site visits also allowed staff members to "recalibrate their ratings" and develop a shared understanding for the future of their program (Fetterman, 1997). In addition, managers who are interviewed as part of the process may think about the IP efforts with a new perspective, having met the external evaluators and learned what other area programs are doing to support IP.

LESSON 4. *IHS staff members involved in the program assessment process were often inspired to make immediate programmatic changes.*

During the interviews conducted during the site visits, program staff members and the external evaluators often identified issues or examples of how a program could be improved immediately following a site visit. Specific ideas were generated and next steps were identified, in part, because of the collaborative nature of the group meetings. For example, the value of developing regular or long-term strategic program plans was discussed, along with a process for incorporating ideas and feedback from area, district, and service unit IPP staff members on an annual basis. Additional ideas discussed included ideas for training workshops or modules that would benefit area, district, or service unit IP. Overall suggestions discussed during site visits were often immediately incorporated into program budget requests submitted to area office staff members for the next year's funding. Although the ideas mentioned during these group or individual interviews were later included in the recommendations identified in the more formal, written area evaluation report, some ideas generated during the data collection process were implemented immediately—that is, prior to the final report being completed. This concept was emphasized by the EA methods popularized in the 1970s (Smith, 1989). The IHS staff and the outside evaluators consider such "real-time" program improvement a positive outcome of the PSDA process, especially since program improvement was a primary purpose of the evaluation.

LESSON 5. *Process evaluation can be more relevant and comprehensive if complete data are provided.*

Assessments of the area IPPs depend on the amount and quality of information—particularly documentation—provided prior to, during, and following the site visits. For the pilot sites (Oklahoma City and Navajo), the collection of all the materials necessary to evaluate the program was limited by the lack of specificity in the document and information requests sent by the evaluators prior to their first site visit. The protocol for document requests was improved as the evaluators gained a better understanding of the type of reports usually available from IHS and tribal IPP staff members. A letter requesting specific information and documents was developed for subsequent area evaluations to specifically request types of documents and information from area IPP staff members. Among the materials sent to area IP specialists prior to a site visit are approximately ten sample table templates that require area IPP staff members to summarize information across years. IP specialists receive (1) *general information,* including the organizational structure of the IHS area, the number, name, and location of tribes served by the area, the organizational structure of the IPP, and resource allocation/accounting (for example, the overall program spending amounts and program spending categories), (2) *information on staff roles and responsibilities,* as well as the names and locations of IPP staff members, (3) *information on training,* such as the training experiences of current staff members, the number and types of area training activities, and a list of specific evaluation projects conducted, (4) *information on program partnerships and collaboration,* including the number and types of collaboration with national, state, and local partners, as well as the number and activity level of tribal/community coalitions, and (5) *program implementation information,* such as the number and types of projects funded and the intervention project focus. For IHS areas assessed after the pilot test, the evaluators requested that the summary tables be completed by area staff members prior to a site visit, if possible, or during and after a visit.

LESSON 6. *The data collection, analysis, and report preparation can be made more efficient during the course of a process evaluation.*

During the pilot site evaluations, the evaluators relied on handwritten notes to document details related to program implementation and structure. The evaluators have since benefited from entering interview notes directly into laptop computer files to record information. This has allowed the evaluators to be more efficient and effective at documenting information and ideas discussed during site visit interviews, focus groups, and field visit observations. After the final reports were completed for the pilot test evaluation sites, the efficiency with which information was summarized from documents, interviews, and site visits was also improved. For example, as a result of having developed a final report format and structure, it was easier for subsequent reports to be completed, as they followed a standardized format that could be adapted to account for the unique needs of each area. More recently, area staff members preparing for a site visit have benefited from reviewing completed evaluation reports from other areas. This has enabled them to learn how contextual factors are described and considered for each evaluation component. In addition, IPP staff members are provided with the opportunity to review a draft of the completed evaluation report to see the content, level of specificity, and tone of the recommendations that are included in the final report.

LESSON 7. *Process evaluation can provide important insights to guide policy and programs at multiple levels.*

The results from this evaluation have application at multiple levels within IHS and tribal IPPs. IHS headquarters IPP staff members are interested in the eventual creation of a profile that describes all twelve IHS area IPPs' stage of development across the twelve evaluation components. Having this information will allow IHS headquarters staff to (1) identify best practices across area programs, (2) prioritize resources on those evaluation components requiring improvement for most areas (for example, strategic planning and program evaluation), and (3) seek continued collaboration between the evaluators and the IHS staff of the various areas, districts, and service units as the recommendations outlined in the stage of development area reports are implemented. The recommendations must be carefully considered by each area program. Area staff members are encouraged to develop a strategic plan and to identify the most relevant and realistic recommendations to pursue in the short and long term. The degree to which higher-level area managers and district and service unit staff members support the process and are interested in improving an area's IPP will determine the extent to which the recommendations from this assessment process are implemented.

LESSON 8. *Empowerment evaluators must possess a wide range of skills.*

An external evaluator conducting an evaluation based on empowerment principles must be a trainer, facilitator, teacher, and advocate—and must be comfortable in such diverse roles (Smith, 1998). Fetterman, Kaftarian, and Wandersman (1996) state that the external evaluator is responsible for ensuring that the evaluation environment is conducive to sharing knowledge and honest beliefs about the program, and he or she must involve multiple stakeholders in the process. In conducting the first six IHS area evaluations, the evaluators met with approximately 100 IHS and 150 tribal representatives, and many of these individuals indicated that the evaluation process felt safe because they trusted that the evaluators were knowledgeable professionals. The evaluators agree with Fetterman, Kaftarian, and Wandersman (1996), who state that two evaluators are likely to be more effective than one. Empowerment evaluation has a social component that is better facilitated with two individuals who bring different personalities and backgrounds to the project.

LESSON 9. *External evaluators provide a valuable outside perspective, but they must also understand the purpose, history, context, and organizational structure of the agency or program under review.*

The same two external evaluators were involved from the beginning in this evaluation project, which made possible the continuity and institutional memory required for the understanding of IHS and tribal concerns and issues related to IPPs. UNC evaluators have expertise in public health principles and practices, including program evaluation, program management, intervention development, training, marketing, advocacy, and effective implementation strategies, such as IP. The evaluators had much to learn, however, about the complexities of the IHS and its historical and current working relationship with tribal entities in the United States. IHS headquarters and area IPP staff members assisted the evaluators as they gained an understanding of the IHS system in general and the IHS IPP specifically. Because the UNC staff worked collaboratively with the IHS staff, the evaluators quickly learned how the IHS IPP is designed, and they developed in-depth knowledge of area contextual factors that were and continue to be important to consider when recommendations are provided to area IPP staff members.

LESSON 10. *Peer review is appropriate and helpful.*

The pilot test of the evaluation approach identified the benefits of developing a peer reviewer system. The external evaluators are now accompanied during the area site visit by another area's IPP staff person—an IP specialist/EH officer from either an area or a district office, who has previously participated in the assessment process in his or her area. The peer review system allows for a sharing of information across all area IPPs. Area IPP staff members often have a limited understanding of how other area IPPs are organized and implemented and what the contextual factors are within other areas—such as their IP priorities or their tribal self-governance. The peer review system has increased understanding among the IHS IPP staff members of conditions in other IHS areas. The peer review process is an excellent way to involve IHS staff members in the process, thus providing another opportunity for peer reviewers to consider issues from multiple perspectives, such as from another area or from IHS's national IPP.

Limitations of the Program Stage of Development Assessment Process

The limitations or challenges in implementing an evaluation using empowerment principles include the time involved and the need to occasionally compromise scientific method (Smith, 1998). For example, the amount of time area staff members devoted to preparing information (such as summary tables) and identifying useful documents for the evaluators prior to a site visit varied widely across the six areas completed to-date. This was due in part to the scheduling challenges of some of the area site visits. As a result, the evaluators occasionally received only minimal information about an area's IPP prior to conducting a site visit. On several occasions, the evaluators waited months following a visit before they received completed tables and other source documents from the area IPP staff. Although this limitation became less significant as the evaluators became more knowledgeable about the IHS IPP (concerning such items as similarities in implementation, organizational structure, and staffing plans), having more information and documents prior to a visit reduced the time required to complete a draft evaluation report. In addition, the development of effective recommendations is a process that requires a lot of personnel time (Hendricks, 1994).

Because the evaluation process did not follow the traditional performance for score model commonly used by the IHS to review its programs, those areas initially participating in the evaluation did not fully understand that the process was designed to be collaborative. Under the more traditional evaluation methods implemented by the IHS, staff members often insulate themselves from the evaluation process and results by telling the evaluators what they think the evaluators want to hear. As IHS staff members in multiple areas became familiar with the collaborative evaluation process, this challenge diminished. The addition of the peer reviewer also increased IHS staff members' understanding of the collaborative nature of the PSDA process.

During the site visits, the evaluators were not always able to interview higher-level managers in the area, as the amount of interest in and support for the area IPP and the evaluation process varied among the managers. There are also some concerns regarding the validity of the information provided to the external evaluators by the program staff. When the evaluators held group interviews, some participants may have understated their concerns about a program, or they may have emphasized only the positive parts of their program. For example, some staff members may not have shared information that would place their IPP in the basic or intermediate range. However, the evaluation process was designed not only to identify challenges but also to facilitate a discussion about the solutions. So the evaluators emphasized that the staff members should share the reality of their IP activities rather than relating what they thought the evaluators wanted to hear.

In addition, there is the possibility that the external evaluators were biased or did not investigate beyond the basic reporting of information to understand more complex contextual factors within an area IPP. Chelimsky (1997) indicates that when a developmental evaluation approach is used, the program staff members and external evaluators are required to collaborate; therefore, close relationships are likely to form. Empowerment or participatory evaluation methods assume that evaluators will develop a vested interest in the program because of the degree of involvement they have with program staff members and other stakeholders. There is the risk that outside evaluators will lose their perspective, sidestep controversial issues, avoid reporting negative findings, and only report or make recommendations that have been supported by program staff members (Hendricks, 1994). Having twelve clearly identified evaluation components and criteria for basic, intermediate, and comprehensive programs reduced the likelihood of bias in identifying the program stage of development for each area.

Implications for Research

The twelve components identified in the PSDA tool should be subjected to tests of construct and predictive validity. Empirical evidence supporting the criteria outlined for the evaluation components is available, based on general program planning principles, best practices in IP, and organizational development theories (Green and Kreuter, 1999; Scheirer, 1994). Although the criteria for the twelve components have face validity, there is the need to determine which components are related, and to what extent they are related, to the effectiveness of an area's IPP. In response to the increased demand for evidence-based evaluation, it will be valuable to extend this current project by designing and implementing an impact evaluation (Dever, 1997; Green and Tones, 1999). It will be easier to design the impact or outcome study after having completed the area IPP PSDA process in all twelve IHS areas.

Summary

This chapter describes a framework for assessing the stage of development and for providing recommendations to improve a national-level IPP that is implemented in twelve IHS areas across the United States to improve the services for, and meet the IP needs of, American Indians and Alaskan Natives. In this chapter, the process used to identify the evaluation components and to develop the PSDA tool has been described. In addition, the evaluators have described how the area evaluation process was guided by empowerment and EA principles, and they have detailed the steps taken to implement this evaluation. Ten lessons learned from this process evaluation are presented and the implications for practice and research are identified. Process evaluation is useful for documenting how a program operates and to what extent best practices are used. The in-depth understanding of a program gained through a process evaluation can lead to specific and timely programmatic improvements.

References

Berger, L., and Mohan, D. *Injury Control: A Global View.* New York: Oxford University Press, 1996.

Bonnie, R., Fulco, C., and Liverman, C. *Reducing the Burden of Injury: Advancing Prevention and Treatment.* Washington, D.C.: National Academy Press, 1999.

Centers for Disease Control and Prevention. "Framework for Program Evaluation in Public Health." *Morbidity and Mortality Weekly Report,* 1999, *48*(RR-11), 1–41.

Centers for Disease Control and Prevention. *Web-Based Injury Statistics Query and Reporting System (WISQARS).* Atlanta, Ga.: National Center for Injury Prevention and Control, 2002.

Chelimsky, E. "The Coming Transformations in Evaluation." In E. Chelimsky and W. Shadis (eds.), *Evaluation for the Twenty-First Century: A Handbook.* Thousand Oaks, Calif.: Sage, 1997.

Christoffel, T., and Gallagher, S. *Injury Prevention and Public Health: Practical Knowledge, Skills, and Strategies.* Gaithersburg, Md.: Aspen, 1999.

Christoffel, T., and Teret, S. *Protecting the Public: Legal Issues in Injury Prevention.* New York: Oxford University Press, 1993.

Dale, R. *Evaluation Frameworks for Development Programmes and Projects*. Thousand Oaks, Calif.: Sage, 1998.

Dever, G. *Improving Outcomes in Public Health Practice: Strategy and Methods*. Gaithersburg, Md.: Aspen, 1997.

Fetterman, D. "Steps of Empowerment Evaluation: From California to Cape Town." *Evaluation and Program Planning*, 1994, *17*(3), 305–313.

Fetterman, D. "In Response." *Evaluation Practice*, 1995, *16*(2), 179–199.

Fetterman, D. "Empowerment Evaluation and Accreditation in Higher Education." In E. Chelimsky and W. Shadish (eds.), *Evaluation for the Twenty-First Century: A Handbook*. Thousand Oaks, Calif.: Sage, 1997.

Fetterman, D., Kaftarian, S., and Wandersman, A. (eds.). *Empowerment Evaluation: Knowledge and Tools for Self-Assessment and Accountability*. Thousand Oaks, Calif.: Sage, 1996.

Green, J., and Tones, K. "Toward a Secure Evidence Base for Health Promotion." *Journal of Public Health Medicine*, 1999, *21*(2), 133–139.

Green, L., and Kreuter, M. *Health Promotion Planning: An Educational and Ecological Approach*. (3rd ed.) Mountain View, Calif.: Mayfield, 1999.

Hendricks, M. "Making a Splash: Reporting Evaluation Results Effectively." In J. Wholey, H. Hatry, and K. Newcomer (eds.), *Handbook of Practical Program Evaluation*. San Francisco: Jossey-Bass, 1994.

House, E., and Howe, K. *Values in Evaluation and Social Research*. Thousand Oaks, Calif.: Sage, 1999.

Indian Health Service. *Trends in Indian Health*. U.S. Department of Health and Human Services, Rockville, Md.: Indian Health Service, 1998–1999.

Kegler, M. C., Twiss, J. M., and Look, V. "Assessing Community Change at Multiple Levels: The Genesis of an Evaluation Framework for the California Healthy Cities Projects. *Health Education and Behavior*, 2000, *27*(6), 760–779.

Learmonth, A. "Utilizing Research in Practice and Generating Evidence from Practice." *Health Education Research*, 2000, *15*(6), 743–756.

Milstein, B., and Wetterhall, S. "A Framework Featuring Steps and Standards for Program Evaluation." *Health Promotion Practice*, 2000, *2*(3), 221–228.

Patton, M. *Utilization-Focused Evaluation*. (2nd ed.) Thousand Oaks, Calif.: Sage, 1986.

Patton, M. *Qualitative Evaluation and Research Methods*. (2nd ed.) Thousand Oaks, Calif.: Sage, 1990.

Pawson, R., and Tilley, N. *Realistic Evaluation*. Thousand Oaks, Calif.: Sage, 1997.

Rivara, F., Grossman, D., and Cummings, P. "Injury Prevention: First of Two Parts." *New England Journal of Medicine*, 1997a, *337*(8), 543–548.

Rivara, F., Grossman, D., and Cummings, P. "Injury Prevention: Second of Two Parts." *New England Journal of Medicine*, 1997b, *337*(9), 613–618.

Safe States Working Group. *Five Components of a Model State Injury Prevention Program and Three Phases of Program Development*. Oklahoma City, Okla.: State and Territorial Injury Prevention Director's Association, 1997.

Scheirer, M. "Designing and Using Process Evaluation." In J. Wholey, H. Hatry, and K. Newcomer (eds.), *Handbook of Practical Program Evaluation*. San Francisco: Jossey-Bass, 1994.

Smith, M. F. *Evaluability Assessment: A Practical Approach*. Boston: Kluwer, 1989.

Smith, M. K. "Empowerment Evaluation: Theoretical and Methodological Considerations." *Evaluation and Programming Planning*, 1998, *21*, 255–261.

Smith, R. *Guidelines: Indian Health Service Injury Prevention Program.* Rockville, Md.: Indian Health Service, 1994.

Smith, R., and Robertson, L. "Unintentional Injuries and Trauma." In E. Rhoades (ed.), *American Indian Health: Innovations in Health Care, Promotion, and Policy.* Baltimore, Md.: Johns Hopkins University Press, 2000.

South, J., and Tilford, S. "Perceptions of Research and Evaluation in Health Promotion Practice and Influences on Activity." *Health Education Research,* 2000, *15*(6), 729–741.

World Health Organization. *Health Promotion Evaluation: Recommendations to Policy-Makers.* Geneva: WHO Regional Office for Europe, 1998.

APPENDIX A: PROGRAM STAGE OF DEVELOPMENT ASSESSMENT TOOL.

COMPONENT	BASIC	INTERMEDIATE	COMPREHENSIVE
1. Mission/Vision—Describes the Mission/Vision of the area's injury prevention program.			
One-year plan exists	Area annual injury prevention plan documented, with goals and objectives.	Plan includes benchmarks (based on limited local data) and responsible parties.	Plan is based on area/district priorities using appropriate local data.
How is the plan developed?	Plan is developed by area injury specialist (AIS) without local data or advice from field staff.	Plan is developed by AIS with limited input from other IHS and tribal injury personnel.	Plan is developed by AIS with significant input from other IHS and tribal injury personnel.
Who develops it?			
How is the plan disseminated?	Plan distribution is limited.	Plan is distributed to all IHS injury personnel.	Plan is distributed to all IHS and tribal injury personnel.
How often is the plan updated?	Plan is reviewed on an annual basis.	Plan is reviewed and updated on an annual basis.	Plan is updated and revised semiannually. Completion of goals and objectives is assessed.
3- to 5-year strategic plan exists	Strategic plan is not developed.	Strategic plan is in process.	Strategic plan for 3–5 years is in place.
2. Resource Allocation/Accounting—Describes resources used to support the area's injury prevention program.			
Resource allocation from area IPP	IHS area funding for injury prevention is limited and minimal.	IHS area funding is fair and equitable.	IHS area funding goes beyond an area's regular share.
Resource allocation to area IPP (internal sources)	IHS funds are provided to SUs and tribes through area IP projects on an _irregular_ basis.	IHS funds are provided to SUs and tribes through area IP projects on _annual_ basis.	IHS funds are provided to SUs and tribes through area IP projects on _annual_ basis based on goals and objectives and previous evaluations.
Control over budget	AIS does not prepare an annual program budget and has no spending authority.	AIS prepares an annual program budget but has limited spending authority.	AIS is involved in budget development and manages and controls IP funds.
External funding sources exist	External funding sources are not developed.	External funding sources provide resources to limited aspects of the IPP. AIS prepares grant and/or contract proposals to secure _some_ external resources for interventions.	External funding sources provide resources for major IP initiatives, including positions. Grant funds allow for more extensive interventions than would be possible from IHS funding. AIS prepares grant and/or contract proposals to secure _significant_ external resources for interventions.

3. Management Support—Describes the Management Support provided to support the area's injury prevention program.

Support for injury prevention	Limited management support exists for injury prevention activities, at the area and field levels.	Implicit management support exists for injury prevention programs and activities.	Formal and explicit support exists at the area and field level for injury prevention, as demonstrated by interest in, performance evaluation criteria relating to, and resource allocation for injury prevention activities.
Authority for program direction	The AIS has limited authority in developing and implementing program direction (i.e., IP elements are in upper management's performance plans only).	The area IP specialist has authority in developing and implementing program direction.	AIS has primary authority for the direction of program, actively networks with states and other agencies on a regional and/or national level to further injury prevention efforts.
Performance standards (associated with quality improvement system)	AIS has no involvement in developing the performance standards and is not consulted in progress reporting.	IP elements are in upper management's performance plans and the area IP specialist drafts the performance standards and progress reports.	IP elements are in the area IP specialist's performance plan. The AIS prepares the performance standards and progress reports.

4. Staffing/Roles and Responsibilities—Indicates the staff roles and responsibilities that support the area's injury prevention program.

Job descriptions exist	AIS job description exists; it outlines injury prevention roles and responsibilities.	Area and district injury prevention job descriptions exist; they outline general injury prevention roles and responsibilities (including training). Area and district staff mentor field EH staff in IP practices.	Area and district injury prevention job descriptions exist; they clearly define specific roles and responsibilities. Area and district staff mentor field EH staff, other IHS, and tribal staff in IP practices (including the provision of training). Assistance is provided to develop tribal IP positions.
Area-level staff: amount of staff time devoted to IP program activities	One staff person is responsible for an area's injury prevention activities for at least half of his or her time, with the remaining half-time devoted to collateral duties.	One staff person is responsible for an area's injury prevention activities for most of his or her time, with the remaining time devoted to collateral duties.	One staff person is responsible for an area's injury prevention activities on a full-time basis.

(Continued)

APPENDIX A: PROGRAM STAGE OF DEVELOPMENT ASSESSMENT TOOL. (CONTINUED)

COMPONENT	BASIC	INTERMEDIATE	COMPREHENSIVE
District/service unit staff: amount of staff time devoted to IP program activities		At least one staff person is responsible for assisting the AIS with district-level injury prevention program activities.	District IP positions are filled and perform IP as their primary duty with input and guidance from area injury specialist. Service unit staff are on board doing injury prevention.
Extent to which EH staff fulfills IP program responsibilities.	Few EH field staff members have active responsibilities related to the area's IP program.	Some EH field staff members have active responsibilities related to the area's IP program.	All EH field staff members have active responsibilities related to the area's IP programs (e.g., studying local injury issues, fostering community IP coalitions, networking with tribal, state, and other agencies, and preparing grant funding to address local IP issues).

5. Training—Describes the training activities conducted and supported by an area's injury prevention program.

COMPONENT	BASIC	INTERMEDIATE	COMPREHENSIVE
Staff training levels	30 percent of the EH staff have completed Level I and II IP training courses.	50 percent of the EH staff have completed Level I and II IP training courses.	70 percent of the EH staff have completed IP Level I and II training courses. Active community injury prevention coalitions have IP-trained members.
Training provided at area—who implements training?	Area training opportunities are primarily available for IHS staff, but only if funds are available. IP training is generally available only through EMB courses.	Area training opportunities are available on an annual basis for IHS staff and tribal personnel. Area injury staff members conduct Level I and II training workshops for IHS staff and tribal personnel.	Area training opportunities are available on a semiannual basis for IHS staff and tribal personnel. Injury and EH staff members coordinate and teach IP training in the area, other areas, and at EMB courses.
Tribal involvement	Tribal participation in IP training courses is limited.	Some tribal members participate in IP training courses.	Many tribal members have taken Level I and II training courses.

Additional trainings	At least 50 percent of the injury prevention program staff have completed the IHS IPP fellowship program.	At least 70 percent of the injury prevention program staff have completed the IHS IPP fellowship program.	All injury prevention program staff members have completed the IHS IPP fellowship program. Out-of-area training opportunities are available on an annual basis for the IHS staff and tribal personnel.
How are trainings reflected in the budget?	Training activities are not reflected in the IP budget.	A minimum amount of resources (funds, staff) for training are reflected in the IP budget.	Extensive support for training (funds, staff time for local trainings, and travel expenses to IHS courses and conferences out of the area) is reflected in the budget.

6. Partnerships/Collaboration—Describes the collaborative relationships developed to support an area's injury prevention program.

What partnerships exist?	Partnerships and collaboration exist only with other IHS programs (e.g., CHR, Health Education, etc.) for injury prevention activities.	Partnerships and collaboration exist with other IHS programs AND state/local entities for injury prevention activities.	Active partnerships and collaboration exist with other IHS programs, state/local AND, national/federal entities for injury prevention activities.
Extent, quality, and results of collaboration	Collaboration is limited to sharing of information at meetings and through newsletters.	Collaborating involves assistance in identifying program goals, objectives, and activities.	Collaboration includes developing, implementing, and evaluating activities that fulfill identified goals/objectives.
How often is contact made?	Injury staff maintains some (e.g., 1–2 times per year) contact with other groups/agencies to share information.	Injury staff maintains periodic contact (e.g., quarterly) with other groups/agencies to share program information.	Injury staff maintains regular contact (e.g., monthly) with other groups/agencies to share program information.
Tribal partners/coalitions	Tribal IP coalitions are formed in some locations.	Community coalitions network with other coalitions and networking opportunities are provided through workshops and meetings. Intertribal coalition networking is fostered at area IP meetings and workshops.	Tribal coalitions network and collaborate with other community coalitions and other agencies to address and resolve local injury issues. Collaboration is documented with meeting minutes, nomination letters, recognition letters, and/or awards.

(Continued)

APPENDIX A: PROGRAM STAGE OF DEVELOPMENT ASSESSMENT TOOL. (CONTINUED)

COMPONENT	BASIC	INTERMEDIATE	COMPREHENSIVE
7. Needs Assessment/Defined Service Population—Describes assessment of needs used to guide an area's injury prevention program.			
Needs assessments are collected	Informal needs assessments are conducted to obtain feedback and/or share information about community concerns and issues.	Semiformal needs assessments are conducted to develop tailored, local-level injury prevention programs in direct response to community member requests.	Formal and extensive local-level needs assessments are conducted to develop and inform goals, objectives, design, and evaluations of injury prevention interventions.
Tribal/community involvement in identifying needs	Tribal/community members are not included in identifying community needs (e.g., attending focus groups and meetings, completing surveys, etc.).	Tribal/community members are usually involved in identifying community needs (e.g., attending focus groups and meetings, completing surveys, etc.).	Tribal/community members are always involved in identifying community needs (e.g., attending focus groups and meetings, completing surveys, etc.).
How it is used	Needs assessments are used to obtain feedback and share information.	Needs assessments are used to plan IP interventions.	Needs assessments are used to plan IP interventions and for determining baseline measures for evaluation of IP interventions.
8. Surveillance Data Collection—Describes the data collection systems used to guide an area's injury prevention program.			
Types of surveillance data collected	Uses existing data reports to examine injury types. Local data are not collected. Uses data on incidence by injury type; limited data on cause of injury. Limited analysis by subgroup	Annually conducts area and district/service unit-level analysis of existing injury hospitalization and death databases (obtains and uses E-coded information).	Annually conducts an area, district/service unit and tribal-level analysis of existing injury databases assessing prehospital, hospitalization, and death databases (obtains and uses E-coded information). Level II data collection (field investigations) is conducted.
Extent to which local data are collected			
What sources are used?	Uses limited sources for injury surveillance data.	Uses several sources for injury surveillance data (e.g., police crash reports, fire reports, emergency provider data).	Uses multiple sources for injury surveillance data (e.g., police crash reports, fire reports, emergency provider data).

How is information disseminated?	Injury data information is not regularly disseminated.	Annually prepares injury surveillance "fact sheets" for each district, service unit, and/or tribes.	Prepares comprehensive reports of injury surveillance at an area, district/service unit and tribal level. Disseminates surveillance data on a regular basis and to a wide audience.
Quality of data and surveillance system	Quality of data surveillance systems is not assessed.	Quality of data and surveillance systems are assessed periodically.	Evaluates quality of surveillance systems on a regular basis and takes steps to improve systems.
Use of advanced technology (e.g., GIS)	Advanced technology not used to link data or track injury events.	Limited use of advanced technology (e.g., GIS system) to link data and/or track injury events.	Extensive use of advanced technology (e.g., GIS system) to link data and/or track injury events.

9. Injury Program Planning and Implementation—Describes the types of interventions conducted by an area's injury prevention program.

Who initiates and how?	Injury prevention program ideas and activities are initiated and implemented by the IHS staff only.	Injury program ideas and activities are initiated and implemented by the IHS staff with the support of tribal/community members.	Injury program ideas and activities are initiated by the IHS staff, with the support of tribal/community members and with collaborators or partners.
Who develops and implements programs? (e.g., tribal involvement)	IP programs are implemented by the IHS staff only. Limited tribal involvement in developing and implementing programs.	Occasional tribal and community input sought in developing and implementing programs.	Tribes and communities determine primary direction of local injury prevention programs.
Intervention types	Program interventions are consistent with best practices in the literature. Injury prevention interventions include those limited to "off-the shelf" style activities (e.g., safety seat activities (e.g., seat-belt campaigns, etc.). Injury prevention interventions include a single-level focus (e.g., individual, vehicle/vector, environmental change).	Program interventions are consistent with best practices in the literature, as well as tribal/community requests, and are directly linked to IP Program goals and objectives. Injury prevention interventions include a single-level focus (e.g., individual, vehicle/vector, or environmental change) using multiple methods (health education, engineering, and policy development and enforcement).	Program interventions are consistent with best practices, tribal/community requests, IP Program goals/objectives, and local data and are culturally appropriate. Injury prevention interventions focus on multiple levels (i.e., individual, vehicle/vector, and environmental change) using multiple methods (health education, engineering, and policy development and enforcement).

(Continued)

COMPONENT	BASIC	INTERMEDIATE	COMPREHENSIVE
Monitoring provided	Monitoring and support of injury program activities is limited (e.g., occasionally conducted from area office by phone, fax, or e-mail).	Monitoring and support of injury program activities are regular (e.g., conducted on a regular basis through phone, fax, and e-mail).	Monitoring and support of injury program activities is conducted on a regular basis through phone, fax, and e-mail, and by in-person contact (through site visits). As a result of this monitoring, program managers make adjustments to program activities, as needed. IHS injury staff and community/tribal members share responsibility for program monitoring (outside experts are identified and consulted, as necessary).

10. Marketing/Advocacy—Describes the marketing/advocacy activities used to promote an area's injury prevention program.

COMPONENT	BASIC	INTERMEDIATE	COMPREHENSIVE
Materials developed	Some materials have been developed to increase public awareness about the problem of injury, in general, and the injury prevention program, specifically.	Materials and communication channels have been specifically developed to increase awareness about the problem of injury, in general, and the injury prevention program, specifically.	Injury program is publicized regularly through the use of multiple channels (radio, newspaper, community events, brochures, other materials).
Staff involvement	Staff members are not actively involved in advocating for attention to injury prevention and control with decision makers.	Staff members provide occasional briefings for decision makers about the importance of injury problem.	Injury staff members advocate at local, tribal, and state levels for policy and environmental changes that might affect injury morbidity and mortality. Injury staff members advocate at multiple levels for attention to funding of injury control activities.

Uses of media to promote awareness	Staff members are not actively involved with the media in promoting the concept of injury prevention and control.	Staff members interact with media to provide information about injury as a problem and local media give occasional attention to the issue.	Injury staff members actively work with media to address injury prevention as an issue in the community and ensure that accurate information is included in news and feature stories about the problem. Injury staff members respond to and initiate opportunities to discuss the problem and programs in public forums (e.g., community meetings, hearings, media events).
Awareness of injury problem	The public is not aware that injury is an important public health problem.	Injury is recognized at the area and local level as an important problem needing attention.	Injury is recognized as a significant problem by tribal leaders, community members, and community groups.

11. Evaluation/Reporting—Describes the reporting and evaluation activities conducted as part of the area's injury prevention program.

Types of interventions conducted and when conducted?	Injury prevention interventions are usually not evaluated, and if so, usually only after a program has been completed.	Process and impact evaluations are usually conducted for injury prevention interventions.	Process, impact, and outcome evaluations are always conducted for injury prevention interventions. Evaluations employ scientific designs and analysis procedures. Outside technical assistance is used, as necessary, to implement evaluations.
Who conducts program evaluations?	Program evaluations are conducted by AIS or other IHS injury staff.	AIS, district injury staff, and tribal personnel are involved in conducting program evaluations.	AIS, district injury staff, tribal personnel, community members, and outside consultants are involved in conducting program evaluations. Outside technical assistance is used as necessary to implement evaluations.

(Continued)

COMPONENT	BASIC	INTERMEDIATE	COMPREHENSIVE
How are program evaluations reported/used?	Report of program evaluations is limited to final project reports.	Project evaluations are reported in project final reports and area injury program annual reports. Midcourse corrections are made to interventions, based on process evaluation measures collected.	Program evaluations are reported in final reports, injury program annual reports, scholarly journals, or at scholarly presentations (i.e., in forums accessible to others wanting to learn from the project and build on experience). Program evaluations are used within the area to share lessons learned and challenges and to inform future program development.

12. Technical Assistance/Building Tribal Capacity—Describes technical assistance activities of an area's injury prevention program.

COMPONENT	BASIC	INTERMEDIATE	COMPREHENSIVE
Training received	A few tribal members have received Level I-II training.	Some tribal members have received Level I-III training in injury prevention.	All tribal injury personnel have received Level I-III and some have received IHS injury fellowship training.
Training provided	Limited IP training is provided to tribal personnel.	Training opportunities are provided on an annual basis to tribal personnel.	Training opportunities are provided on a semi-annual basis to tribal personnel.
Assistance to tribes in obtaining IP funding.	IHS injury personnel do not assist tribes in obtaining external/special funding for injury prevention programs/projects.	IHS injury personnel occasionally assist tribes in obtaining external/special funding for injury prevention programs/projects.	IHS injury personnel regularly assist tribes in obtaining external/special funding for injury prevention programs/projects.
Needs assessment data collection	Tribal members are not involved with the collection and use of IP needs assessment data.	Tribal members are usually involved with the collection and use of needs assessment data to plan IP interventions.	Tribal members are always involved with the collection and use of needs assessment data to plan IP interventions and evaluations.

| Injury program planning, implementation, and evaluation; Other assistance provided to tribal personnel
• coalitions
• data sharing | There is limited tribal involvement in developing, implementing, and evaluating injury prevention programs.
Tribal IP coalitions are formed in some locations. | There is occasional tribal involvement in developing, implementing, and evaluating injury prevention programs.
Intertribal coalitions networking is fostered at area IP meetings and workshops.
Injury surveillance "fact sheets" are prepared annually for tribes. | Tribes determine primary direction for and are directly involved with the implementation and evaluation of injury prevention programs.
Tribal coalitions network with other coalitions and agencies to address and resolve local injury issues.
Comprehensive reports of injury surveillance data are provided regularly to tribes. |

Unique/Other Program Aspects

Information about unique or other program aspects or activities would be recorded using this tool, such as contributions to other areas, how area IP programs have handled specific barriers, and work on national or international projects/activities.

CHAPTER THIRTEEN

Tracking the Process and Progress of the National Folic Acid Campaign

Katherine Lyon Daniel, Christine E. Prue,
and Michele Volansky

The discovery in the early 1990s that the B vitamin folic acid could prevent many serious birth defects of the brain and spine was the most remarkable breakthrough in birth defects prevention since the discovery of the rubella vaccine (Medical Research Council, 1991; Czeizel and Dudas, 1992). This simple information, so important to prospective parents, seemed to be an easy sell. However, the fact that women needed to consume folic acid in the days before conception and in the earliest days of pregnancy became a health communication challenge, especially in the United States, where about half of all pregnancies are unplanned or mistimed (Abma and others, 1997; Henshaw, 1998). When intervention efforts began, professional organizations such as the American Academy of Pediatrics and the American College of Obstetricians and Gynecologists, as well as advocacy groups like the National March of Dimes Birth Defects Foundation and the Spina Bifida Association of America (SBAA), collaborated with the CDC to petition the federal Food and Drug Administration (FDA). These organizations wanted the FDA to require food manufacturers to add folic acid to fortified ("enriched") foods in sufficient amounts to prevent serious birth defects, also called neural tube defects (NTDs) (Food and Drug Administration, 1996).

The authors wish to thank the National March of Dimes Birth Defects Foundation, Westat, and the Spina Bifida Association of America. In particular, the assistance of Judith Gooding, Mary Iodice, Sharon Hammond, Katherine Treiman, and Erika Reed was invaluable to this project.

This passive environmental intervention was expected to reduce the incidence of devastating birth defects by 50 to 70 percent. However, there arose the concern that fortifying at high enough levels may harm some vulnerable populations, such as young children, who might get "too much" folic acid. When the fortification level was set at 140 micrograms (mcg) per 100 grams of grain product, it was estimated that women of childbearing age might increase their average daily consumption of folic acid by only 100 mcg per day, which falls short of the amount recommended for most women to avoid birth defects, which is 400 mcg per day. The next public health challenge was to determine how to communicate to all reproductive women that they should actively ensure that they are consuming enough folic acid to prevent these serious birth defects.

Partners Join Forces to Reach Women

The approximately sixty million women of childbearing age in the United States (U.S. Census Bureau, 2000) have differing beliefs and motivations regarding preventive health behaviors and pregnancy (Henshaw, 1998). Reaching women with messages that promote folic acid use has become the new challenge for professional organizations, advocacy groups, and the CDC. To optimize the unique strengths and resources of each partner and to formalize each partner's role and responsibilities, the National Council on Folic Acid (NCFA) was formed in 1997 (see Table 13.1).

TABLE 13.1. LIST OF FOUNDING PARTNERS ON THE NATIONAL COUNCIL ON FOLIC ACID.

American Academy of Family Physicians
American Academy of Pediatrics
American College of Obstetricians and Gynecologists
American College of Physicians—American Society of Internal Medicine
American Dietetic Association
American Nurses Association
American Pharmaceutical Association
Association of Maternal and Child Health Programs
Association of State and Territorial Health Officials
Association of State and Territorial Public Health Nutrition Directors
Association of Women's Health, Obstetric, and Neonatal Nurses
Centers for Disease Control and Prevention
National Coalition of Hispanic Health and Human Services Organizations (currently
    the National Alliance for Hispanic Health)
National Healthy Mothers, Healthy Babies Coalition
National March of Dimes Birth Defects Foundation
Shriner's Hospital for Children
Spina Bifida Association of America
U.S. Department of Agriculture

The mission of the NCFA is to reduce the number of NTD-affected pregnancies by recommending that women of childbearing age consume 400 mcg of folic acid daily from fortified foods and/or supplements, in addition to consuming food folate from a varied diet (Centers for Disease Control and Prevention, 1992; Institute of Medicine, 1998). The NCFA outlined several strategies to be used to accomplish this goal:

• Increase the proportion of women who understand that consuming folic acid daily can help prevent birth defects
• Make folic acid awareness a routine and standard part of the delivery of preventive health care services to women
• Increase the level and availability of folic acid in food
• Evaluate the effectiveness of folic acid projects and programs and share lessons learned

Important approaches to accomplishing these strategies included (1) a commitment to conducting a broad-based public health education campaign through all available media, (2) partnering with corporations to increase exposure to the folic acid message, (3) developing, demonstrating, and evaluating model programs that reach reproductive women of various social and economic groups, and (4) conducting behavioral research to identify barriers to the use of supplements.

Early in the partnership, NCFA members delineated their roles in the campaign, which were based on the resources and capabilities of their respective organizations. The CDC had the resources and expertise to conduct the formative (audience-focused), process, and outcome research for the campaign; therefore, the CDC provided the leadership for these activities. The March of Dimes and other advocacy groups had the capacity and infrastructure to disseminate materials, once they were developed. The health care professional organizations, such as nursing and physician groups, had the capacity to provide their members with information about folic acid. Other partners had expertise regarding Hispanic health issues, because Hispanic women have had one and a half times the rate of births affected by NTDs that Caucasian women have had and three times the rate of such births that African American women have had (Shaw, Velie, and Wasserman, 1997). The NCFA served as a steering group, making decisions and broad directives, and ad hoc committees were formed to tackle specific projects identified during the planning process. Following principles of the CDCynergy health communication planning framework (Centers for Disease Control and Prevention, 1998b), the NCFA partners followed a series of steps that were felt to be necessary for effective communication program planning, implementation, and evaluation:

1. Define and describe the problem
2. Analyze the problem, looking for effective solutions

3. Begin communication program planning
4. Map out implementation and evaluation efforts
5. Conduct implementation and evaluation efforts
6. Reflect on lessons learned

Overview of the National Folic Acid Campaign

The national folic acid campaign itself focuses on the education of reproductive women through partners and the health care system. Some of the key tenets of performing effective health communication include segmenting audiences, doing formative research with audience members and key stakeholders, developing creative concepts that deliver a "key promise," testing those concepts with the audience for understanding and motivation, formulating the educational materials (including those of the mass media), and testing messages with their intended audiences (Maibach and Parrott, 1995). Several influential theories of effective health promotion targeted toward behavior change include attitudes of the recipient as a key filter for health messages (Prochaska, DiClemente and Norcross, 1992; Rosenstock, Strecher, and Becker, 1988; Bettman, 1979). This means identifying a message that each recipient finds appealing and personally motivating. A message must also be delivered to the audience in a manner and context that optimizes receipt of the message and the likelihood of action. The CDCynergy framework encourages public health practitioners to perform many types of evaluation, including formative evaluation (to ensure that the intervention—in this case, communication—is appropriate to the audience and outcome), process evaluation (to ensure that the program is implemented as planned), and outcome evaluation (to measure the effects of the intervention). Although the complete evaluation plan for the national folic acid campaign includes formative, process, and outcome measures (such as knowledge, awareness, the reported consumption of folic acid, blood folate levels, and, ultimately, birth defect case surveillance), this chapter focuses on the campaign process evaluation efforts.

Campaign Objectives

The folic acid campaign is designed to encourage women of reproductive age to act on the 1992 U.S. Public Health Service Recommendation (Centers for Disease Control and Prevention, 1992), which states that all women capable of becoming pregnant consume 400 mcg of folic acid daily. This recommendation was later updated by the Institute of Medicine to specify that the 400 mcg of folic acid should come from synthetic sources, as in supplements or fortified foods

(Institute of Medicine, 1998). The communication objectives for the campaign were to increase

- Awareness about folic acid
- Knowledge that folic acid reduces the risk of birth defects
- Knowledge that folic acid should be taken before pregnancy
- The number of women who daily take a multivitamin containing folic acid

The national folic acid campaign relies on multiple communication channels, including mass-reach media such as television and radio, and interpersonal channels such as group presentations and counseling. Each of these channels has unique advantages. Mass media interventions, particularly television public service announcements (PSAs), have enormous potential to reach many people, whereas interpersonal interventions, such as group presentations, are not so far-reaching but can be very powerful and persuasive. The application of media advocacy (the strategic use of news media to advance a public policy initiative) can also be an effective means of influencing policy on many important health issues (Wallack, Dorfman, Jernigan, and Themba, 1993). NCFA partners worked together to carry out the campaign at the national and community levels, using a variety of mass media and interpersonal communication channels. For example, March of Dimes chapters throughout the country have primary responsibility for placing PSAs on television, on the radio, and in the print media and have been equally involved in distributing educational materials, making informational presentations to community groups, and giving scientific lectures to health care professionals across the country.

Audience Segmentation

The CDC's research team reviewed many data sources to identify the factors that are most influential regarding the target behavior of taking folic acid every day, and these sources included several national surveys and databases (Maibach, Maxfield, Ladin, and Slater, 1996; National Center for Health Statistics, 1996; Abma and others, 1997; Centers for Disease Control and Prevention, 1998a; Colley, Shulman, Fischer, and Rogers, 1999; March of Dimes, 2000). The CDC also worked with Westat, an evaluation contractor, to conduct extensive audience research with women, health providers, and families affected by NTDs (Hammond, Volansky, Treiman, and Child, 1998). This led to the design and production of appealing and motivational messages for two unique audience segments: women planning a pregnancy in the next year (called pregnancy contemplators) and women not planning a pregnancy in the next year (called pregnancy precontemplators). Because Hispanic women are at increased risk, formative research was also conducted with this important audience, which eventually led to the production of culturally appropriate Spanish-language messages and materials. The methods and results of this component of the campaign and process evaluation are not presented in this publication but they are generally parallel with those of the English-language national campaign.

After identifying key target audiences, focus groups were convened to determine which approaches to folic acid health education would work best. The key message that appealed to women contemplating becoming pregnant within approximately one year focused on healthy, beautiful babies: "Make sure [you] get enough folic acid every day, because the time to prevent birth defects is *before* you know you're pregnant." The message that appealed to women not contemplating pregnancy in the near future emphasized that even though a woman has a lot to do before motherhood, she should take folic acid today—and everyday—so that "your body's ready when you are."

Campaign Implementation

Preparation for the campaign launch began in January 1999 with a national conference and training activities for NCFA partner organizations. The campaign began nationally in May 1999 with many communities planning activities around Mother's Day. The first phase of the campaign targeted pregnancy contemplators with the "Before You Know It" PSA. The second phase of the campaign targeted pregnancy precontemplators. This "Ready . . . Not" PSA was distributed in September 1999.

Process Evaluation Approach

Members of the NCFA conducted the campaign and evaluation in accordance with their agency's priorities, capacities, and resources. The CDC's birth defects prevention program (supplemented with funds awarded by a CDC-wide competition for evaluation funds) was the major contributor to the process evaluation. To measure the implementation and effectiveness of this voluntary partnership-driven public education effort, research questions were developed for the process evaluation of the campaign. To measure dissemination of the campaign's messages as proxy measures of audience reach (media dose delivered) the following questions were asked:

- How widely were folic acid messages disseminated through different media channels?

- How frequently were the campaign and other PSAs aired on television and the radio?
- How frequently did PSAs appear in newspapers and magazines?
- How many news stories related to folic acid or including folic acid messages appeared on television, on the radio, and in the print media?

To ensure that campaign messages were delivered as intended (fidelity), the following questions were asked:

- What was the nature of the news stories related to folic acid?
- Were the stories accurate, or did they carry misinformation?
- To what extent did the stories include key campaign messages, such as, "Folic acid should be taken before pregnancy" and "Multivitamins contain the recommended amount of folic acid"?

To assess the degree to which the campaign was implemented overall (nonmedia dose delivered), the following questions were asked:

- How many people were potentially exposed to folic acid messages through non-media channels?
- Specifically, how many brochures and other materials were distributed?
- How many people participated in community-based events such as presentations?

To assess the variability of the campaign implementation in different markets (variance), the following questions were asked:

- How did the extent of message activity and message dissemination vary from one media market to the next?
- In which markets was message dissemination highest and lowest?

To provide the NCFA with feedback on any needed campaign refinements (dose received), the following questions were asked:

- How were women of reproductive age exposed to and affected by campaign messages?
- Specifically, what do women recall about folic acid?
- Where do women report seeing, hearing, or reading folic acid messages?

CDC researchers wanted to make a comparison of the evidence for campaign implementation and preliminary effectiveness between geographic areas that had fully implemented the campaign and areas that had not. However, because the campaign was voluntary on the state and local levels, the CDC could not control where implementation efforts took place. Therefore, as in a natural experiment, the evaluation team planned to collect data wherever possible and then select geographic areas or "media markets" from the top 10 percent and bottom 10 percent of the exposure range. Telephone surveys gauging the target audience's exposure, recall, and reaction to campaign messages were then conducted (along with surveying measures of knowledge, attitudes, and behaviors—often called KABs). Data were compared between areas representing the highest and lowest implementation efforts.

Key participants of evaluation efforts included CDC staff members and research fellows, employees of Westat (the primary evaluation contractor), Prospect Associates (the creative contractor), and the March of Dimes (the key partner and administrative leader of the NCFA). The methods employed to monitor implementation of and exposure to the national campaign were intended to provide an overall picture of the campaign activities delivered and received.

Process Evaluation Methods

To measure the implementation and preliminary effectiveness of this education effort, process measures were applied in the following five areas: (1) monitoring of media coverage, (2) content analysis of news media, (3) monitoring of nonmedia activities (such as local events and presentations), (4) use of media and nonmedia measures to create exposure indices, and (5) tracking recall of messages from an outcome survey. Table 13.2 presents an overview of the various methods used to conduct the process evaluation.

Measures of reach help determine the number of people potentially exposed to messages about folic acid by examining information such as the number of people who have seen messages on TV or read materials containing messages about folic acid. However, measuring actual exposure to messages is difficult and costly; thus, estimations or proxy measures are frequently used instead (Flay and Cook, 1989). In the case of the NCFA campaign, the number of times PSAs were aired, the number of news stories printed, and the number of people in attendance at lectures or presentations were used as proxy measures of potential exposure.

Monitoring of Media Coverage

To track the dissemination of the folic acid campaign through the mass media, the evaluation team contracted with several professional media monitoring services to monitor all PSAs, news stories, and commercial advertising related to folic acid on television, on the radio, and in print. Companies chosen offered

TABLE 13.2. SUMMARY OF PROCESS EVALUATION METHODS.

Media Activities

Public Service Announcements	News Coverage	Commercial Product Advertising	Exposure Indices*
• Television • Radio (Spanish Only) • Print	• Television • Radio (English Only) • Print • Content Analysis	• Television • Radio • Print	✓ ✓ ✓

Nonmedia Activities

Material Distribution	Lectures and Presentations	
• March of Dimes (MOD) activities • CDC State Contacts activities • Requests from the CDC National Folic Acid Clearinghouse • Activities of key National Council on Folic Acid (NCFA) partners (e.g., Spina Bifida Association of America [SBAA], Healthy Mothers, Healthy Babies)	• MOD activities • CDC State Contacts activities • Requests from the CDC National Folic Acid Clearinghouse • Activities of key NCFA partners (e.g., SBAA and Healthy Mothers, Healthy Babies)	✓ ✓ ✓ ✓

Outcome Survey

Process Evaluation Questions	
1. Have you ever heard, read, or seen anything about folic acid? 2. Where did you learn about folic acid?	Not applicable

*Indices were created to examine campaign exposure in each checked area—for example, television news, PSAs, and advertisements—in order to examine exposure levels within each of the selected fifty-eight media markets.

extensive monitoring of print publications and broadcast media within the project budget. Burrelle's monitors more than eighteen thousand print publications and has readers who scan publications for designated key words and phrases. Video Monitoring Services (VMS) records television and radio news and advertisements and also has readers scan segments for designated key words. TVAccess and NewsWorld Television/Potomac Television had Sigma-encoded copies of the respective PSAs, which allows electronic detection and tracking of airplay for videos distributed to TV stations and broadcast and cable networks through satellite data. Both VMS and Burrelle's were given specific search terms in order to identify media coverage regarding folic acid and the national education campaign (see Table 13.3).

Although campaign efforts were national in scope, process evaluation efforts were limited to select markets for several reasons. First, media monitoring services do not collect data in every media market in the United States. A media market is a geographic area defined in terms of television viewing patterns and originating television broadcast stations. For this process evaluation, fifty-eight media markets were selected on the basis of area coverage by professional media monitoring services and wide geographic distribution. Second, although every effort was made to collect uniform data across all fifty-eight media markets, this was not always possible. Data collected on media activity was limited because professional monitoring services do not routinely monitor all channels in all markets at all times. For example, radio programs are typically monitored during *drive times* (defined here as 7 to 10 a.m., 11 a.m. to 1 p.m., and 4 to 7 p.m.) and were not monitored in all fifty-eight media markets. Table 13.3 shows the types of media channels that were monitored (including television, radio, and print) and the number of markets in which each channel was monitored.

Because the national folic acid campaign is a three-year, nationwide effort, year-round media monitoring was not feasible, because of budgetary constraints. The evaluation team collected process evaluation data during an initial three-month monitoring period (August 1 through October 31, 1999), with subsequent monitoring occurring primarily during times when NCFA partners were actively engaged in educational outreach efforts. Costs for media monitoring for the three-month period in the selected media markets totaled approximately $2,500. Table 13.3 includes a breakdown of the costs according to each monitoring service.

Content Analysis of News Media

After collecting and quantifying data on the media hits in each media market, a content analysis was conducted of print, television, and radio news stories about folic acid that ran during the monitoring period. The content analysis goal was to assess the degree to which news stories and bylines included the communication objectives of the campaign, defined as increasing the number of women who (1) are aware of folic acid, (2) know that folic acid can prevent birth defects, (3) know that folic acid should be taken before pregnancy, and (4) take the recommended amount of folic acid daily. Researchers assessed whether the news content included key campaign messages (for example, that folic acid is needed before pregnancy) and whether they included any inaccurate information or miscommunicated the campaign messages.

TABLE 13.3. MONITORING SERVICES USED, TYPE OF MEDIA MONITORED, NUMBER OF MARKETS MONITORED, AND COSTS OF MONITORING FOR ENGLISH-LANGUAGE MEDIA EFFORTS.

Monitoring Service	Type of Media Monitored	Number of Monitored Markets (N = 58)	Cost of Service	Total Cost Over Three-Month Period[1]
Video Monitoring Services (VMS) of America, L.P., News Services[2]	Television news and radio news	Television 43 Radio 16	$7 per broadcast segment related to folic acid	$959 (137 related news segments found)
	Television and radio commercial advertisements	National network television stations and selected radio stations	$400 per month to track up to 5 ads in 5 local markets	$600 (minimal costs due to lack of related ads)
TVAccess[3]	Television public service announcements (PSAs) produced by CDC ("Before You Know It"; "Ready . . . Not")	58	**Donated** (courtesy of March of Dimes)	**Donated** (courtesy of March of Dimes)
NewsWorld Television/ Potomac Television[3]	Television PSAs produced by the Spina Bifida Association of America (SBAA) ("Hillary Clinton" PSA and "Babies" PSA)	52	**Donated** (courtesy of the SBAA)	**Donated** (courtesy of the SBAA)
Burrelle's[2]	Print news (newspapers and magazines) Print PSAs produced by CDC ("Before You Know It"; "Ready . . . Not") Print (newspapers and magazines) Ads	58	$230 per month plus $1.45 per clip	$1010 (221 related clips found)

[1]Does not include labor costs to evaluate and analyze collected data.

[2]VMS and Burrelle's were given the following search terms in order to identify media coverage related to folic acid and the national education campaign: (1) folic acid and birth defects, (2) folic acid and pregnancy/pregnant, (3) folic acid and baby or babies, (4) folic acid and the March of Dimes, (5) folic acid and the CDC, and (6) (after reviewing initial stories) folic acid and women of childbearing age.

[3]TV Access and NewsWorld Television/Potomac Television used Sigma-encoded copies of the respective PSAs, tracked through satellite data.

Fourteen content/message variables were identified (see Table 13.4), and a codebook was developed to ensure consistency between coders. Researchers reviewed the complete, original print news articles and had a brief summary format of radio and television news stories. Content/message variables were selected when they contained (1) key campaign messages (content/message variables such as "Take folic acid before pregnancy" and "Multivitamins/supplements are a source of folic acid"), (2) news coverage of the national and local campaign activities and those of campaign partners (content/message variables such as mentioning the National Council on Folic Acid and local campaign events), or (3) featured or breaking news stories related to folic acid (content/message variables such as "Folic acid prevents heart disease" and "Folic acid prevents Down's syndrome").

Monitoring of Nonmedia Activities

Nonmedia activities were an important part of campaign efforts to disseminate messages about the benefits of folic acid. Research shows that an effective way

TABLE 13.4.   CONTENT/MESSAGES OF ALL NEWS STORIES, ALL MARKETS COMBINED (*N* = 341 NEWS STORIES).

Content/Message Variables	Number of News Stories, Including Content/Message (n = 341)	Percentage of News Stories with Content/ Message (n = 341)
Prevents neural tube defects or birth defects in general	199	58 %
Multivitamins/supplements are sources of folic acid	169	50 %
Women should take folic acid	166	49 %
Prevents Down's syndrome	156	46 %
Other sources of folic acid (e.g., food)	151	44%
Take folic acid before pregnancy	118	35%
Mentions campaign partners	87	26 %
Health care providers as a source of information	.78	23 %
Folic acid prevents heart disease/has other health benefits	32	1 %
Mentions CDC	29	< 1%
Mentions National Council on Folic Acid	24	< 1%
Mentions local campaign events	21	< 1%
Mentions Hispanic women	14	< 1%
Recommends to contact/see your doctor	1	< 1%

to stimulate behavior change is to supplement the mass media with nonmedia activities such as interpersonal communication (Brown and Einsiedel, 1990). The persuasive conveying of complex messages is more likely to occur through interpersonal channels, especially those with small, select audiences (Rogers and Kincaid, 1981). NCFA partners accessed interpersonal channels by distributing materials at community events, giving presentations, and counseling women for healthy pregnancy outcomes. This included efforts tailored to reach special risk groups (such as Hispanic women) or influential groups (such as health care providers).

CDC's partners provided information on their nonmedia activities during the three-month time frame. Using a brief questionnaire, they elicited information about the distribution of educational materials, types of educational materials distributed (for example, brochures and fact sheets), and the number of lectures/presentations and attendees at those functions. Respondents were asked to confine their responses to their respective media markets so that data collected from the monitoring of nonmedia activities would be comparable to that collected from media monitoring. However, state and local campaign organizations typically represent either an entire state or a specific city and therefore do not cover the same boundaries as media markets defined for media tracking purposes. Quantifying the reach of such expansive activities strictly within the selected media markets proved difficult to accomplish with a high degree of accuracy. Consequently, information about activities for which audience reach crossed media markets was analyzed along with any other qualitative information provided by NCFA partners.

Individuals and organizations that had requested materials from the CDC's National Clearinghouse on Folic Acid anytime during the year preceding the campaign kickoff were also contacted to learn more about how these materials were distributed and used. The clearinghouse maintains a variety of educational materials on the subject of folic acid, ranging from brochures and posters to videotapes. The CDC contacted requesters by using a standardized telephone questionnaire specifically designed to elicit information from the requester regarding the number of materials that had been distributed, the audience to whom the materials had been distributed, and whether materials had been distributed within the defined media markets. Table 13.2 includes the type of nonmedia information that was elicited to help ensure a successful process evaluation.

Use of Media and Nonmedia Measures to Create Exposure Indices

Data collected from the media and nonmedia tracking efforts were aggregated to create exposure indices for each media market to determine which media markets had higher levels of campaign exposure and which markets had lower levels of exposure. Areas of higher and lower message activity would then be used for sampling the target audience to determine not only their recall of campaign messages but also their overall KABs related to folic acid.

Development of the Media Exposure Index. Data collected from all media monitoring activities were recorded in a media exposure index that was developed by the research team to track all media activity in each of the fifty-eight media markets. This index or grid listed all fifty-eight media markets, the month during which the coverage occurred, the type of media channel used (for example, television or print) and the type of media activity (for example, PSA or news) that occurred within each market. Because some types of media hits included news coverage that aired on national programming (for example, *Good Morning America*), these hits were recorded on the grid in the "national" category and were not counted in the totals of any of the individual fifty-eight markets. The media exposure index represents the total number of media hits, which is the number of times messages about folic acid were detected by the systems tracking media channels, with one news story or one thirty-second PSA airing counted as one hit.

Development of the Nonmedia Exposure Index. The nonmedia exposure index was developed by totaling activity reports from partners. This included all members of the NCFA as well as commercial sources and CDC contacts, and it contained data representing the number of materials distributed and the number of people potentially exposed to lectures, presentations, and other community-based activities within defined media markets.

Combined Communication Exposure Index. The media and nonmedia exposure indices were then examined to assess the potential exposure to messages about folic acid in each selected media market. This tool (referred to as the combined communication exposure index [CEI]), allowed for an integrated yet separate comparison of these communication approaches. In other words, media and nonmedia measures were ranked separately, and high ratings in both categories were necessary to achieve high exposure status. In addition to examining the number of media and nonmedia hits, other factors included (1) market characteristics, such as population size, (2) the number and types of communication channels used, and (3) the time of day in which broadcast coverage aired (known as *daypart*). The information yielded by the CEI would serve as the basis for subsequent sampling of the target audience in markets with higher and lower levels of campaign message activity for the outcome survey, and it would allow process evaluation measures to be linked to outcome data across all the women surveyed.

Tracking Recall of Messages from an Outcome Survey

As a final process measure, women responding to the surveys in the outcome evaluation phase were also asked to report their recall of exposure to the public health education campaign. The outcome evaluation component consists of a series of telephone surveys that have been designed to measure the effects of the campaign on changes in KABs related to folic acid as well as audience recall of the campaign.

The first surveys of the target audience were conducted in selected geographic areas in Winter 2000, approximately nine months after the initial campaign launch. To obtain information about campaign exposure, the target audience members were asked the following five research questions:

- Have you ever heard, read, or seen anything about folic acid?
- What have you heard, read, or seen about folic acid?
- Where did you learn about folic acid?
- You said you learned about folic acid on television. Was this an advertisement or PSA, news program, or some other type of program?
- Where did you hear, read, or see the advertisement or PSA?

Process Evaluation Results

Research Question 1: How Widely Were Folic Acid Messages Disseminated Through Different Media Channels?

Table 13.5 summarizes the media-monitoring findings for all channels and for all markets combined. The total number of media hits was 3,403; of these, 3,062 (90 percent) were PSAs. For English-language media, 74 percent of the hits overall were CDC-produced PSAs and 16 percent were PSAs produced by the SBAA. A total of 337 English-language news stories were identified in print and on television and radio channels, accounting for only 10 percent of all English-language hits. The largest quantity of news stories identified were print stories (n = 200), 95 percent of which were published in newspapers, with radio broadcast news stories being the fewest in number (n = 10).

This result has implications for the future implementation of campaign activities. Campaign partners were able to place PSAs in various media—primarily television. News coverage, although an important part of the media, was used in the campaign at a much smaller proportion. This suggests that the message was in fact provided to a variety of media so that it could be delivered but that the uptake or response of television was the primary medium in this campaign.

TABLE 13.5. OVERVIEW OF ENGLISH-LANGUAGE MEDIA MONITORING RESULTS FOR ALL FIFTY-EIGHT MEDIA MARKETS, AUGUST–OCTOBER 1999.

Media Type	Number and Percentage of Media Hits
News Coverage	
Television	127 (4%)
Radio	10 (<1%)
Print	200 (6%)
Total news coverage	337 (10%)
Public Service Announcements (PSAs)	
Television	
(CDC-produced)	2,512 (74%)
(Spina Bifida Association of America-produced)	533 (16%)
Radio (CDC-produced)	Not monitored
Print (CDC-produced)	17 (<1%)
Total PSAs	3,062 (90%)
Commercial Advertisements	
Television and print	4 (<1%)
Total hits	3,403 (100%)

The television reach to the target audience in the higher markets was approximately 30 to 40 percent, which is about average for a PSA campaign (Snyder and Hamilton, 2001).

Research Question 2: What Was the Nature of the News Stories Regarding Folic Acid?

The campaign messages that were most widely covered in news stories were that (1) folic acid prevents birth defects—either NTDs or birth defects in general (58 percent of stories), (2) multivitamins and B complex supplements are a source of folic acid (50 percent), and (3) women should take folic acid (49 percent). Other campaign messages received less coverage. For example, the message that folic acid should be taken before pregnancy was mentioned in just 35 percent of the stories (see Table 13.4).

Few news stories mentioned the campaign itself or the campaign partners. For example, less than 1 percent (n = 21) of news stories mentioned local campaign events, even in areas where nonmedia tracking indicated that events were occurring. The minimum number of stories that mentioned local campaign events may be explained in part because the types of low-circulation community newspapers likely to cover such campaign events were not tracked during most of the monitoring period. Only newspapers with a circulation of more than a thousand were monitored for the first ten weeks. Likewise, the monitoring of radio news, which might cover local events, was limited; for example, radio news was monitored in only sixteen markets during limited times.

During the first monitoring period, the evaluation team found minimal misinformation about folic acid in the news media; the evaluation team more frequently encountered cases in which news stories contained some key campaign messages but not all. Despite the low frequency of inaccurate news stories or misinformation in the news media in this case, the CDC and the campaign partners plan to remain vigilant to ensure a prompt response to any misleading or inaccurate news stories that could undermine the national campaign efforts.

Research Question 3: How Many People Were Potentially Exposed to Folic Acid Messages Through Nonmedia Channels?

Findings from the nonmedia monitoring activities—for example, materials distribution, lectures, and presentations—indicate that the distribution of educational materials was a frequently used approach for disseminating messages about the benefits of folic acid. Although women of childbearing age are the primary target audience for the campaign, nonmedia activities reached the general public as well. Many materials distribution efforts targeted either the general public or persons involved in educating and treating women, such as health care providers, counselors, and teachers. Data regarding nonmedia activities also indicate that education and outreach are occurring in a variety of settings, ranging from Women, Infants, and Children (WIC) program clinics to churches, local high schools, and grocery stores.

In reviewing and summarizing nonmedia monitoring findings, it is also important to note the limitations of the data collection process. First, the short time frame for collecting this data did not allow for the collection of in-depth information that would more accurately capture the extent of nonmedia activities occurring at the local level. Second, data collection was hampered by the retrospective nature of this effort; the evaluation team was required to rely on respondents' recall of past outreach events and activities to determine levels of nonmedia activity in each market. In the future, a prospective tracking system, in which campaign partners keep monthly logs or journals of their nonmedia activities, would greatly improve the collection of data.

Research Question 4: In Which Markets Was Message Dissemination Highest and Lowest?

Appendix A shows the CEI with the number of media and nonmedia hits in the four media markets with the highest exposure to the folic acid education campaign and the four media markets with the lowest exposure to the campaign. As previously mentioned, media and nonmedia coverage were weighted equally in determining which of the fifty-eight monitored media markets had the highest exposure levels to the campaign and which had the lowest exposure levels. Market characteristics (such as population size), viewership numbers, and the type of communication channels were also considered for use in weighing the data within each media market. But there was a lack of support in the current body of communication literature for the use of such approaches. Nielsen Media Research (1998), however, supported the concept that television PSAs aired during late night television (1 a.m. to 5 a.m.) would have the least number of viewers, particularly within the target audience for this campaign. As a result, the time of day in which the television PSAs aired (daypart) was used in selecting higher- and lower-exposure markets. Thus, only those television PSAs that aired between 5 a.m. and 12:30 a.m. were counted toward determining exposure levels for this process evaluation.

Research Question 5: How Were Women of Reproductive Age Exposed to (and Affected by) Campaign Messages?

A total of 2,807 women responded to the English-language survey conducted after the campaign and monitoring period. The average age of the respondents was twenty-eight years, 55 percent were married, and more than half had received some education beyond high school. Fifty-five percent were employed full-time and most had a household income of more than $30,000. Of the respondents, 72 percent categorized themselves as "white," 10 percent as "black," and 6 percent as "Native American," "Pacific Islander," or "Asian"; 15 percent reported that they were of Hispanic ethnicity.

Responses to the questions regarding whether respondents had heard about folic acid, as well as the questions concerning the source of exposure to the folic acid message, are presented in Table 13.6. Overall, about 65 percent of respondents in higher-exposure areas had heard about folic acid, compared with 63 percent in lower-exposure areas; this difference was not statistically significant. The source of information for women in the higher and lower markets varied, and areas that had the largest saturation of media did not have a higher level of media recall. Overall, the survey responses indicate that the dose received in the higher-exposure areas did not differ significantly from the dose received in the lower-exposure areas.

TABLE 13.6.   ENGLISH-LANGUAGE FOLIC ACID COMMUNICATION SURVEY
RESPONDENTS: NUMBER AND PERCENTAGE OF WOMEN WHO
HAVE HEARD, READ, OR SEEN SOMETHING ABOUT FOLIC
ACID AMONG WOMEN IN HIGHER- AND LOWER-EXPOSURE
MARKETS, AND SOURCE OF INFORMATION.

| | E-FACES (N = 2,807) | |
	Higher Exposure (n = 1,405) Number (%)	Lower Exposure (n = 1,402) Number (%)
Women who have heard, read, or seen anything about folic acid	907 (65)	886 (63)
Source of Information		
Television	232 (17)	253 (18)
Physician	243 (17)	218 (16)
Magazine	180 (13)	165 (12)
School/college	74 (5)	83 (6)
Other	113 (8)	98 (7)
Don't know	65 (5)	69 (5)
Have not heard about folic acid	498 (35)	516 (37)

However, when examined by reported pregnancy intention (data not shown), more respondents who were pregnancy contemplators had heard, read, or seen something about folic acid than had respondents who were precontemplators (73 percent of contemplators and 63 percent of precontemplators, $p < .05$). This suggests that the impact of message exposure on women may have been affected by personal feelings or plans about pregnancy, and it confirms that efforts to influence behavior change may be filtered through the recipient's attitudes and beliefs (Prochaska, DiClemente, and Norcross, 1992; Rosenstock, Strecher, and Becker, 1988; Bettman, 1979). Thus, for the majority of women (about 80 percent are not currently planning a pregnancy), this pregnancy-focused message may not have been appealing, memorable, or personally relevant.

Discussion

The process evaluation demonstrated that CDC and partners successfully implemented most campaign activities. However, the process measures included in the outcome survey also indicated that this level of implementation did not result in measurable change in knowledge or behavior among respondents. We were, however, able to rule out an important rival hypothesis and we determined that the intervention was delivered as planned. The question then became What can we do to ensure that the messages were received and acted upon?

There were a number of strengths to this process evaluation effort. The national folic acid campaign was comprehensive and enabled the evaluation team to thoroughly analyze and identify exposure markets in which to conduct the outcome evaluation surveys. Unlike experimental designs, where message exposure is manipulated to artificially designate higher- and lower-exposure-level media markets, the measurement of the national folic acid campaign was conducted as a natural experiment: all members of the target audience potentially had the opportunity to receive the public health message. Thus, the results of the process evaluation data revealed markets in which a limited amount of PSA message activity took place, compared with markets in which no message activity occurred. This indicates there may not have been sufficient variation in exposure levels across market areas to support hypothesis testing about women's KABs, with regard to folic acid and birth defects. For example, the highest media outreach areas in this study achieved a reach of between 30 and 40 percent, typical for a PSA campaign (Snyder and Hamilton, 2001). By comparison, three mass media campaigns designed to prevent smoking among adolescents in the southeastern United States reached 79 to 94 percent of the target audience through a combination of radio and television PSAs (Bauman and others, 1991). A commercial advertisement campaign may strive to reach 80 to 90 percent of its target audience. Without the detailed process evaluation results, the relative disadvantage of the folic acid campaign's reach may not have been understood.

Another strength of this evaluation was the procurement of solid baseline data. Because the CDC had identified baseline KABs of folic acid-related health status, the process evaluation measures were able to identify which needed improvement, and they identified real differences following the campaign. For example, the CDC was able to identify significant differences in the sources of folic acid information for Spanish- versus English-speaking women and between pregnancy contemplators and precontemplators. The survey outcome instrument itself was a reliable measure that had been conducted on a national level for several years by the March of Dimes and the Gallup Organization. The process questions that were added reflected actual exposure to the campaign messages, and these questions were also tested and piloted with the target audience prior to implementation. A further strength was the set of rigorous communication research methods (Fishbein and others, 2002; Flay and Cook, 1989) that were applied to both the development and the implementation of the campaign and were included in all discussions of the process evaluation plans and implementation.

This project was also subject to several limitations. It was challenging to integrate the results from different data collection sources, concatenate the data, and weight the data by the appropriate variables, such as accuracy, reliability, and reach. This was an evolving process that was accomplished by an experienced team of researchers; nevertheless, a different group might have come up with another method, approach, or set of weights for the data. One of the challenges was in defining the relative importance or weight of a "personal" (face-to-face) encounter with a trained medical worker, such as a nutritionist, versus passively viewing one or more PSAs on television. Despite differing numbers of each, the team decided to treat media and nonmedia exposures as equal contributors to the overall success of a campaign. Using this method, a market area with good media exposure but no organized nonmedia efforts was not eligible to be considered a high-exposure market. However, this may not reflect the "real-life" weight of these exposures.

Another limitation was the inability to track targeted, or specialized, interventions from the national level. Efforts by community partners to reach community leaders, health professionals, or important target groups (for example, women trying to get pregnant) may have been so minimal that any change would be diluted by the overall population and would become undetectable by the process measures we applied. In addition, the summative reports (measuring reported exposure to the message) are subject to a reporting bias. Specifically, it is unknown whether women who answered no to the question "Have you heard, read, or seen anything about folic acid?" were truly unexposed or whether they were exposed but either did not attend to the message or forgot the exposure over the six-month time span between potential exposure and request for recall. These self-reports are therefore limited in what they reveal about the *fact* of exposure (dose delivered) and tell more about the *effectiveness* of the exposure (dose received).

While interpreting the media monitoring data, it is essential to keep in mind that monitoring was not uniform across all markets and channels. For example, although television PSAs were monitored in all media markets, the monitoring of broadcast news story coverage was not possible in all markets. In addition, without consistent monitoring data for radio PSAs, it is difficult to see how this exposure may have influenced the outcome. Overall, the media monitoring results suggest that during this early phase of the national campaign, the public was more likely to hear about folic acid through campaign PSAs than through news stories or commercial advertisements.

Perhaps the major limitation of the process evaluation is that the results are dependent on the ability of the evaluators to ascertain what has been accomplished that was not in their control. Tracking one's own work is relatively easy—especially with forethought. It is much more difficult, however, particularly on a national level, to track the activities of other individuals and organizations, some of whom are informal partners and all of whom have their own independent networks, sponsors, ideas, resources, and volunteers.

As outlined in Snyder and Hamilton (2001), several factors may explain why the hypothesized differences in reported exposure between higher and lower markets were not found. The level of campaign activity in higher markets may not have been high enough to make a discernible difference in KABs or campaign exposure. The monitoring time frame of three months may have been too short to measure true exposure levels, or the design of the survey questions may have prevented the detection of true differences. Finally, concurrent or "background" exposure to the folic acid message through nonmonitored commercial or education sources across all markets may have obscured the effects of the NCFA campaign in higher-exposure markets by an unmeasured secular trend.

Lessons Learned About Process Evaluation

LESSON 1. *Working with partners is both a strength and a challenge.*

The nature of this campaign was such that many individuals, groups, and organizations were conducting folic acid education in a way that perhaps was not even connected with the campaign. Measuring the process of all of these exposures is important in making informed decisions about higher- and lower-exposure areas. To do so, however, means collecting process evaluation data from a wide variety of sources and making requests of organizations with their own program goals and efforts in progress. Forging immediate and strong relationships with community groups and asking those groups for help is an important factor. At times, time lines and objectives were altered to accommodate the majority of partners.

LESSON 2. *Studying any intervention at the national level presents unique challenges.*

Financing national campaigns is expensive; evaluating them is also costly. For example, although national studies typically benefit from large sample sizes, it is expensive to collect enough data to do subgroup analyses. A particular problem for a communication campaign is ensuring that there are enough resources in reserve to respond to "breaking news" and to adapt to unforeseen or emerging issues. When conducting such a broad process evaluation, careful planning should always include a budget sufficient to cover unanticipated expense.

LESSON 3. *Measuring communication exposure is complicated.*

Building systems for conducting evaluation and pioneering new ways to collect data can be time-consuming and expensive. Collecting and building a "uniform" dataset for a national campaign when the data have not been collected uniformly or universally is especially challenging. In particular, coordinating with hundreds of partners in all fifty states and in dozens of organizations on documentation requests required extensive effort. More prospective planning would have allowed researchers access to better data through community-based participatory research methods (Israel, Schulz, Parker, and Becker, 1998) or empowerment evaluation (Fetterman, 2001).

LESSON 4. *Process evaluation of a national-level communication campaign produces huge amounts of data.*

Consultants to the CDC who were retained at the planning phase cautioned against directing too much effort toward documenting the specific details of smaller-level exposures. These consultants instead recommended spending time and resources with a big-picture view. A systematic approach to categorizing the data and determining its relevance and utility was critical to maintaining an overall perspective, not to mention team morale. Because the team had been unable to identify any previous studies that tracked efforts with this level of detail, members felt it necessary to collect everything, "just in case." In future iterations, selecting proxy measures in advance for each category that might reflect the overall level of activity without generating huge amounts of data would be more efficient. For this campaign, tracking only summative rating measures of television PSAs and print news media (with nondetailed content analysis or analysis of a sample of stories) as measures for media tracking, as well as collecting reports of nonmedia community interventions by magnitude (such as community events that were attended by more than five thousand people or materials distributed in quantities of more than a thousand), would have pointed toward the same conclusions about higher- and lower-exposure areas. Conducting surveys afterward, if possible, can provide valuable information.

Conclusion

This study makes several contributions to the process evaluation literature on communication campaigns. First, it outlines one method for integrating media and nonmedia communication data and discusses issues of comparing and interpreting these data. Second, it presents an outline of the resources necessary to conduct a rigorous process evaluation of a national campaign. Third, it introduces a discussion of the special issues involved in communication campaigns, especially those that do not have sufficient resources to guarantee exposure to the intervention (in this case, media and nonmedia messages), along with presenting a model index for standardizing assessment of communication exposures. Finally, the study includes an assessment of challenges of conducting process evaluation of partnership-based activities on a national level.

Whether or not a campaign implemented differently would have resulted in greater differences in the higher and lower exposure areas is unknown. Whether or not these process evaluation measures had the rigor to detect all effective means of getting the folic acid message to women is also unknown (for example, personal communications between health care providers and their patients were not measured). Assuming that all else is equal, we can conclude that a three-month voluntary media campaign was not sufficient to produce significant measurable differences among the majority of the target audience. Results from this process evaluation were important to the documentation, continued development, and effectiveness of the folic acid intervention. In addition, these results will be used to plan and evaluate future CDC efforts that include both paid media outreach and community partnerships sustained over a longer period of time.

References

Abma, J. C., and others. "Fertility, Family Planning, and Women's Health: New Data from the 1995 National Survey of Family Growth." *Vital Health Statistics,* 1997, *23*(19), 1–114.

Bauman, K. E., and others. (1991). "The Influence of Three Mass Media Campaigns on Variables Related to Adolescent Cigarette Smoking: Results of a Field Experiment." *American Journal of Public Health,* 1991, *81,* 597–604.

Bettman, J. R. *An Information Processing Theory of Consumer Choice.* Reading, Mass: Addison-Wesley, 1979.

Brown, J., and Einsiedel, E. "Public Health Campaigns: Mass Media Strategies." In J. Ray and L. Donohew (eds.), *Communication and Health: Systems and Applications.* Hillsdale, N.J.: Erlbaum, 1990.

Centers for Disease Control and Prevention. "Recommendation for the Use of Folic Acid to Reduce the Number of Cases of Spina Bifida and Other Neural Tube Defects." *Morbidity and Mortality Weekly Report,* 1992, *41,* 1–14.

Centers for Disease Control and Prevention. *Behavioral Risk Factor Surveillance System Guide.* Atlanta, Ga.: Centers for Disease Control and Prevention, National Center for Chronic Disease Prevention and Control, 1998a.

Centers for Disease Control and Prevention. *CDCynergy: A Tool for Planning, Implementing, and Evaluating Public Health Communication Programs.* Atlanta, Ga.: Centers for Disease Control and Prevention, Office of Communication, 1998b. CD-ROM.

Colley, G. B., Shulman, H. B., Fischer, L. A., and Rogers, M. M. "The Pregnancy Risk
    Assessment Monitoring System (PRAMS): Methods and 1996 Response Rates from
    Eleven States." *MCH Journal*, 1999, *3*(4), 199–209.

Czeizel, A. E., and Dudas, I. "Prevention of the First Occurrence of Neural-Tube Defects by
    Periconceptional Vitamin Supplementation." *New England Journal of Medicine*, 1992, *327*,
    1832–1835.

Fetterman, D. M. *Foundations of Empowerment Evaluation.* Thousand Oaks, Calif.: Sage, 2001.

Fishbein, M., and others. "Avoiding the Boomerang: Testing the Relative Effectiveness of
    Anti-Drug Public Service Announcements Before a National Campaign." *American Journal
    of Public Health*, 2002, *92*(2), 238–245.

Flay, B. R., and Cook, T. D. "Three Models for Summative Evaluation of Prevention
    Campaigns with a Mass Media Component." In R. E. Rice and C. K. Atkin (eds.),
    Public Communication Campaigns (2nd ed.) Thousand Oaks, Calif: Sage, 1989.

Food and Drug Administration. "Food Standards: Amendment of Standards of Identity for
    Enriched Grain Products to Require Addition of Folic Acid (21 CFR Parts 136, 137, and
    139)." *Federal Register*, 1996, *61*, 8781–8797.

Hammond, S. L., Volansky, M., Treiman, K., and Child, W. *Folic Acid and Birth Defects Preven-
    tion: Focus Group Research with Women at Risk* (Task order no. 927650). Rockville Md.: Westat,
    1998.

Henshaw, S. K. "Unintended Pregnancy in the United States." *Family Planning Perspectives*,
    1998, *30*, 24–29.

Institute of Medicine. "Dietary Reference Intakes: Folate, Other B Vitamins, and Choline."
    In *Dietary Reference Intakes for Thiamin, Riboflavin, Vitamin B6, Folate, Vitamin B12, Pantothenic
    Acid, Biotin, and Choline.* Washington, D.C.: National Academy Press, 1998.

Israel, B. A., Schulz, A. J., Parker, E. A., and Becker, A. B. "Review of Community-Based
    Research: Assessing Partnership Approaches to Improve Public Health." *Annual Review of
    Public Health*, 1998, *19*, 173–202.

Maibach, E. W., and Parrott, R. L. (eds.). *Designing Health Messages: Approaches from Communica-
    tion Theory and Public Health Practice.* Thousand Oaks, Calif.: Sage, 1995.

Maibach E. W., Maxfield, A., Ladin, K., and Slater, M. "Translating Health Psychology into
    Effective Health Communication: The American Healthstyles Audience Segmentation
    Project." *Journal of Health Psychology*, 1996, *1*(3), 261–277.

March of Dimes. *Folic Acid and the Prevention of Birth Defects: A National Survey of Pre-Pregnancy
    Awareness and Behavior Among Women of Childbearing Age—1995–2000.* (Publication
    31–1404–00). White Plains, N.Y.: March of Dimes, 2000.

Medical Research Council, Vitamin Study Research Group. "Prevention of Neural Tube
    Defects: Results of the Medical Research Council Vitamin Study." *Lancet*, 1991, *338*,
    131–137.

National Center for Health Statistics. *The Third National Health and Nutrition Examination Survey
    (NHANES III, 1988–94): Reference Manuals and Reports.* Hyattsville, Md.: National Center
    for Health Statistics, 1996.

Nielsen Media Research. *1998 Report on Television.* New York: Nielsen Media Research, 1998.

Prochaska, J. O., DiClemente, C. C., and Norcross, J. C. "In Search of How People Change:
    Applications to Addictive Behaviors." *American Psychologist*, 1992, *47*, 1102–1114.

Rogers, E. M., and Kincaid, D. L. *Communication Network: Toward a New Paradigm for Research.*
    New York: Free Press, 1981.

Rosenstock, I. M., Strecher, V. J., and Becker, M. H. "Social Learning Theory and the Health Belief Model." *Health Education Quarterly,* 1988, *15,* 175–183.

Shaw, G. M., Velie, E. M., and Wasserman, C. R. "Risk for Neural Tube Defect-Affected Pregnancies Among Women of Mexican Descent and White Women in California." *American Journal of Public Health,* 1997, *87*(9), 1467–1471.

Snyder, L. B., and Hamilton, M. A. "A Meta-Analysis of U.S. Health Campaign Effects on Behavior: Emphasize Enforcement Exposure and New Information and Beware the Secular Trend." In R. Hornick (ed.), *Public Health Communication: Evidence for Behavior Change.* Hillsdale, N.J.: Erlbaum, 2001.

U.S. Census Bureau. *Census 2000 Summary File 1, Matrices P13 and PCT12.* [http://factfinder.census.gov]. Feb. 2002.

Wallack, L., Dorfman, L., Jernigan, D., and Themba, M. *Media Advocacy and Public Health: Power for Prevention.* Thousand Oaks, Calif.: Sage, 1993.

APPENDIX A: COMBINED COMMUNICATION EXPOSURE INDEX, FOLIC ACID CAMPAIGN.

| | MEDIA COVERAGE | | | | | | | | | | | NON-MEDIA COVERAGE | | |
| | PSA COVERAGE | | | | | | NEWS COVERAGE | | | ADS | TOTALS | | | | |
Market Ranking	CDC TV PSAs	% shown in dayparts of choice[1]	SBAA TV PSAs	% shown in dayparts of choice[1]	Radio PSAs	Print PSAs	TV News	Radio News	Print News	Print Ads	Total Media Hits	Total TV PSA Hits in dayparts of choice	Materials Distributed	Presentation Attendance	Other Activities
Media Market 1	204	80.4%	3	100.0%	no monitoring	0	3	no monitoring	8	0	218	167.0	12,600	1,623	—
Media Market 2	348	97.1%	26	30.8%	no monitoring	0	3	0	6	0	383	346.0	19,800	0	Materials sent to DPH officers across state
Media Market 3	142	41.5%	67	100.0%	no monitoring	0	7	0	7	0	223	126.0	22,350	180	Billboard; outreach to grocery stores
Media Market 4	140	38.6%	2	0.0%	no monitoring	0	2	0	0	0	144	54.0	27,345	20	—
Media Market 55	0	0.0%	0	0.0%	no monitoring	0	1	no monitoring	0	0	1	0.0	0	0	—
Media Market 56	4	50.0%	0	0.0%	no monitoring	0	no monitoring	no monitoring	1	0	5	2.0	0	0	—
Media Market 57	0	0.0%	0	0.0%	no monitoring	0	1	0	0	0	1	0.0	1,125	459	Written information sent to 5–10 public health newsletters
Media Market 58	0	0.0%	0	0.0%	no monitoring	0	no monitoring	no monitoring	3	0	3	0.0	250 (+1-5000)	0	—

[1]Dayparts of Choice: Early morning (5 am–8:30 am);   Daytime (10 am–4:30 pm);   Early Fringe (4 pm–7:30 pm);   Prime Time (8 pm–10 pm);   Late Evening (10:30 pm–12:30 am)

NAME INDEX

A

Abma, J. C., 358, 362, 381
Abrams, D. B., 7, 21, 156, 158, 177, 179, 184, 185, 200, 201
Addy, R. C., 209
Agro, A. D., 63, 76
Ahluwalia, J. S., 250, 252, 267
Alleyne, E., 210, 238
Altpeter, M., 270, 285
Ammerman, A., 115
Amonette, M. D., 59, 76
Anderson, C., 2, 10, 21
Arthey, S., 63, 74
Atkins, L. A., 34, 56
Atkins, R., 90, 108
Atkinson, J., 31, 57
Augustyniak, R., 294, 320

B

Babb, S., 294, 320
Babsin, C., 31, 56
Bak, S. M., 63, 75
Baker, S. L., 249, 266
Bandura, A., 118, 140, 185, 200, 210, 213, 214, 237, 250, 266

Barab, S. A., 118, 140
Baranowski, T., 2, 4, 8, 10, 13, 14, 21, 23, 178, 179, 213, 237, 249, 250, 252, 253, 254, 264, 266, 267, 269, 270, 280, 281, 285
Barth, R., 210, 238
Bartholomew, L. K., 8, 21, 270, 285
Basch, C. E., 5, 21, 118, 140, 213, 214, 215, 237, 270, 285
Basen-Engquist, K., 209, 210, 212, 214, 215, 217, 233, 234, 237
Bauman, K .E., 377, 381
Becker, A. B., 250, 267, 380, 382
Becker, M. H., 361, 376, 383
Beilin, L. J., 249, 266
Bempong, I., 115, 140
Benedict, S., 184
Benson, P., 32, 56
Berger, L., 324, 345
Bernstein, E., 85, 90, 109
Bernstein, I., 71, 76
Bert, M. S., 184, 201
Bettman, J. R., 361, 376, 381
Bibeau, D., 2, 22, 118, 140, 185, 201
Bickel, W. E., 314, 320

Biener, L., 158, 163, 178, 179, 294, 320
Blaine, T. M., 20, 293
Block, G., 249, 266
Blum, H. L., 293, 320
Bogenschneider, K., 32, 56
Boles, S. M., 12, 14, 22, 59, 65, 75
Bone, L. R., 119, 139, 141
Bonnie, R., 324, 345
Borland, R., 59, 74
Botvin, G. J., 215, 217, 234, 237, 238
Braithwaite, R. L., 250, 252, 267
Brannigan, R., 13, 22
Brasfield, T. L., 210, 238
Brawley, O. W., 115, 140
Brousard, B. A., 268, 285
Brown, J., 370, 381
Buller, D. B., 59, 74
Bush, P. J., 215, 237

C

Caballaro, B., 269, 270, 285
Cacioppi, J. T., 194, 201
Campbell, M. K., 184, 188, 189, 200

SUBJECT INDEX

A

Acceptability survey, *126*

Accountability, 41, 47, 294

Action plan implementation, 41–51

Action plan worksheets, 41, *42–43*

Activity Closeout Form, 162, *183*

Adolescent Social Action Program (ASAP): background on, 83–85; conclusions on, 106–108; description of, 85–92; lessons learned from, 100–105; limitations of, and opportunities for learning, 107–108; process evaluation in, 92–97; results in, 97–100; review of, 27; sample forms from, 110–113; strengths of, 106

Adoption, 60, 69, 74

Adoption patterns, elucidating, 284

Alpha testing, 306–307

American Academy of Family Physicians, *359*

American Academy of Pediatrics, 358, *359*

American Cancer Society, 58, 59, 74, 115, 140

American College of Obstetricians and Gynecologists, 358, *359*

American College of Physicians— American Society of Internal Medicine, *359*

American Dietetic Association, *359*

American Nurses Association, *359*

American Pharmaceutical Association, *359*

Analytic strategies, employing, 10, 20

Annie E. Casey Foundation, 31, 56

Application forms, 65, 67, 68

Archives, 10

Are We Almost There?, *48*

ASAP Session Observation Form, 111–113

Asset-based approach, 32, 44

Association of Maternal and Child Health Programs, *359*

Association of State and Territorial Health Officials, *359*

Association of State and Territorial Public Health Nutrition Directors, *359*

Association of Women's Health, Obstetric, and Neonatal Nurses, *359*

Attendance logs, 10, *94, 95,* 106, 272, 273

Attitude, 228, *229,* 361

Audio-and-video tapes, 10, 133

"Avoiding Type III Errors in Health Education Program Evaluations: A Case Study" (Basch and others), 5

Awareness, 162, 165–166, 171, *172*

B

Barriers: definition of, 8; focus on, 190, 199; lack of focus on, 284

Barriers and facilitators, focus on, 84, 254, *255,* 263

Baseline prevalence, 169–170

Baseline surveys, 63, *124,* 131, 187

Behavior change theories, 156, 161, 185, 187, 361. *See also specific theories*

Behavioral guidelines, 277, *278*

Behavioral priority, tailoring to, 188, 198